DEATH AND CHRONIC ILLNESS IN THE FAMILY

What does it mean to be 'present and accounted for' when a family member is facing chronic illness or death? How does one define a self in relation to the ill or dying member and the family? Rooted in Murray Bowen's family systems theory, this edited volume provides conceptual ideas and applications useful to clinicians who work with families facing chronic illness or the death of a member.

The text is divided into four parts: Part I provides a detailed overview of Bowen's theory perspectives on chronic illness and death and includes Murray Bowen's seminal essay "Family Reaction to Death." In Parts II and III, chapter authors draw upon Bowen theory to intimately explore their families' reactions to and experiences with death and chronic illness. The final part uses case studies from contributors' clinical practices to aid therapists in using Bowen systems perspectives in their work with clients.

The chapters in this volume provide a rich and broad range of clinical application and personal experience by professionals who have substantial knowledge of and training in Bowen theory. *Death and Chronic Illness in the Family* is an essential resource for those interested in understanding the impact of death and loss in their professional work and in their personal lives.

Peter Titelman, PhD, maintains a private practice in Northampton, Massachusetts, specializing in Bowen family systems therapy. He is the founder of the Northampton Seminar on Bowen Theory and its Applications.

Sydney K. Reed, MSW, is in private practice specializing in Bowen family systems therapy. She is the co-founder and senior faculty of the Center for Family Consultation in Evanston, Illinois.

DEATH AND CHRONIC ILLNESS IN THE FAMILY

Bowen Family Systems Theory Perspectives

Edited by
Peter Titelman
Sydney K. Reed

Routledge
Taylor & Francis Group
NEW YORK AND LONDON

First published 2019
by Routledge
711 Third Avenue, New York, NY 10017

and by Routledge
2 Park Square, Milton Park, Abingdon, Oxon, OX14 4RN

Routledge is an imprint of the Taylor & Francis Group, an informa business

Library of Congress Cataloging-in-Publication Data
Names: Titelman, Peter, editor. | Reed, Sydney K., editor.
Title: Death and chronic illness in the family : Bowen family systems theory perspectives / edited by Peter Titelman, Sydney K. Reed.
Description: New York, NY : Routledge, 2019. | Includes bibliographical references and index.
Identifiers: LCCN 2018018210 | ISBN 9781138200180 (hbk : alk. paper) | ISBN 9781138200197 (pbk : alk. paper) | ISBN 9781315515052 (ebk)
Subjects: LCSH: Family psychotherapy. | Chronic diseases—Psychological aspects. | Death—Psychological aspects.
Classification: LCC RC488.5 .D3715 2019 | DDC 616.89/156—dc23
LC record available at https://lccn.loc.gov/2018018210

ISBN: 978-1-138-20018-0 (hbk)
ISBN: 978-1-138-20019-7 (pbk)
ISBN: 978-1-315-51505-2 (ebk)

Typeset in Bembo
by Apex CoVantage, LLC

From *Peter Titelman*

To the memories of my parents, mentor, teacher, friend, and colleague

Lory, d. 1977 and Leonard Titelman, d. 1993

Murray Bowen, d. 1990

William Norris, d. 2014

Dick Miller, d. 2016

Loretta Nowakowski, d. 2017

From *Sydney K. Reed*

For teaching me what it means to be family:

Dr. Bowen for his theory and his challenging teaching style

My nuclear family: David, Mathew, Amy, Justin, Nicole, Zeiler, and Zaria

My family of origin: Eva and Joe Zeiler, Joe and Linda Zeiler,

Jacque and Jim Ruegamer

All members of my extended family: the Streckers and the Zeilers

TITLES OF RELATED INTEREST

Titelman (ed.)—*The Therapist's Own Family: Toward the Differentiation of Self*

Titelman (ed.)—*Clinical Applications of Bowen Family Systems Theory*

Titelman (ed.)—*Emotional Cutoff: Bowen Family Systems Theory Perspectives*

Titelman (ed.)—*Triangles: Bowen Family Systems Theory Perspectives*

Bregman & White (eds.)—*Bringing Systems Theory to Life: Expanding the Horizons for Bowen Family Systems Theory*

Titelman (ed.)—*Differentiation of Self: Bowen Family Systems Theory Perspectives*

CONTENTS

FOREWORD

The consideration of death, especially of one's own mortality, has been a preoccupation of humans since the evolution of the wondrous primate brain allowed for the awareness of the future and so of one's end. The reality of death is never far from consciousness. Along with the effort to understand life and how it came to be, the human has struggled to comprehend death and its meaning. It is a subject many seek to avoid considering, and yet in one form or another it influences our daily lives.

The reality of death involves more than the concern about our own mortality. Few life experiences are more difficult than the death of one we love. Its impact persists for some time as we attempt to adjust to and accept the loss of one to whom we are deeply attached. At some level, either consciously or unconsciously, we are also aware of the degree to which our well-being depends on our important others. A significant illness or potential loss of those we are most connected to is a source of anxiety. A threat to their health and safety can be experienced as a threat to our own self.

Loss and the grieving process have been central subjects in psychology and pastoral care. Their impact on the health and well-being of individuals is well known. For the greater part of the past century a significant focus in psychotherapy has been on the impact of a major loss on an individual's current functioning. The grieving process has been principally seen as a psychological phenomenon influencing the individual psyche, and the recovery from loss has been viewed as an intrapsychic process, the resolution of which requires time and the support of others.

The development of a family systems theory by Murray Bowen represented a radical shift in understanding human behavior. To many in the helping professions, Bowen's family systems theory represents one of a number of therapeutic approaches the practitioner might apply with an individual or family in psychotherapy or counseling. It is often thought of as a school of thought entailing a transgenerational approach. Ideas entailed in the theory may be selected and "integrated" with other approaches perceived to fit with one's personal point of view, but the profound shift in thinking required to grasp Bowen theory is often overlooked.

The death or threatened loss of a family member or loved one highlights differences between Bowen theory and other conceptual approaches. The concepts of the family emotional system and differentiation of self provide a significantly different perspective on how one views and experiences the impact of death and loss on individuals and families.

Conventional thinking for the most part focuses on the feelings, the subjective reaction to a death. The awareness and exploration of one's feelings and their open expression are seen as central to the resolution of a loss.

A figure-ground shift occurs when a loss is seen as occurring in the context of the family emotional system. Its impact is no longer seen as an individual process, but one that occurs amidst the interdependent relationship system of the family. The emotional reverberations occurring in the family must also be considered as members respond not only to their own loss, but also to the reactions to loss of others they are connected to. The chain reactions to a loss in the family affect all in varying degrees. Knowledge of one's functional position in the family, that of others, and of the member who died is an important aspect of resolving a loss. The functioning of each family member influences the functioning of those they are connected to as the experience of loss reciprocally influences those in the family system. Knowledge of the impact on the functioning of family members and one's relationship with them provides a broader view of the impact of a loss on self.

The concepts of differentiation of self and the multigenerational family emotional process can aid one to see the degree of emotional interdependence at play in oneself and in others. This knowledge can add a clarity that a focus on the subjective feeling states alone cannot. The loss of a family member is an important event and in general is a time in which the family is in a state of flux. It represents a time in which one can potentially learn more about the family and an opportunity to develop a more personal relationship with important others.

During such periods, Bowen theory can serve as a guideline in coming to know the predictable shifts that occur in a family's functioning. It is not uncommon, for example, that the loss of an important family member can lead to an increase in emotional distance among some members and/or an increase in family stuck-togetherness. Bowen theory can assist individuals in navigating through such automatic emotional responses in a manner that can contribute to a more open and resilient system.

Death and Chronic Illness in the Family: Bowen Family Systems Theory Perspectives represents an important collection exhibiting the value of Bowen theory in understanding the impact of a loss and its resolution. Death and chronic illness are a part of every family's heritage. Each loss has the potential to affect the adaptiveness of a family, contributing to an increase or decrease in its functioning. The chapters in this volume provide a rich and broad range of theory, application, and personal experience by professionals who have considerable experience in developing a knowledge of Bowen theory.

Sydney Reed and Peter Titelman bring their own long-standing study of this family systems theory in contributing to and editing this important work. Murray Bowen's "Family Reaction to Death," included in this volume, represented a milestone in understanding loss from a systems perspective. *Death and Chronic Illness in the Family* provides another resource for those interested in understanding the impact of death and loss in their professional work and in their personal lives.

Robert J. Noone, PhD
Co-founder and Faculty
Center for Family Consultation
Evanston, Illinois

PREFACE

This edited volume on death and chronic illness is based on the perspective of Murray Bowen's family systems theory, particularly its view of the family as an emotional unit or system. The focus of this book is on the experience within the family when one of its members has a chronic illness or dies.

Death and chronic illness are the most significant nodal events that can shake the equilibrium of the family emotional unit. Chronic illness and death are losses, generating a range of sadness, grief, and/or relief for the family. The levels of chronic anxiety, stress, and differentiation of self of individuals in the family, as well as for the family as a whole, play a large part in the way families—nuclear and extended—manage death along a continuum of emotional stability.

Bowen developed a continuum of profiles in order to describe the variation in differentiation of self. The family's level of differentiation consists of the aggregate of the level of differentiation of all its members: nuclear family, family of origin, and extended family members. Differentiation is based on the balance of the forces of togetherness and individuality. Differentiation in a family is based on the beliefs, values, levels of chronic anxiety, levels of reactivity, and the emotional process in relationships between family members. A family that functions at a higher level of differentiation is very likely to maintain its stability or can likely draw on its resilience to stabilize itself following a death. A family that functions at a lower level of differentiation is likely to become destabilized and may take a long period of time to restabilize itself. And some families that are at the lowest levels of differentiation may not be able to restabilize the family system at all.

This book describes how some individuals or entire families may be more resilient and others less so. Readers will learn how the family as an emotional unit responds to chronic illness and death. They will gain an understanding of what Bowen described as being "present and accounted for" when family members are relating to the chronically ill or dying family member. They will read examples of the authors' experiences of their own efforts to define themselves in relation to chronic illness and/or death in their own families and in families they see in their clinical work. The book provides conceptual ideas that can be useful for professionals who lend a hand to those families facing chronic illness or death of a family member.

Fourteen of the contributors had training or direct personal experience with Murray Bowen. Three other contributors have had training at the Bowen Center for the Study of the Family in Washington, DC All the contributors in this volume have studied and applied Bowen theory in dealing with chronic illness and/or death in their families and in their clinical practice.

The first part of the book focuses on a Bowen theory perspective on death. The second part focuses on death in the therapist's own family. The third part focuses on chronic illness in the therapist's own family. The fourth part focuses on death in the therapist's clinical practice. The last chapter describes a young man's effort to define himself during the last two weeks of his father's life. Materials drawn from clinical cases presented in this book have been modified to protect the confidentiality of the individuals discussed in their families.

Each contributor has his or her perspective on death and chronic illness. It is our belief that the volume as a whole is consonant with Bowen's conception of the family reaction to death and chronic illness.

Chapter 1, the cornerstone of this book, is a reprint of Murray Bowen's chapter, "Family Reaction to Death." It was initially printed in 1976, in *Family Therapy: Theory and Practice*, edited by Phil Guerin and published by Gardner Press, Inc. Two years later the chapter was reprinted in Bowen's classic book, *Family Therapy in Clinical Practice* (1978), published by Jason Aronson, Inc. Bowen died in 1990. Unlike most conventional psychiatric and psychological books and articles written on the individual in relation to death, Bowen focused on how the family emotional unit experiences and deals with the interlocking relationships in the family emotional unit at the time of a death. There are three main parts in his chapter: The first part describes the problem of the closed communication system within the interlocking triangular relationships between the patient, the family, and physicians. Bowen describes family therapy methods that have been in managing some of the anxiety that creates the closed communication system. The second section deals with the "emotional shock wave" that is present in a significant percentage of families following a death. The final section describes the impact of funerals on a family and how the professional person can lend a hand to help the surviving relatives to maintain or improve the emotional stability of the family unit by calmly managing their anxiety while confronting death.

In Chapter 2, Peter Titelman describes the relationship between death and differentiation in the family from a Bowen perspective. The first part describes Bowen's own experience of exposure to mortality from his earliest youth to adulthood. The second part describes Bowen's natural systems perspective on death. The third part provides a framework for understanding death and differentiation in the family from a Bowen perspective. There are also clinical sections on principles, concepts, and rituals regarding death. The fourth part describes examples of variations in the way families at different levels of differentiation face death. The fifth part describes a clinical application for addressing chronic illness and death in the family.

In Chapter 3, Anne S. McKnight discusses a historical perspective on death from individual thinking to family systems theory. In 1918, Sigmund Freud theorized that the only way to overcome grief was to focus on the emotions triggered by the death of a loved one. Elizabeth Kubler-Ross elaborated on the idea. She proposed that an individual needs to go through five stages of grief. Through extensive research, George Bonanno found a natural resilience in people to carry on despite their loss. Murray Bowen proposed that the impact of a death varied according to the family's capacity for managing changes in the interdependence around the loss.

In Chapter 4, Stephanie Ferrera looks at mortality as a biological fact, reviews the history of the human experience with death, and describes systems of belief that humans have embraced in coping with loss. She suggests that a biological and historical perspective can lead to greater objectivity toward the emotion-laden challenge of mortality; this, in turn, can guide one in defining the beliefs and values by which one lives and dies.

In Chapter 5, Sydney K. Reed describes the deaths of both of her grandmothers. In 1972 she was not present at the funeral when her maternal grandmother died. Three years later she was present at the funeral when her paternal grandmother died. She contrasts these two events, suggesting a shock wave occurred in the first death that might have been handled differently had she been "present and accounted for" and known more about the "emotional shock wave" pattern as happened in the second death. She examines the process of the emotional shock wave as her family experienced it and also describes how being present at nodal events offers an opportunity to work on differentiation of self.

In Chapter 6, Kent E. Webb illustrates and accounts for the significant amount of disruption and dysfunction that occurred within the nuclear family after the father's early death and how it took decades for the family to achieve equilibrium. The phenomena of emotional shock wave and emotional aftershocks are demonstrated through examples of the family's response to the father's death.

In Chapter 7, Anthony J. Wilgus describes how a way of thinking rooted in Bowen theory guides the way of being for a man whose family member abruptly committed suicide in the wake of some major life shifts. Thoughtfulness emanating from this perspective can assist others to function with a little more clarity and planning while addressing the numerous pragmatic decisions that demand attention following a sudden death.

In Chapter 8, Catherine M. Rakow asks the question, "Does the past influence the present?" The death of a family member and the ensuing emotional shock wave were the catalyst to investigate the connection to the chronic anxiety in the family. This chapter came from facts of a family history and family events, years of observations in relationships, and a persistent curiosity in understanding "the bigger picture." It sheds light on interlocking triangles across four generations as unfinished emotional issues from the past play out in one mother–daughter–grandson relationship.

In Chapter 9, Anonymous describes how territorial behavior can be observed as the possession and disposition of property within and between generations. The property may be real estate, cash, personal property, or investments. This chapter uses territorial behavior as one important clinical tool for the assessment of emotional process. Territorial behavior and family emotional process reciprocally influence one another over generations. The chapter demonstrates the value of observing territorial behavior among family members as a way of monitoring and modifying emotional process in the context of death. The author's efforts at differentiation of self over several years are reported.

In Chapter 10, Eileen B. Gottlieb presents a systems view of chronic illness. She focuses on three ideas derived from Bowen family systems theory in an effort to understand the origin, expression, and impact of this chronic illness that includes the role of the relationship system and family emotional process. She describes chronic illness as a multigenerational process. Finally, she posits that chronic illness may be unpreventable. The management of the relationships around it becomes significant to the next generation.

In Chapter 11, Selden Dunbar Illick describes her continuing efforts to resolve degrees of unresolved emotional attachment with her parents at the time of their illnesses and deaths (two and a half weeks apart). The focus of her chapter is on how chronic illness and death provide an opportunity for further resolving degrees of unresolved attachment in the family system, in particular with her mother and her father. She also describes how the degrees of unresolved emotional attachment played a part in her marriage and continues in her interactions with her adult children.

In Chapter 12, Peter Titelman describes his effort to define himself in his relationship with his father when his father had Alzheimer's disease. He also describes his sister's Alzheimer's diagnosis and the reaction in her nuclear family, the Alzheimer's of his first cousin, and his own anxiety that he may end up with Alzheimer's disease. The final section provides reflections on Alzheimer's disease and ways that family members can relate to the one with the disease when it occurs in the family.

In Chapter 13, Susan W. Graefe describes her experience of having polio. She credited the success of her struggle with polio—that she has dealt with since age seven—to the fact that her mother gave her lots and lots of love, and no sympathy. A determined mother and a steady and dependable father helped her to face life's challenges.

In Chapter 14, Laura Havstad describes the principles of a clinical approach based on Bowen theory when severe symptoms in family members follow a death in the family.

In the shock wave following death, family patterns intensify and family members in vulnerable positions become symptomatic. A clinical example is used to illustrate the positive results of coaching a family member to get out of relationship patterns impairing the symptomatic one, while working towards differentiation of self.

In Chapter 15, Michael J. Sullivan describes how families vary in response to death. Some collapse into a regression, never to regain their predeath equilibrium. Chronic debilitating symptoms persist across the family network for decades. Others experience an initial period of disruption, marked by acute symptoms typically with the most vulnerable members, followed by a gradual realignment. Still other families experience a period of bereavement, move forward, and thrive. This chapter will describe these different adaptive trajectories from a Bowen systems theory perspective and emphasize the importance of the underground emotional "aftershocks" in the symptoms clinical families typically present.

In Chapter 16, David S. Hargrove and Elizabeth Grady describe how family emotional process influences the experience of death in the system. Both the dying person and the surviving family are subject to the impact of chronic anxiety as it is experienced by family members, medical staff seeking to care for the dying person, and collateral personnel who may be involved in the dying process. Expression of anxiety follows the structure exemplified in the concepts contained in Bowen family systems theory.

In Chapter 17, Andrea Maloney Schara reports on a ten-year project (1983–1993) to consider many variables around the AIDS epidemic. She asked the question: Could Bowen family systems psychotherapy be useful? Symptoms appeared in one person who was isolated from his family. As people reengaged, there was an initial increase in symptoms among family members, but an increase in the health status of those living with AIDS. If the family is an emotional unit, then reconnecting could alter the direction of anxiety. As people were in more thoughtful contact, many were less vulnerable to symptoms.

In Chapter 18, Kendall Baker wrote a journal during the last two weeks of his father's life. It includes Baker's description of the dying process as well as the interactions of family members as they prepared for the loss of this significant family leader. Katharine Baker contributes an introduction to the journal, framing the family experiences in the context of Bowen theory.

ACKNOWLEDGEMENTS

Peter Titelman

I thank all the contributors for the effort and quality that went into each of their chapters. I learned from them; I have enjoyed working with them. They are my colleagues and friends.

I thank Elizabeth Utschig for her creative and excellent graphic design work for our family diagrams, and for editing my chapters and those of the other contributors. She has been an important member of our team.

I thank Stephanie Ferrera for reading and making suggestions for one of my chapters.

I thank my co-editor, Sydney K. Reed, for asking me to join her in creating this book, and for our good collaboration.

I thank my wife, Katharine Gratwick Baker, for her clarity and kindness in reading my two chapters and putting up with me through all the many years when I have been editing books on Bowen theory.

Sydney K. Reed

I, too, would like to thank our contributors for their thoughtful rendering of Bowen family systems theory and family emotional process as they have observed and studied both for many years. Friends and colleagues all. I have learned much for each of them over the years and in their chapters in this book:

In addition to Elizabeth Utschig's creative work as a graphic designer, which has made the book visually pleasing, I thank her for her encouraging words throughout the many years of working together.

I thank my colleagues at the Center for Family Consultation for 40 years of intellectual adventures and shared learning.

Carol Moran, Dorothy Jones, and Leslie Fox were gracious in their time and suggestions after reading my chapter. Thank you.

Thank you to David, Mathew, Justin, Amy, and Nicole, my close family members, who were supportive and encouraging in this process.

I'm grateful that Peter Titelman was up for a sixth book. Without him, this book would not have happened.

ABOUT THE EDITORS

Peter Titelman, PhD, maintains a private practice in clinical psychology, specializing in Bowen family systems therapy and consultation, in Northampton, Massachusetts. Dr. Titelman has been leading a consultation group on the professional's own family for 35 years as a founder and faculty of the Northampton Seminar on Bowen Theory and Its Applications. He is also a founding member of the New England Seminar on Bowen Theory in Worcester, Massachusetts. He is the editor of *The Therapist's Own Family: Toward the Differentiation of Self* (Jason Aronson, Inc., 1987); *Clinical Applications of Bowen Family Systems Theory* (Haworth Press 1998, now published by Routledge/Taylor & Francis); *Emotional Cutoff: Bowen Family Systems Theory Perspectives* (Haworth Press, 2003); *Triangles: Bowen Family Systems Theory Perspectives* (Haworth Press, 2008, now published by Routledge/Taylor & Francis); and *Differentiation of Self: Bowen Family Theory Perspectives* (Routledge/Taylor & Francis, 2014). Dr. Titelman was on the faculty of Leadership in Ministry in Newton, Massachusetts. He was a co-founder and clinical director of the Family Living Consultants of the Pioneer Valley in Northampton, Massachusetts. Dr. Titelman has taught and supervised graduate students as an adjunct faculty member at Antioch New England Graduate School, Keene, New Hampshire; Massachusetts School of Professional Psychology, Newton, Massachusetts; St. Joseph's College, West Hartford, Connecticut; and Smith College of Social Work, Northampton, Massachusetts. He has given presentations and training events nationally and internationally, including teaching Bowen family systems theory at the Society of Family Consultants and Psychotherapists in Moscow, Russia, and he presented a seminar at An-Najah University in the West Bank of

Palestine. Dr. Titelman has presented papers at the following Centers in the Bowen theory network: the Bowen Center of the Study of the Family, Washington, DC; the Center for Family Consultation, Evanston, Illinois; the New England Seminar on Bowen Theory, Worcester, Massachusetts; the Princeton Family Center for Education, Princeton, New Jersey; the Vermont Family Center, Burlington, Vermont; and the Western Pennsylvania Family Center, Pittsburgh, Pennsylvania. His current research interests, in addition to chronic illness and death, include the concepts of differentiation of self and emotional process in society, specifically the Israeli-Palestinian conflict from a Bowen theory perspective.

Peter Titelman received a BA degree from Earlham College and received a PhD in clinical psychology from Duquesne University.

Sydney K. Reed, MSW, has a private practice in psychotherapy specializing in Bowen family systems therapy. She is the co-founder and senior faculty of the Center for Family Consultation in Evanston, Illinois, a center for postgraduate training and continuing education for health professionals, clergy, and businesspersons in Bowen family systems theory and therapy. For 37 years she worked for the Family Service Center of Wilmette as senior clinical staff and supervisor of social work interns. She was a consultant to Care Communications in Chicago where she consulted with their staff and taught in their professional training courses for health care specialists. She provided workshops and consultation to professional women as a faculty member of the Women's Leadership Institute in Chicago. For the last 25 years she has provided training for clergy—as individuals, groups, or in workshops—interested in understanding how Bowen theory applies to churches and congregations.

She published a chapter in *Clinical Application of Bowen Family Systems Theory* (Titelman, 1987, Jason Aronson) and articles for several Bowen family systems journals.

Family reaction to death as described by Bowen theory was one of her first interests as important deaths in her family occurred within the first years of meeting Dr. Bowen. She has continued to study and teach about this subject over the last 40 years.

Ms. Reed is a graduate of Oberlin College and received her MSW at the University of Illinois.

CONTRIBUTORS

Anonymous

Katharine Gratwick Baker, PhD, LICSW
Private Practice
Northampton, MA

Kendall Baker, MFA
Artist/Fine Arts Professor
Caldwell University
Caldwell University, NJ

Murray Bowen, MD (1913–1990)
Founder of the Georgetown Family Center
Washington, DC

Stephanie J. Ferrera, MSW, LCSW
Co-Founder and Faculty, Center for Family Consultation
Private Practice
Oak Park, IL

Eileen B. Gottlieb, MEd
Director, The Family Center
Delray Beach, FL
Education Director, Florida Family Research Network
Delray Beach, FL
Senior Faculty, Bowen Theory South Florida
Delray Beach, FL

Elizabeth Grady, DO
Internal Medicine, Palliative Care and Hospice Health Center
East Boston Neighborhood Health Center
East Boston, MA

Susan W. Graefe, ACSW, LICSW, BCD
Private Practice
Warwick, RI

David S. Hargrove, PhD
Faculty, The Bowen Center for the Study of the Family
Washington, DC

Laura Havstad, PhD
Director, Programs in Bowen Theory
Private Practice
Sebastopol, CA

Selden Dunbar Illick, LCSW
Private Practice
Vero Beach, FL
Director Emeritus, Princeton Family Center
Board Member, Princeton Family Center for Education
Princeton, NJ

Anne S. McKnight, LCSW, EdD
Director, The Bowen Center for the Study of the Family
Washington, DC

Catherine M. Rakow, MSW, ACSW
Private Consultant
Independent Researcher
Confluence, PA
Faculty, Western Pennsylvania Family Center
Pittsburgh, PA

Andrea Maloney Schara, LCSWA
Private Practice

Faculty, Navigating Systems
Washington, DC

Michael J. Sullivan, LMSW
Private Practice
Traverse City, Michigan

Kent E. Webb, MSW, LCSW
Private Practice
Denver, CO

Anthony J. Wilgus, MA, MSW
Professor of Social Work, Emeritus
The University of Findlay
Findlay, OH
Trainer and Consultant in Bowen theory
Oberlin, OH

I

BOWEN THEORY PERSPECTIVES ON DEATH IN THE FAMILY

1

FAMILY REACTION TO DEATH[1]

Murray Bowen

Direct thinking about death, or indirect thinking about staying alive and avoiding death, occupies more of man's time than any other subject. Man is an instinctual animal with the same instinctual awareness of death as the lower forms of life. He follows the same predictable instinctual life pattern of all living things. He is born, he grows to maturity, he reproduces, his life force runs out, and he dies. In addition, he is a thinking animal with a brain that enables him to reason, reflect, and think abstractly. With his intellect he has devised philosophies and beliefs about the meaning of life and death that tend to deny his place in nature's plan. Each individual has to define his own place in the total scheme and accept the fact that he will die and be replaced by succeeding generations. His difficulty in finding a life plan for himself is complicated by the fact that his life is intimately interwoven with the lives about him. This presentation is directed to death as a part of the total family in which he lives.

There are no simple ways to describe man as part of the relationship around him. Elsewhere (Bowen, 1978, p.2), I have presented my own way of conceiving of the human as an individual and, also, as part of the emotional-social amalgam in which he lives. According to my theory, a high percentage of human relationship behavior is directed more by automatic instinctual emotional forces than by intellect. Much intellectual activity goes to explain away and justify behavior being directed by the instinctual-emotion-feeling complex. Death is a biological event that terminates a life. No life event can stir more emotional directed thinking in the individual and more emotional reactiveness in those about him. I have chosen the concept of "open" and "closed" relationship systems as an effective way to describe death as a family phenomenon.

An "open" relationship system is one in which an individual is free to communicate a high percentage of inner thoughts, feelings, and fantasies to another who can reciprocate. No one ever has a completely open relationship with another, but it is a healthy state when a person can have one relationship in which a reasonable degree of openness is possible. A fair percentage of children have a reasonable version of this with a parent. The most open relationship most people have in their adult lives is in a courtship. After marriage, in the emotional interdependence of living together, each spouse becomes sensitive to subjects that upset the other. They instinctively avoid the sensitive subjects, and the relationship shifts toward a more "closed" system. The closed communication system is an automatic emotional reflex to protect self from the anxiety in the other person, though most people say they avoid the taboo subjects to keep from upsetting the other person. If people could follow intellectual knowledge instead of the automatic reflex and gain some control over their own reactiveness to anxiety in the other, they would be able to talk about taboo subjects in spite of the anxiety, and the relationship would move toward a more healthy openness. But people are human, the emotional reactiveness operates like a reflex, and by the time the average person recognizes the problem it can be impossible for two spouses to reverse the process themselves. This is the point at which a trained professional can function as a third person to work the magic of family therapy toward opening a closed relationship.

Chief among all taboo subjects is death. A high percentage of people die alone, locked into their own thoughts, which they cannot communicate to others. There are at least two processes in operation. One is the intrapsychic process in self [that] always involves some denial of death. The other is the closed relationship system: People cannot communicate the thoughts they do have, lest they upset the family or others. There are usually at least three closed systems operating around the terminally ill person. One operates with the patient. From experience, every terminally ill patient has some awareness of impending death and a high percentage have an extensive amount of private knowledge they do not communicate to anyone. Another closed system is the family. The family gets its basic information from the physician, which is supplemented by bits of information from other sources and is then amplified, distorted, and reinterpreted in conversations at home. The family has its own carefully planned and edited medical communiqué for the patient. It is based on the family interpretation of the reports and modified to avoid the patient's reactiveness to anxiety. Other versions of the communiqué are whispered within the hearing of the patient when the family thinks the patient is sleeping or unconscious. Patients are often alert to whispered communications. The physician and the medical staff have another closed system of communication, supposedly based on medical facts, which is influenced by emotional reactivity to the family and within the staff. Physicians attempt to do factual reports to the family, which are distorted by the medical emotionality and the effort to put the correct emphasis on the "bad news" or "good news." The more reactive the physician, the more likely he is to put in medical jargon [what] the family does not hear or to become too simplistic in his efforts to communicate in lay language. The more anxious the physician, the more likely he is to do too much speechmaking and too little listening, and to end up with a vague and distorted message and little awareness of the family misperception of his message. The more anxious the physician, the more the family asks for specific details the physician cannot answer. Physicians commonly reply to specific questions with overgeneralizations that miss the point. The physician has another level of communication to the patient. Even the physician who agrees with the principle of telling the patient "facts" can communicate them with so much anxiety that the patient is responding to the physician instead of the content of what is being said. Problems occur when the closed communication system of medicine meets the age-old closed system between the patient and the family, and anxiety is heightened by the threat of terminal illness.

My clinical experience with death goes back some 30 years to detailed discussions about death with suicidal patients. They were eager to talk to an unbiased listener who did not have to correct their way of thinking. Then I discovered that all seriously ill people, and even those who are not sick, are grateful for an opportunity to talk about death. Over the years I have tried to do such discussions with seriously ill people in my practice, with friends and people I have known socially, and with members of my extended families. I have never seen a terminally ill person who was not strengthened by such a talk. This contradicts former beliefs about the ego being too fragile for this in certain situations. I have even done this with a spectrum of comatose patients. Terminally ill people often permit themselves to slip into coma. A fair percentage can pull themselves out of the coma for important communications. I have had such people come out long enough to talk and express their thanks for the help and immediately slip back. Until the mid-1960s, a majority of physicians were opposed to telling patients they had a terminal illness. In the past decade the prevailing medical dictum about this has changed a great deal, but medical practice has not kept pace with the changed attitude. The poor communications between the physician and the patient, between the physician and the family, and between the family and the patient are still very much as they were before. The basic problem is an emotional one, and a change in rules does not automatically change the emotional reactivity. The physician can believe he gave factual information to the patient, but in the emotion of the moment, the abruptness and vagueness in the communication, and the emotional process in the patient, the patient failed to "hear." The patient and the family can pretend they have dealt clearly with each other without either being heard through the emotionality. In my family therapy practice within a medical center, I am frequently in contact with both the patient and the family, and to a lesser extent with the physicians. The closed system between the patient and the family is great enough, at best. I believe the poor communication between the physician and the family and between the physician and the patient is the greatest problem. There have been repeated situations in which the physicians thought they were communicating clearly, but the family either misperceived or distorted the messages, and the family thinking would be working itself toward malpractice anger at the physician. In all of these, the surgical and medical procedures were adequate, and the family was reacting to terse, brief speeches by the physician who thought he was communicating adequately. In these, it is fairly easy to do simple interpretations of the physician's statements and avert the malpractice thinking. I believe the trend toward telling patients about incurable illness is one of the healthy changes in medicine, but closed systems do not become open when the surgeon hurriedly blurts out tense speeches about the situation. Experience indicates that physicians and surgeons have either to learn the fundamentals of closed system emotionality in the physician-family-patient triangle, or they might avail themselves of professional expertise in family therapy if they lack the time and motivation to master this for themselves. A clinical example of closed system emotionality will be presented later.

Family Emotional Equilibrium and the Emotional Shock Wave

This section will deal with an order of events within the family that is not directly related to open and closed system communications. Death, or threatened death, is only one of many events that can disturb a family. A family unit is in functional equilibrium when it is calm and each member is functioning at reasonable efficiency for that period. The equilibrium of the unit is disturbed by either the addition of a new member or the loss of a member. The intensity of the emotional reaction is governed by the functioning level of emotional integration in the family at the time or by the functional importance of the one who is added to the family or lost to the family. For instance, the birth of a child can disturb the emotional balance until family members can realign themselves around the child. A grandparent who comes for a visit may shift family emotional forces briefly, but a grandparent who comes to live in a home can change the family emotional balance for a long period. Losses that can disturb the family equilibrium are physical losses, such as a child who goes away to college or an adult child who marries and leaves home. There are functional losses, such as a key family member who becomes incapacitated with a long-term illness or injury which prevents his doing the work on which the family depends. There are emotional losses, such as the absence of a lighthearted person who can lighten the mood in a family. A group that changes from lighthearted laughter to seriousness becomes a different kind of organism. The length of time required for the family to establish a new emotional equilibrium depends on the emotional integration in the family and the intensity of the disturbance. A well-integrated family may show more overt reactiveness at the moment of change but adapt to it rather quickly. A less integrated family may show little reaction at the time and respond later with symptoms of physical illness, emotional illness, or social misbehavior. An attempt to get the family to express feelings at the moment of change does not necessarily increase the level of emotional integration.

The "Emotional Shock Wave" is a network of underground "aftershocks" of serious life events that can occur anywhere in the extended family system in the months or years following serious emotional events in a family. It occurs most often after the death or the threatened death of a significant family member, but it can occur following losses of other types. It is not directly related to the usual grief or mourning reactions of people close to the one who died. It operates on an underground network of emotional dependence of family members on each other. The emotional dependence is denied, the serious life events appear to be unrelated, the family attempts to camouflage any connectedness between the events, and there is a vigorous emotional denial reaction when anyone attempts to relate the events to each other. It occurs most often in families with a significant degree of denied emotional "fusion" in which the families have been able to maintain a fair degree of asymptomatic emotional balance in the family system. The basic family process has been described elsewhere (Bowen, 1978).

The "Emotional Shock Wave" was first encountered in the author's family research in the late 1950s. It has been mentioned in papers and lectures, but it has not been adequately described in the literature. It was first noticed in the course of multigenerational family research with the discovery that a series of major life events occurred in multiple, separate members of the extended family in the time interval after the serious illness and death of a significant family member. At first, this appeared to be coincidence. Then it was discovered that some version of this phenomenon appeared in a sufficiently high percentage of all families, and now a check for the "shock wave" is done routinely in all family histories. The symptoms in a shock wave can be any human problem. Symptoms can include the entire spectrum of physical illness from an increased incidence of colds and respiratory infections to the first appearance of chronic conditions, such as diabetes or allergies, to acute medical and surgical illnesses. It is as if the shock wave is the stimulus that can trigger the physical process into activity. The symptoms can also include the full range of emotional symptoms from mild depression, to phobias, to psychotic episodes. The social dysfunctions can include drinking, failures in school or business, abortions, and illegitimate births. An increase in presence of the shock wave provides the physician or therapist with vital knowledge in treatment. Without such knowledge, the sequence of events is treated as separate, unrelated events.

Some examples of the shock wave will illustrate the process. It occurs most often after the death of a significant family member, but it can be almost as severe after a threatened death. An example was a grandmother in her early sixties who had a radical mastectomy for cancer. Within the following two years, there was a chain of serious reactions in her children and their families. One son began drinking for the first time in his life, the wife of another son had a serious depression, a daughter's husband failed in business, and another daughter's children became involved in automobile accidents and delinquency. Some symptoms were continuing five years later when the grandmother's cancer was pronounced cured. A more common example of the shock wave follows the death of an important grandparent, with symptoms appearing in a spectrum of children and grandchildren. The grandchild is often one who had little direct emotional attachment to the grandparents. An example: After the death of a grandmother, a daughter appeared to have no more than the usual grief reaction to the death but reacted in some deep way, transmitting her disturbance to a son who had never been close to the grandmother but who reacted to the mother with delinquent behavior. The family so camouflages the connectedness of these events that family members will further camouflage the sequence of events if they become aware the therapist is seeking some connectedness. Families are extremely reactive to any effort to approach the denial directly. There was a son in his mid-thirties who made a plane trip to see his mother who had had a stroke and who was aphasic. Before that time, his wife and children were leading an orderly life, and his business was going well. His effort to communicate with his mother, who could not speak, was a trying experience. En route home on the plane, he met a young woman with whom he began the first extramarital affair in his life. During the subsequent two years, he began living a double life, his business was failing, and his children began doing poorly in school. He made a good start in family therapy, which continued for six sessions; then I made a premature connection between his mother's stroke and the affair. He canceled the subsequent appointment and never returned. The nature of the human phenomenon is such that it reacts vigorously to any such implications of the dependence of one life on another.

Other families are less reactive and they can be more interested in the phenomenon than reactive to it. I have seen only one family who had made an automatic connection between such events before seeking therapy. This was a father who said, "My family was calm and healthy until two years ago when my daughter was married. Since then it has been one trouble after another, and the doctor bills have become exorbitant. My wife had a gall bladder operation. After that, she found something wrong with each house where we lived. We have broken three leases and moved four times. Then she developed a back problem and had a spinal fusion. My son had been a good student before my daughter married. Last year, his school work went down and this year he dropped out of college. In the midst of this, I had a heart attack." I would see this as a family with tenuously balanced emotional equilibrium in which the mother's functioning was dependent on her relationship with the daughter. Most of the subsequent dysfunction was in the mother, but the son and father were sufficiently dependent on the mother that they too developed symptoms. The incidence of the emotional shock wave is sufficiently prevalent that the Georgetown Family Section does a routine historical check for it in every family history.

Knowledge of the emotional shock wave is important in dealing with families on death issues. Not all deaths have the same importance to a family. There are some in which there is a fair chance the death will be followed by a shock wave. Other deaths are more neutral and are usually followed by no more than the usual grief and mourning reactions. Other deaths are a relief to the family and are usually followed by a period of better functioning. If the therapist can know ahead of time about the possibility of an emotional shock wave, he can take some steps toward its prevention. Among the deaths most likely to be followed by a serious and prolonged shock wave are the deaths of either parent when the family is young. This not only disturbs the emotional equilibrium, but also removes the function of the breadwinner or the mother at a time when these functions are most important. The death of an important child can shake the family equilibrium for years. The death of the "head of the clan" is another that can be followed by a long-term underground disturbance. It can be a grandfather who may have been partially disabled but who continued some kind of decision-making function in family affairs. The grandmothers in these families usually lived in the shadow of their husbands, and their deaths were less important. The family reaction can be intense following the death of a grandmother who was a central figure in the emotional life and stability of the family. The "head of the clan" can also be the most important sibling in the present generation. There is another group of family members whose deaths may result in no more than the usual period of grief and mourning. They may have been well liked, but they played peripheral roles in family affairs. They are the neutral ones who were neither "famous nor infamous." Their deaths are not likely to influence future family functioning. Finally, there are the family members whose deaths are a relief to the family. This includes the people whose functioning was never critical to the family, and who may have been a burden in their final illness. Their deaths may be followed by a brief period of grief and mourning, which is then followed by improved family functioning. A shock wave rarely follows the death of a dysfunctional family member unless that dysfunction played a critical role in maintaining family emotional equilibrium. Suicides are commonly followed by prolonged grief and mourning reactions, but the shock wave is usually minor unless the suicide was an abdication of an essential functional role.

Therapy at the Time of Death

Knowledge of the total family configuration, the functioning position of the dying person in the family, and the overall level of life adaptation is important for anyone who attempts to help a family before, during, or after a death. To attempt to treat all deaths as the same can miss the mark. Some well-functioning families are able to adapt to approaching death before it occurs. To assume that such families need help can be an inept intrusion. Physicians and hospitals have left much of the problems about death to chaplains and ministers with the expectation they know what to do. There are exceptional clergymen who intuitively know what to do. However, many young chaplains or clergymen tend to treat all death as the same. They operate with their theology, a theory about death that does not go beyond the familiar concepts of grief and mourning, and they tend to aim their help at the overt expression of grief. This may provide superficial help to a majority of people, but it misses the deeper process. The popular notion that expression of grief through crying may be helpful to most complicates the situation for others. It is important for the physician or therapist to know the situation, to have his own emotional life under reasonable control without the use of too much denial or other extreme mechanisms, and to respect the denial that operates in the family. In my work with families, I carefully use direct words, such as death, die, and bury, and I carefully avoid the use of less direct works, such as passed on, deceased, and expired. A direct word signals to the other that I am comfortable with the subject, and it enables others to also be comfortable. A tangential word may appear to soften the fact of death; but it invites the family to respond with tangential words, and the conversation soon reaches the point that one wonders if we are talking about death at all. The use of direct words helps to open a closed emotional system. I believe it provides a different dimension in helping the family to be comfortable within themselves.

The following is a clinical example that illustrates an effort to open the communication with a terminally ill patient, her family, and the medical staff. As a visiting professor in another medical center, I was scheduled to do a demonstration interview with the parents of an emotionally disturbed daughter. En route to the interview room, I learned the mother had a terminal cancer, that the surgeon had told the father, and the father had told the family therapist, but that the mother did not know about it. In my own practice, it would have been automatic to discuss this issue with the family, but I was reluctant to take this course when follow-up interviews would not be possible. A large group of professional people and trainees observed the interview. I elected to avoid the critical issue. The beginning of the interview was awkward, difficult, and sticky. I decided the cancer issue had to be discussed. About ten minutes out, I asked the mother why she thought her surgeon, her family, and the others had not told her about her cancer. Without the slightest hesitation, she said she thought they were afraid to tell her. She calmly said, "I know I have cancer. I have known it for some time. Before that, I was afraid of it, but they told me it was not cancer. I believed them for a time, thinking it was my imagination. Now I know it is cancer. When I ask them and they say 'No,' what does it mean? It either means they are liars or I am crazy, and I know I am not crazy." Then she went into detail about her feelings, with some moderate tears, but with full control of herself. She said that she was not afraid to die for herself, but she would like to live long enough to see the daughter have a life for herself. She hated the responsibility of leaving the daughter the responsibility of the father. She spoke with deep feeling but few tears. She and I were the calmest people in the room. Her therapist wiped away tears. The father reacted by joking and kidding about the mother's vivid imagination. To prevent his reaction from silencing her, I made a few comments to suggest he not interfere with his wife's serious thoughts. She was able to continue, "This is the loneliest life in the world. Here I am, knowing I am going to die, and not knowing how much time I have left. I can't talk to anyone. When I talk to my surgeon, he says it is not a cancer. When I try to talk to my husband, he makes jokes about it. I came here to talk about my daughter and not about myself. I am cut off from everyone. When I get up in the morning, I feel terrible. I look at my eyes in the mirror to see if they are jaundiced and the cancer has spread to my liver. I try to act cheerful until my husband goes to work, because I don't want to upset him. Then I am alone all day with my thoughts, just crying and thinking. Before my husband returns from work, I try to pull myself together for his sake. I wish I could die soon and not have to pretend any longer." Then she went into some background thoughts about death. As a little girl she felt hurt when people walked on graves. She had always wished she could be buried above ground in a mausoleum, so people would not walk on her grave. "But," she said, "We are poor people. We can't afford a mausoleum. When I die, I will be buried in a grave just like everyone else." The technical problem in this single interview was to permit the mother to talk, to keep the father's anxiety from silencing her, and to hope the regular therapist could continue the process later. It is impossible to do much toward opening an emotionally closed relationship of this intensity in a single session, although the father said he would try to listen and understand. The patient was relieved to be partially out of the closed system in which she had lived. The therapist said she had known about the cancer but had been waiting for the mother to bring it up. This is a common posture for mental health professionals. The therapist's own emotionality had prevented the wife from talking. At the end of the interview, the mother said, smiling through her tears, "We have sure spent an hour walking around on my grave, haven't we?" As I said goodbye to them in the hall, the mother said, "When you go home tonight, thank Washington for sending you here today." The less expressive father said, "We are both grateful." There were a few minutes with the audience who had observed the interview. Part of the group had been moved to tears, most were silent and serious, and a few were critical. The criticism was expressed by a young physician who spoke of hurting the wife and having taken away her hope. I was pleased at having decided to take up this issue in this single demonstration interview. En route home, my thoughts went to the differences in audience response and the problems of training young professional people to contain their own emotionality sufficiently to become more objective about death. I guessed it would be easier to train those who cried than those who intellectualized their feelings. This is an example of a good result in a single session. It illustrates the intensity of a closed relationship system between the patient, the family, and the medical staff.

The Function of Funerals

Some 25 years ago, I had a clinical experience that illustrates the central point of the next section of this chapter. A young woman began psychoanalysis with, "Let me bury my mother before we go on to other things." Her mother had been dead six years. She cried for weeks. At the time, I was practicing within the framework of transference and intrapsychic dynamics. The patient's statement was used later as a way of describing systems theory about the unresolved emotional attachments between people that remain viable for life, that attach to significant future relationships, and that continue to direct the course of a life. There is a way to utilize the funeral to more completely "bury the dead at the time of death." Few human events provide as much emotional impact as serious illness and death in resolving unresolved emotional attachments.

The funeral ritual has existed in some form since man became a civilized being. I believe it serves a common function of bringing survivors into intimate contact with the dead and with important friends, and it helps survivors and friends to terminate their relationship with the dead and to move forward with life. I think the best function of a funeral is served when it brings relatives and friends into the best possible functional contact with the harsh fact of death and with each other at this time of high emotionality. I believe funerals were probably more effective when people died at home with the family present, and when family and friends made the coffin and did the burial themselves. Society no longer permits this, but there are ways to bring about a reasonable level of personal contact with the dead body and the survivors.

There are numerous present-day funeral customs that function to deny death and to perpetuate the unresolved emotional attachments between the dead and the living. It is most intense in people who are anxious about death and who use the present form and content of funerals to avoid the anxiety. There are those who refuse to look at a dead body because, "I want to remember them as I knew them." There is the anxious segment of society that refers to funerals as pagan rituals. Funeral custom makes it possible for the body to be disposed of from the hospital without the family ever having personal contact with it. Children are commonly excluded from funerals to avoid upsetting them. This can result in a lifetime of unrealistic and distorted fantasies and images that may never be corrected. The private funeral is another custom that avoids the emotionality of death. It is motivated by family anxiety to avoid contact with emotionality in others. It denies the friendship system an opportunity to terminate their relationship with the dead, and it deprives the family of the supportive relationships from friends.

I believe that professional support to a family at the time of death can help the family members toward a more helpful funeral than would be possible if they listened to advice from anxious relatives and friends. In 20 years of family practice, I have had contact with several thousand families, and I have been in the background "coaching" families through hundreds of deaths and funerals. I urge family members to visit dying family members whenever possible and to find some way to include children if the situation permits. I have never seen a child hurt by exposure to death. They are "hurt" only by the anxiety of survivors. I encourage involvement of the largest possible group of extended family members, an open casket, and the most personal contact that is possible between the dead and the living prompt obituary notices; and the notification of relatives and friends, a public funeral with the body present, and the most personal funeral service that is possible. Some funeral services are highly ritualized but it is possible to personalize even the most ritualized service. The goal is to bring the entire family system into the closest possible contact with death in the presence of the total friendship system and to lend a helping hand to the anxious people who would rather run than face a funeral.

The following is an example of coaching friends from the background. It involved neighbors rather than people in my professional practice. The young parents in their early thirties and their three children ages ten, eight, and five, had come to live with her widowed mother in preparation for the husband's going overseas on a prolonged assignment. On a Sunday one month before his scheduled departure, the young mother died suddenly of a heart attack. The entire community was shocked. That evening, I spent some three hours with the father. He and his wife had been very close. He had dozens of questions about how to handle the present emergency, the funeral, the future of the children, and his own life. He wondered if the children should go to school the next day, what he should tell the teachers, and if he should seek release from his overseas work. In the afternoon, he had tried to tell the children about their mother's death, but he started to cry and the children responded, "Please don't cry, Daddy." He said he simply had to have another mother for the children, but he felt guilty saying this only eight hours after his wife had died. During the visit, I outlined what I would consider to be the ideal course of action for him. I suggested he take as many of the ideas as were consistent with himself, and if they made sense to him, to use them as far as he could go. I suggested that the ability of children to deal with death depends on the adults, and the future would be best served if the death could be presented in terms the children could understand and they could be realistically involved in the funeral. I warned him of adverse emotional reactions of friends and to be prepared for criticism if he decided to involve the children. In the first hours after the death, the children had been responding to his emotionality rather than to the fact of the mother's death. In this kind of situation, it is common for the children to stop talking and deny the death. I suggested that he get through this block by mentioning the death at frequent intervals during the coming days, and, if he started to cry, to reassure the children that he was all right and not to worry about him.

I wanted to keep the channel open for any and all questions they might have. I suggested that the children decide whether or not they wished to go to school the next day. On the issue of involving the children with the dead mother, I suggested that he arrange a time before the funeral to take the children to the funeral home, to remove all other people from the room, and for him and the children to have a private session with their dead mother. I reasoned that this would help the children adapt to the reality of the mother's death, and that it could work if anxious members of the extended family were excluded. On Tuesday evening, I spent an hour in the bedroom with the father in a chair and the three children in his lap. He could cry, and they could cry, and the children were free to ask questions. He told them about the plan to go to the funeral home the following afternoon. The five-year-old son asked if he could kiss Mommie.

The father looked to me for an answer. I suggested that would be between the son and his mother. Later, in the living room, I announced to the relatives and friends that the father would take the children to the funeral home the next afternoon, that it was to be private, and that no one else could be present. Privately, I considered it unwise to expose the children to the emotionality in that family. The father's mother said, "Son, that will be too hard on you." The father replied, "Mother, shut up. I can do it." On Wednesday evening, I visited the funeral home. The entire family friendship system was present. The maternal grandmother, who had been calm through these days, said, "Thank you very much for your help." The father did a detailed account of the children's visit in the afternoon. The children went up to the casket and felt their mother. The five-year-old son said, "If I kissed her, she could not kiss back." All three spent some time inspecting everything, even looking under the casket. The eight-year-old son got under the casket and prayed that his mother could hold him in her arms again in heaven. Some family friends came while the father and children were in the room. The father and children withdrew to the lobby while the friends went into the room. In the lobby, the youngest son found some polished pebbles in a planter. He was the one who found objects to give his mother as "presents." He took a small pebble into the room and placed it in his mother's hand. The other children also got pebbles and put them into their mother's hand. They then announced, "We can go now Daddy." The father was much relieved at the outcome of the visit. He said, "A thousand tons were lifted from this family today." The following day I attended the funeral. The children did well. The ten-year-old daughter and eight-year-old son were calm. During the service, the eight-year-old whispered to the father, "Daddy, I sure am going to miss Mommie." The five-year-old clung to the father with some tearfulness.

There was some criticism about the father involving the children in the funeral, but he did well with it and the criticism turned to admiration after the funeral home visit. I was in close contact with the family the following year. The father continued to mention the mother's death. Within a week the children were talking about the mother in the past tense. The children stayed with their grandmother. There was none of the usual complications usually seen after a death of this kind. The father took an assignment closer to home, so he could return if he was needed.

The following year, the father remarried and took the children with him and his new wife to another city. It has now been 12 years since the death and the family adjustment has been perfect. I am still in periodic contact with the family, which now includes three grown children from the first marriage and younger children from the second marriage. Some years after the death, the father wrote his version of the experience when the first wife died, entitled, "My God, My Wife Is Dead." He described his initial shock, his efforts to get beyond self-pity, his resolution to make his own decisions when anxiety was high, and the emotional courage that went into his plan in the critical days before the funeral and burial. This illustrates what I would consider an optimum result from a traumatic death that could have had lifelong sequelae; but this father had more inner strength than any other relative I have seen under stress of this intensity.

Summary

Family systems theory provides a broader perspective of death than is possible with conventional psychiatric theory, which focuses on death as a process within the individual. The first part of this chapter deals with the closed relationship system between the patient, the family, and physicians, and family therapy methods that have been helpful in overcoming some of the anxiety that creates the closed system communication. The second section deals with the "Emotional Shock Wave" that is present to some degree in a significant percentage of families.

Knowledge of this, which is the direct result of family research, provides the professional person with a different dimension for understanding emotional interdependence and the long-term complications of death in a family. The final section deals with the emotional impact of funerals and ways the professional person can help surviving relatives to achieve a better level of emotional functioning by calmly facing the anxiety of death.

NOTE

1 This chapter was first published in *Family Therapy: Theory and Practice*, edited by Phillip J. Guerin. New York: Gardner Press, 1976. (Reprinted with permission).

REFERENCE

Bowen, M. (1978). *Family reaction to death: Family therapy in clinical practice.* Jason Aronson: New York and London.

2

DEATH AND DIFFERENTIATION IN THE FAMILY

Peter Titelman

There are many books and journal articles on illness and death, but for the most part they focus on the individual who is chronically ill or the individual who is dying or has died. This edited book is different. It is based on Bowen family systems theory and its paradigm of the family as an emotional unit. This approach views the death of a family member as an important nodal event as the family seeks to maintain equilibrium in its emotional unit or system. In Bowen theory the family consists of the nuclear family as well as the extended families.

Murray Bowen's classic chapter on this subject is "Family Reaction to Death" (1978, pp. 321–335). It is the cornerstone of this book. Each author is grounded in Bowen theory but brings to the topic his or her own experience, perspective, and thinking, creating what we might call a collection of individual "I-Statements."

Bowen's Experience With Mortality: From Youth to Adulthood

Looking at the facts of Murray Bowen's life can shed some light onto the development of Bowen theory and Bowen's ability to take a new theoretical stance on death and loss. Murray Bowen was the oldest of his siblings and a natural leader in his family of origin. His father owned and ran a funeral home in Waverly, Tennessee. His involvement with the family funeral home put him in touch with death as a natural part of the human life cycle and taught him that life and death are inevitably linked together. Bowen saw death beginning in his youth, and death did not make him anxious.

He grew up on the family farm in contact with the world of animals and other forms of nature. He saw animals being born and dying, and this experience undoubtedly played a part in his later interest in natural systems.

As an adolescent, Bowen worked on an ambulance taking sick or injured patients to the hospital. Seeing an adolescent male die in the confusion of the hospital was a nodal event, one strand that led him to studying medicine and surgery before choosing to become a psychiatrist.

Before studying psychiatry Bowen spent four years as a physician, stationed in England during World War II. Undoubtedly, this was another experience of dealing with trauma and death.

During his psychiatric residency at the Menninger Institute after the war, Bowen interviewed suicidal patients and had communication that was open and straightforward. In every interview Bowen had with patients regarding death, they spoke directly and openly about it. It was a reciprocal process, one that was initiated by Bowen's lack of anxiety and fear of death. That set up the potential for having an "open system" conversation about death. Bowen was among the first in psychiatry and medicine to address chronic illness and death directly.

Bowen's Natural Systems Perspective on Death

Bowen wrote that:

> Man . . . follows the same predictable instinctual life pattern of all living things. He is born, he grows to maturity, he reproduces, his life force runs out, and he dies.
>
> (1978, p. 321)

Man is more preoccupied with death or with staying alive than with any other subject. Death is universal. The human is like all biological organisms in that all lives end in death. If one did not die, one would have never lived. There never could be a beginning of life, if there is not also an end to life.

Bowen Theory Provides a Framework for Understanding Death in the Family

This chapter includes the following sections: 1) The Family Is an Emotional System, 2) Differentiation of Self in Relation to Death in the Family, 3) The Solid Self and the Pseudo Self in Relation to Death in the Family, 4) Basic and Functional Levels of Differentiation of Self in Relation to Death in the Family, 5) Differentiation of Self and Chronic Anxiety in Relation to Death in the Family, 6) Emotional Reactivity and Differentiation of Self in Relation to Death in the Family, 7) The Continuum of Differentiation in the Family in Relation to Death, 8) Variation in Differentiation and Family Reaction to Death, and 9) A Clinical Application for Chronic Illness and Death in the Family: Talk to the Person Behind the Dysfunction.

The Family Is an Emotional System

In the 1950s there was a beginning shift in focus from the individual to a family focus as the unit of study. Bowen was one of several investigators who initiated the family therapy movement at that time.

Bowen's initial theoretical description of "the family as a system" took place in 1955, at the beginning of a paradigm shift from an individual to a family focus for the *emotional unit* of psychotherapy, theory, and research in a small nationwide group of psychotherapists and researchers. Bowen and other family therapists initially used the phrase "the family as the unit of treatment," and the shorthand phrase became "the family as a unit" in the context of clinical practice.

Bowen's natural systems theoretical version of the new paradigm was that the family is an *emotional system.* He thought of the family as "a combination of 'emotional' and 'relationship' systems." The term "emotional system" refers to the force that motivates the system, and "relationship system" refers to the way it is expressed (1978, p. 158).

The following are key components of Bowen's paradigm of the family as an emotional unit.

1. The family is a *multigenerational emotional system* that consists of the individuals in the family, the nuclear family, the family of origin,

and the extended family. It includes all living members of the family, usually involving three generations, and sometimes more.

2. *The forces of togetherness and individuality* in the emotional system drive relationships in the family unit. These forces are expressed through the emotional process in the relationship system.
3. *Family emotional process* is the emotional activity or reactivity that occurs between two or more individuals in the family. Bowen described emotional process as "the emotional responsiveness by which one family member responds automatically to the emotional state of another . . . It operates during periods of conflict and periods of calm harmony" (1978, pp. 66–67).
4. The family system is held together like an emotional magnet. The term *emotional fusion* describes the behavioral expression of the emotional stuck-togetherness, or emotional oneness, that is found along a continuum in all parts of the multigenerational emotional family.
5. The family system includes the interlocking, *reciprocal functioning* in the relationship system. It includes compensatory change in two persons in the nuclear family; or compensatory change in a segment of the nuclear family; or compensatory change in one or other parts of the family of origin, the extended family, and compensatory reciprocal functioning in multiple generations.
6. *Overadequate-inadequate reciprocity*, which later was renamed *underfunctioning-overfunctioning reciprocity*, is the borrowing and lending of self in the reciprocal functioning between two family members. When this occurs, both selves are compromised, at least to some degree (Titelman, 2014, p. 22).
7. *Functioning position* refers neutrally to the position an individual occupies in the family system in relation to the reciprocally determined positions of the other family members. Bowen took the term "function" from biology to describe the behavior of an individual, a part of the family system, or the family as a whole (Titelman, 2014, p. 22).

The Concept of Differentiation of Self

Differentiation of self is the cornerstone concept in Bowen family systems theory. *Differentiation of self* is an automatic, natural process, and *defining a self* is an intentional process in the human species (Titelman, 2014, p. 24).

Bowen wrote:

> The term "differentiation of self" was chosen as one that most accurately describes this long-term process in which the child slowly disengages from the original fusion with his mother and moves toward his own emotional autonomy.
>
> (1972, p. 74)

> The concept of differentiation of self deals with the degree to which a person becomes emotionally "differentiated" from the parent. In a broad sense the infant is physically separated from the mother at birth, but the process of emotional separation is slow and complicated, and at best incomplete. Originally, it has to do more with factors in the mother and her ability to permit the child to grow away from her, than with factors in the infant.
>
> (1972, p. 74)

This author suggests that the father also may or may not have the capacity to allow the child to grow way from him.

Both the natural process of differentiation of self and the intentional process of defining a self refer to an individual's capacity, or lack of capacity, to separate instinctually driven emotional reactivity from thoughtful, goal-directed activity (Titelman, 2014, p. 24).

Bowen wrote that "[t]he core of my theory had to do with the degree to which people are able to distinguish between the *feeling* and the *intellectual* process" (1978, p. 355).

This author wrote:

> The essence of the continuum of differentiation/undifferentiation is the degree of emotional stuck-togetherness, emotional oneness, or emotional fusion of the members of a family. Bowen originally described this as *the undifferentiated family ego mass*, and later as the *nuclear family emotional system* . . . . Differentiation of self can also be described as the variation in an

> individual's capacity to be a separate self while functioning as part of a family or group.
>
> (Titelman, 2014, p. 25)

Bowen postulated that there are two forces underlying differentiation of self: *togetherness* and *individuality*, [He] described them as residing in the emotional system. Although there is no scientific proof that these instinctual forces exist, Bowen theorists and clinicians have documented empirically—through clinical and nonclinical observation—the behaviors that clearly express these phenomena.

> The instinct for *togetherness* propels an individual to be connected, dependent, and an indistinct part of a couple, family, or nonfamily group. The force for *individuality* propels the individual to be a separate, independent, and distinct entity, following his/her own directives. Differentiation of self, natural, or modified by an individual's efforts, is the balancing of these two instincts in the intellectual system. The more emotion dominates the balance of the two forces, the lower an individual's level of differentiation of self. The more intellect dominates the balance of the two instincts, the higher an individual's level of differentiation of self.
>
> (Titelman, 2014, pp. 25–26)

The Solid Self and the Pseudo Self in Relation to Death in the Family

This author wrote:

> *Solid self* and *pseudo-self* represent two separate modes of functioning that run along a continuum, with pseudo-self at the lower end of functioning and solid self at the higher end of differentiated functioning. The balance of pseudo-self and solid self depends upon which of the two is more prominent . . . The solid self is made up of defined beliefs, convictions, and life principles that are not given up in the face of pressure from the other. Bowen wrote: "Each belief and principle is consistent with the others and [solid] self will

> take responsible action on the principles even in situations of high anxiety" (1978, p. 406). The solid self is expressed through taking I-positions. This is where an individual stands against the pressure of the family (or significant nonfamily members) to bend to the forces of togetherness, and to adapt to the other(s)' views or behaviors in which the self does not believe . . . The pseudo self is a "pretend" self. It is both acquired by and can be changed by emotional pressure from others. Bowen described the pseudo self in the following way: "It is made up of random and discrepant beliefs and principles, acquired because they were required, it is the right thing to believe or to do, or to enhance self image in the social amalgam" (1978, p. 406).
>
> (Titelman, 2014, p. 28)

Families facing the death of a family member, and whose levels of differentiation are moderate to higher, are those who have more solid selves. These families, consisting of the aggregate of their members, are individuals who are not emotionally fused in their family unit. They can be emotionally close, but they are able to maintain their individuality as solid selves. The individuality force is more dominant than the togetherness force. If it is the leader who has died, a new leader emerges and the family accepts and supports him or her. New leadership functions may be distributed in maintaining the stability of the family unit. Families with higher levels of differentiation can be emotionally close, but they are able to maintain their individuality as solid selves.

Families with low levels of differentiation are those that have pseudo selves. They are dominated by the togetherness force over the individuality force. The aggregate members of these families are more undifferentiated and they are more emotionally fused together. Bowen called this emotional oneness and, originally, the undifferentiated ego mass. When family members at low levels of differentiation face death in the family, particularly the death of a leader or significant member, they are more unlikely to be able to maintain the stability of the family emotional unit. It is as if the family leader has been torn away from the family unit, leaving its energy stuck and destabilized.

Basic and Functional Levels of Differentiation of Self in Relation to Death in the Family

It is extremely difficult to assess and conceptualize the discrepancy between the basic and functional levels of individuals, and even more difficult, of the family. The difficulty is that humans have both a solid self and a pseudo self, as was described in the previous section. When an individual is "borrowing" and "lending self" in his or her relationships with family members and significant nonfamily members, through the process of fusion or undifferentiation, she or he will present as having a higher or lower level of functional differentiation compared to her or his basic level of differentiation.

Bowen wrote:

> The degree of pseudo self varies so much it is not possible to make a valid estimate of solid self except from estimating the life patterns over long periods of time . . . With all the variables, it is possible to do a reasonably accurate estimate of the degree of differentiation of self from the fusion patterns in past generations and from the over-all course of a life in the present. (1978, p. 306)

Facing death in a family is one of, if not the most, harsh nodal event(s) in human life. It often raises tremendous stress, acute and chronic anxiety, and reactivity. Bowen wrote: "The real test of the stability of the differentiation comes when the person is again subjected to chronic severe stress" (1978, p. 371).

Differentiation of Self and Chronic Anxiety in Relation to Death in the Family

Although *differentiation of self* is the cornerstone concept of Bowen's theory, differentiation of self is both a concept and a variable. The two main variables in the theory are the continuum of differentiation of self and the range of chronic anxiety. In Bowen theory acute anxiety is the individual's psychological and/or physiological response to a real threat. It is usually time-limited. Chronic anxiety is a response to a perceived or imagined threat that is usually unlimited over time.

Kerr wrote "[S]pecific events or issues are usually the principal generators of acute anxiety. The principal generators of chronic anxiety are people's reactions to a disturbance in the balance of a relationship system" (Kerr and Bowen, 1988, p. 113).

On the continuum of differentiation, higher levels of chronic anxiety are associated with lower functional levels of differentiation of self. Lower levels of chronic anxiety are associated with higher functional levels of differentiation.

Facing death in the family raises acute anxiety for family members and the family as a whole. Those at lower levels of differentiation are more likely to enter a state of chronic anxiety. Families in the mid-range or higher levels of differentiation are unlikely to continue in a state of chronic anxiety and the family tends to emotionally stabilize itself.

Emotional Reactivity and Differentiation of Self in Relation to Death in the Family

This author (2014) wrote that:

> *Emotional reactivity* is the behavioral and physiological expression of anxiety, acute or chronic, in response to another individual. It initially occurs in the family relationship system, and then later in other nonfamily relationships. Reactivity in one family member triggers reactivity in another. Chronic reactivity, in the context of chronic anxiety, leads to a disturbance in the balance of a relationship.
>
> The intensity of emotional reactivity, like that of chronic anxiety, is also linked to the level of differentiation. The lower the level of differentiation, the more frequent the episodes of emotional reactivity, and they are more frequent at higher levels of intensity. At higher levels of differentiation of self, there are less frequent episodes of reactivity and the levels of emotional reactivity are less intense.
>
> (Titelman, 2014, pp. 29–30)

When stress, reactivity, and chronic anxiety are high, the level of differentiation is at a lower level. When a family at the lower level is dealing with death in the family but not confronting it directly, the family emotional unit may become destabilized. And, conversely, when stress, chronic anxiety, reactivity, and adaptiveness are low, the level of differentiation is high, and the family openly and directly communicates regarding death. Adaptiveness is the capacity of the individual and the family to regulate their anxiety and emotional reactiveness in order to maintain or stabilize the emotional equilibrium in the family emotional unit.

The Continuum of Differentiation in the Family in Relation to Death

The capacity to define self in the face of death of family members is a significant factor in Bowen's profile of the continuum of differentiation. Families that have the aggregate of members with moderate and higher levels on the continuum of differentiation are more able to be realistic about communicating and dealing with chronic illness and/or death in the family. Families that have an aggregate of members who are at the lower level of differentiation are more likely to be in denial regarding facing death. They are less likely to be able to communicate openly about these subjects and more likely to have psychological, physical, or social symptoms relating to the loss of their family member.

Based on the aggregate of the family members' emotional stuck-togetherness, emotional oneness, or emotional fusion, the differentiation of family members lies along a continuum of instability/stability at the time of death.

It is essential to understand variation in a family's level of chronic anxiety, stress, and adaptiveness in reaction to chronic illness or death. Families at the lower end of the continuum are more likely to experience more intense "emotional shock waves" (Bowen, 1978) within their nuclear and extended families over multiple generations. Their resilience is weak, and stabilizing the family unit after death is much more difficult. Families functioning at the moderate and higher levels of differentiation are more likely to be able to maintain or stabilize the family emotional unit when facing chronic illness and death. Families' levels of differentiation are crucial variables in responding to death, according to Bowen theory.

Variation in Differentiation and Family Reaction to Death

Low Differentiation in the Family	High Differentiation in the Family
Closed communication in the family	Open communication in the family
Triangles Triangles increase with chronic illness and death in the family; more blaming	**Triangles** Less triangling; dealing one-to-one with members in the family
Nuclear Family • Less stable • More emotional fusion • More unresolved attachment • More grieving	**Nuclear Family** • More stable • Less emotional fusion • Less unresolved attachment • Less grieving and more resilience
The Family Projection Process More blame and scapegoating	**The Family Projection Process** More responsibility for self
Emotional Cutoff More distancing, tearing away	**Emotional Cutoff** Autonomous connection
Multigenerational Emotional Process More intensity, chronic anxiety, and more family members experience greater impact from shock waves	**Multigenerational Emotional Process** Less intensity, chronic anxiety, and family members are less impacted by emotional shock waves
Societal Process Less involvement with extended family, friends, and community when dealing with chronic illness and death.	**Societal Process** Dealing directly with death with family, friends, and community
Emotional Shock Waves • More emotionally significant shock waves • More instability between couples and between couples and families • More likely to lead to health, work, and education problems, and issues in couples or larger families	**Emotional Shock Waves** • Fewer emotional shock waves • Will tend to have more stability couples and families • More likely to not have health, work, and education problems and issues in couples or larger families

Figure 2.1 Variation in differentiation and family reaction to death

Bowen's Clinical Approach to Death: Principles, Concepts, and Rituals

The Denial of Death in the Family

Bowen's clinical approach involved his effort to deal directly with individuals and family members regarding chronic illness and death. He had two principles for both his clients and his own family, friends, and colleagues: 1) being "present and accounted for" when a family member, friend, or colleague is seriously chronically ill, dying, or dead; and 2) facing death directly, without denial, and approaching death in a manner of "easy come, easy go," not denying death but also not overfocusing on death.

Bowen respected the denial that operates in the family. However, he was comfortable and not anxious in using direct words: "death," "die," and "bury." He avoided using less direct words such as "passed on," "deceased," and "expired." Bowen believed it helped the dying person and his or her family members to be more open and realistic about death (1978, p. 329).

The Context of "Open" and "Closed" Systems in Relation to Death

Bowen (1978) wrote:

> An "open" relationship system is one in which an individual is free to communicate a high percentage of inner thoughts, feelings and fantasies to another who can reciprocate. No one ever has a completely open relationship with another, but it is a healthy state when a person can have a relationship in which a reasonable degree of openness is possible . . . The "closed" communication system is an automatic emotional reflex to protect self from the anxiety in the other person, though most people say they avoid the taboo subjects to keep from upsetting the other person.
>
> (p. 322)

The "closed system" is particularly prevalent in the process of communicating about dying and death. Bowen describes the interlock between three closed systems. Each of these

> systems plays a part in the closed communications system. The three closed processes are: 1) the individual patient's intrapsychic denial of death in his or her closed system; 2) the family's closed system in denial of the dying family member, and 3) the physician's anxiety that drives his denial and lack of clarity in describing death to the patient and his or her family interlock. It can be described as a "closed triangle communication process" that leaves the dying patient in the outside position, and the patient's family and the treating physician in the inside positions. However, each leg of the triangle is in the dark. Each side of the triangle cannot communicate clearly and openly in relation to the other two sides. Bowen described poor communication between the physician and the family and between the physician and the patient as the greatest problem.
>
> (1978, p. 324)

> Open and closed systems in communicating about death and grieving vary along a continuum of differentiation. The continuum includes levels of chronic anxiety and the range of differentiation of self for patients, families, and physicians in reaction to death.

The Emotional Shock Wave and Death

This section describes Bowen's auxiliary concept, the emotional shock wave, that occurs in many families dealing with death. It describes how some families, with lower or medium levels of differentiation of self, develop symptoms (psychological, physical, and social as well as accidents, among other problems) in reaction to a family member having a chronic illness or death. The shock waves can move through multiple generations over time or can be contained in the nuclear family. Depending on the degree of intensity and levels of differentiation, families with higher levels of differentiation of self tend to have less intense emotional shock waves with fewer symptoms. If they do have them, they last a shorter time than families with lower levels of differentiation.

> A family unit is in functional equilibrium when it is calm and each member is functioning at reasonable efficiency for that

> period. The equilibrium of the unit is disturbed by either the addition of a new member or the loss a member. The intensity of the emotional reaction is governed by the functioning level of emotional integration in the family at the time, or by the functional importance of the one who is added to the family or lost to the family.
>
> (Bowen, 1978, pp. 324–325)

Bowen (1978) also wrote:

> The "Emotional Shock Wave" is a network of underground "after-shocks" of serious life events that can occur anywhere in the extended family system in the months or years following serious emotional events in a family. It occurs most often after the death or threatened death of a significant family member, but it can occur following losses of other types.
>
> (p. 325)

In summary, emotional shock waves have five components: 1) levels of differentiation in the family; 2) levels of chronic anxiety in the family; 3) a chronic illness, death, or an addition in the family; 4) denial of emotional fusion in the family; and 5) higher levels of the intensity in shock waves can produce a multigenerational transmission of shock waves in extended families over several generations.

Bowen believed that the emotional shock wave was present, to some degree, in a significant percentage of families. According to Bonanno's research (2005; Bonanno, Westphal & Mancini, 2011), a high percentage of families show resilience following the death of a family member. It may be that this is true for the population Bonanno has studied. However, he did study individuals rather than families in his research, and he therefore did not observe the emotional shock waves and disequilibrium in wider family systems after the serious chronic disease or death of a family member.

Functioning Position and Death

Functioning position is an auxiliary Bowen concept. It is a component in several concepts in Bowen theory (*triangles, the nuclear family, the family projection process, the multigenerational transmission process, sibling position, emotional cutoff, and societal emotional process*). *Functioning position* refers neutrally to the position an individual occupies in the family system in relation to the reciprocally determined positions of the other family members.

According to Bowen, when a family member dies, the functioning positions of the living family members will shift, and that will modify the family's functioning in terms of stability or instability. The negative impact on the family is much more powerful with the death of the family leader such as a father, mother, or grandparent. If death involves a "special child," a suicide, or loss of an individual at an early age, the impact on the family is also very powerful. If the family member holds a functioning position of less importance in the family, there is less impact on the family. Examples of lower-impact death and chronic illness are 1) if the dying person has had a lengthy chronic illness and has not been active in the family system for a long period of time, 2) if an individual has a less important position in the family, or 3) if his or her physical or mental functioning is hampered to the degree that he or she makes limited contributions to the functioning of the family as a whole.

Death Rituals in the Family

Human beings are the only species that ponder and reflect upon their own death through an awareness of the past, present, and future. "A ritual is a set of actions, religious or secular, that generates symbolic meaning. Individuals, groups, or entire communities can enact them, publicly or privately, in formal or informal settings" (Titelman, 2014, p. 134). Humans have always had a variety of rituals, religious or secular, depending on their cultures and philosophies. They are mostly related to the traditions of their families, tribes, states, or countries, based on their level of emotional attachment to their parents and extended families. Death rituals and particularly burial grounds permit families to recognize their territorial origins and their continuing history in the past and future. While humans are primarily emotional beings, they do have the capacity to reflect on the meaning of life and death, and this is often expressed through traditional rituals.

Death rituals allow the family and larger social networks to acknowledge death without denial and without isolating the family from the community. Bowen described the universal importance of ritual in dealing with death:

> The best function of the funeral is served when it brings relatives and friends into the best possible functional contact with the harsh fact of death and with each other at this time of high emotionality.
>
> (1978, p. 331)

This author (2014) wrote:

> Family death rituals . . . are enacted along the continuum of differentiation of self in the family. At the lower end of the continuum the ritual will be more inflexible, more rote, and will involve a higher level of emotional reactivity. At higher levels on the continuum, family rituals are more flexible and less emotionally reactive—that is, less impulsive and out of control. They are more expressive of the individuality of family members, rather than being driven by emotional fusion in the family or by societal patterns and expectations.
>
> (p. 134)

This author (2014) also wrote:

> The function of rituals applies equally to religious, secular, traditional, and nontraditional death rituals. The advantages of certain ancient traditional rituals, or newly created ones, depend on the levels of differentiation and chronic anxiety that undergird the way those rituals are expressed and experienced by families and communities.
>
> (p. 134)

Variation in Levels of Differentiation for Families Facing Death

The quandary is in conceptualizing the discrepancy between basic and functional differentiation of self:

> When an individual is "borrowing" and "lending" self in his or her relationships with spouse, children, parents, extended family, and significant or nonfamily members—through the process of emotional fusion or undifferentiation—he or she will present having a higher or lower level of functional differentiation in comparison to his or her basic level of differentiation.
>
> (Titelman, 2014, p. 32)

Bowen wrote:

> The real test of the stability of the differentiation comes when the person [or family] is . . . subjected to chronic severe stress.
>
> (1978, p. 371)

Facing death in the family is a significant event for all humans. It tests the level of solid self. Although death is a very significant factor, it is only one factor that constitutes the profiles of the differentiation of self of the families and the individuals in the family.

The following four examples of families' reaction to death include one family where the information is based on public sources. The other three include a clinical family and two families that are personally known to the author. The four examples provide a variety of family reactions to death in reflecting their level of differentiation.

Conflict of Life and Death: A Family at a Low Level of Differentiation

This example of a family with a low level of differentiation of self is drawn from public sources. Terri Schiavo's death became a right-to-die legal case that lasted from 1990 to 2005. In 1990 she collapsed with cardiac arrest in her apartment in Florida, and her husband called 911.

Extreme dieting and massively overconsuming fluids apparently caused her condition. Family reactions in response to Terri's irreversible vegetative state were extremely intense.

Terri was born in 1963 in Moreland Township, Montgomery County, Pennsylvania, a suburb of Philadelphia. Her parents were Robert and Mary Schindler, and her younger siblings were Bobby and Suzanne. As an adolescent Terri was 5-foot-3 and weighed 200 pounds. She met Michael Schiavo in 1982, and they married in 1984.

Immediately following Terri's collapse in 1990, the relationship between her husband and her parents was amicable. Michael even lived rent-free in the Schindlers' condominium from 1990 to 2003. During that period, up until 1993, Michael sought many forms of treatment for his wife. In the middle of 1993, Michael requested a "do not resuscitate" (DNR) order, after Terri contracted a urinary tract infection (Wikipedia, 2017).

Terri's parents wished to keep her endlessly alive, and her husband wished to end her life as she was in a vegetative state. The conflict went on from 1993 to 2005. The parents struggled to keep their daughter "alive," even though she was in a lifeless condition. Discussion of this case in religious, judicial, legal, and political arenas, including U.S. President George W. Bush's return to Washington, DC, to sign legislation moving the case to the federal courts, added to the emotional reactivity of the conflict between Terri's parents and husband.

Family and societal reactions were extremely emotional and intense.

Terri's father said: "I'm numb, I'm just totally numb. This whole thing, it's hard to believe it." Schiavo's husband Michael Schiavo said he was outraged that the congressional leaders were intervening in the contentious right-to-die battle. He had battled for years with his wife's parents over whether she should be permitted to die or kept alive through the feeding tube . . . Bob Schindler visited his daughter late Sunday and he said he noticed the effects of dehydration on her. He said she appeared to be getting tired, but eventually responded to his teasing by making a face to him . . . Brian Schiavo, Michael's brother, said he spent Sunday afternoon with his brother and Terri at the hospice, but Terri did not move or make any noises.

> "Anybody that thinks that she talks and responds, they need to have a mental health examination," he said. (Bush Signs Schiavo Legislation, 2005)

When the family's conflicts involve many interlocking triangles, it is unlikely that a rational outcome can ever be achieved. The triangle between Terri's parents, her husband, and Terri herself was a "mental construct triangle."[1] The unconscious third party (Terri) could not be present in her permanently unconscious state, and therefore without Terri being able to participate, the situation could not be detriangled. However, in 2000 the federal court recorded that Terri "had made reliable oral declarations that she would have wanted the feeding tube removed" (Wikipedia). The feeding tube was removed and she died in March 2005.

Bowen theory would suggest that this family was at the low level of the continuum of differentiation, expressed by the amount of emotional fusion between the parents and the child. The parents had a need for emotional togetherness that was extremely intense, even when they could never again have a living relationship with Terri.

Functioning Positions and After-Shock Waves Over Three Generations Following a Death: A Family at the Moderate Level on the Continuum of Differentiation

The following is an example of *functioning positions* that were transmitted across three generations in reaction to a significant death in the first generation. The oldest daughter found her father locked in the kitchen and she smelled gas. Her mother and younger sister were not at home so she ran to her cousin who lived next door. However, her father was already dead. His suicide spread an emotional shock wave through the family.

The oldest daughter implicitly took on a functioning position of *rescuer* in her adult work system. Likely in response to her father's suicide, she joined the Red Cross and worked on national and international disasters in order to save lives.

The younger daughter in her adulthood became an educator with a focus on the emotional, social, and educational development of children. When she married and had children, her functioning position became that of the *anxious overfunctioner* in the family in relation to her son, who *underfunctioned* as an anxious, slow-developing academic. The son's underfunctioning was related to his mother's perception of male fragility in her family.

When the son grew up, he became a psychologist. When he visited his parents, who had moved to France when he was a young adult, he realized that his mother was anxious about his father's depression. In a talk between mother and son, the mother expressed anxiety by saying that she felt uncomfortable about taking a business trip to England, feeling that her husband might be suicidal, and not wanting to leave him alone. The son shared his opinion that his father was depressed, but that he was not suicidal. The mother felt relieved and was able to take the trip to carry out the consultation. The mother's concern seemed to have come from the seed that transmitted the emotional shock wave from her father's suicide to herself, and further on to her husband and son.

The three generations of functioning positions in this family produced overfunctioning and underfunctioning, in response to what Bowen described as the initial shock wave following the father's suicide and the way it operated "on an underground network of emotional dependence of family members on each other" (1978, p. 325).

This family had a closed communication system in regard to death and was unable to speak openly about family members who had died. They also had few death rituals that included family and friends.

The following are eight examples of the family's anxiety and denial about death:

1. The younger daughter and her husband avoided death rituals.
2. When the younger daughter's son was eight years old, his maternal grandmother died in Los Angeles from a heart attack. He sensed that his parents were upset and asked them how his Granny was doing at the hospital. His parents at first told him that his grandmother was okay, but soon after both parents told him that she had died. The next day the father drove with his son to the hospital to pick up his grandmother's possessions. The eight-year old boy sat in the car and wondered what his father was doing in the hospital. Later the remains of the grandmother's ashes were sent to Philadelphia and buried at her husband's gravesite in Philadelphia.

3. At age 28, the son went to his first funeral, for his 97-year-old paternal grandmother. His father chose not to go to his mother's funeral.
4. The son's mother knew that her father had committed suicide, but she did not tell her son until he was 30 years old.
5. In 1975, in France, at a family dinner at a restaurant, the son decided to speak directly to his mother and aunt regarding his grandfather's death. They talked about their father, but his aunt said to her nephew that his maternal grandfather had died of a heart attack, denying his suicide. However, his mother said their father had committed suicide. The lack of full openness left no clarity about the death of the maternal grandfather.
6. The mother died in a hospital in London, England, in 1977. She chose to be cremated. The son was at his mother's cremation, but his father and sister did not attend it. However, his father spent several hours sitting with his dead wife in the hospital. Later in the summer of 1977, the son and father buried his mother's ashes under a cherry tree in France where the parents were living. His sister did not come. Once again a memorial of family, friends, and colleagues did not happen. However, following the mother's death, the father received nearly a hundred meaningful letters of condolence from family, friends, and colleagues. Eventually he sent them to his son who shared some of them with his sister. The father put together a luncheon gathering for his dead wife at the teacher's college in New York, where she was co-director of the elementary school. Neither her daughter, living in England, nor her son attended the luncheon.
7. The son's father died in 1993, after having Alzheimer's disease for 11 years. Like his wife, he chose to be cremated. The son was present at the cremation of his father, as he had been for his mother. Both the son and daughter saw their father's body prior to his cremation. The daughter preferred not to attend her parents' cremations. The son, daughter, and their father's partner of 15 years buried his ashes under a second cherry tree, where the mother had been buried 16 years earlier in the garden at their home in France.
8. The family's closed communication system continued when the daughter wrote the obituaries for both their mother and father in the *New York Times*. These were unfortunately short. The son

and daughter did not write obituaries for newspapers in either England, where the daughter lived, or in a small city in New England, where the son lived.

Not having funerals or memorials for their parents and lacking the presence of some of the nuclear family and the extended family, friends and colleagues continued the closed communication system regarding death within this three-generational family. There were circumstances such as moving and living in foreign countries that made it difficult to relate to relatives, friends, and colleagues. Nevertheless, the lack of substantial death rituals was unfortunate. The third generation continues to live with some murmur of an underground emotional shock wave that had started in 1928, following the suicide of the maternal grandfather.

The parents appeared to be at a moderate level on the continuum of differentiation of self, specifically in relation to the way they indirectly dealt with dying and death in the family.

Many years after the deaths of the parents and aunt, the son, who had kept some ashes from each of their cremations, organized a memorial at which the ashes were strewn in the ocean at a special place for the family. It seems this third generation was able to move toward a more "open communication system" in facing and honoring death with their family and friends. They continue to be secular in their beliefs regarding death, but they have tried to create secular death rituals that have meaning for them.

A Dying Grandfather Defines Self in His Relation to His Granddaughter: A Family at a Moderate Level on the Continuum of Differentiation

This vignette highlights a dance between a granddaughter and her grandfather who recognized the end of his life was imminent:

Granddaughter (age 48): [As I slowly rose from the chair, the weight of knowing this could truly be our last goodbye was heavy. Should I pretend as if it were like many past exchanges or should I say something meaningful or possibly profound to him? Gramp (84) was a simple man,

	expressing his love and affection in actions and rarely in words as such. Flowery or deep would not do.]
Granddaughter:	"Okay, Gramp. I'm going to head out."
Grandfather:	"Okay."
Granddaughter:	"So I might be down next weekend. I'll see you then?"
Grandfather:	"I don't think so, honey."
Granddaughter:	"You don't think so? Why is that?"
Grandfather:	"I'm tired."
Granddaughter:	"I know, Gramp. There's nothing you need to do. Just take it easy."
Grandfather:	"I miss Barbara." [Barbara being his wife who had died four years earlier.]
Granddaughter:	"I miss her, too."
Grandfather:	A deep sigh. "I'm tired. I'm ready to die." [His eyes wet with tears.]
Granddaughter:	"I know you are tired. But what if I'm not ready for you to die?" [My voice was catching in my throat.]
Grandfather:	[He looked up to me, with absolute clarity in his eyes and a steeliness in his voice.] "It isn't about you anymore."
Granddaughter:	[My eyes started to fill with tears yet I knew he would want me to be strong in our last moments together, of that I was certain. I took in a deep breath and leaned down to kiss and hug him. As I pulled away from our embrace, I asked him,] "You know I love you, Gramp, right?"
Grandfather:	[He looked up to me with a smile and said:] "Same here," [his trademark retort to me saying, "I love him."]
Granddaughter:	[With that, I nodded and smiled, tears now slowly wetting my cheeks.] "Same here, Gramp," [and I walked away.]

Although both grandfather and granddaughter felt and expressed sadness, they both intentionally accepted the outcome. This indicates a medium- to high-functioning level of differentiation and openness in the defining of two selves in a family.

A Three-Generation Family Confronting Death Intentionally: Moderate to Good on the Continuum of Differentiation

A number of deaths in the G family have been what one might call "intentional." Grandfather Harry G gradually developed extremely crippling arthritis when he was in his early 60s, back in the 1930s, and was in constant pain, unable to move or function as the strong, happy man he had been in his prime. One night he and his wife invited their dear friend, a local doctor, for dinner. After dinner, the doctor told Grandmother G that he would put Harry to bed. He carried him off to the bedroom, got him settled down in bed, and by mutual agreement gave him a shot of something that would help him sleep. The next morning Grandfather G did not wake up.

His niece, Penelope, also decided when she was ready to end her life. She was close to 80, her beloved husband had died, she could no longer farm or tend to the animals, and so one day she went to bed, stopped eating and drinking, and died about 10 days later.

Harry's son, M, was 82 when he died. He was arthritic, had been having difficulty getting around, and had suffered some mental deterioration after a series of small strokes. He also had congestive heart failure. His wife, B, took care of him but needed to do some errands one afternoon, so she arranged for a young man to come and have lunch with her husband. At lunch he told the young man, "If I were to die today, I would feel I had led a good life. I love my wife and children, but I'm ready to go." After lunch M went into the living room to take a short nap. The young man cleared the table and began to wash up the dishes, but a minute later he heard a "clunk" from the living room. When he went there to find out what had happened, he found M dead on the living room floor.

B lived until she was almost 85. She, too, had arthritis and congestive heart failure but managed to lead a happy, engaged life after M died, and she looked forward greatly to a visit with her younger brother in California. Before she left her home in Philadelphia, she gave her oldest son (who lived nearby) power of attorney, and he became a cosigner of her bank account, "just in case anything happens," she said. In California, her brother gave her a wonderful social visit and took her to an Arabian horse farm, which she loved. When they returned from the farm, she said she wanted to take a rest. She lay down in her bedroom, went into a coma, and never got up again. Her brother called her five children, and four of them flew to California to be with her in the intensive care unit (ICU) where doctors had intubated her, trying to decide what treatment she should receive, since they had diagnosed her with spinal meningitis. Her oldest son chose not to come but sent his support for whatever the others decided. The four siblings arrived in her hospital room where she was plugged into many life-sustaining machines. Each of her children carried a copy of her living will in which she stated she wanted no treatment to prolong her life if she were in a vegetative state. The doctors told them that if one of her children had objected, they would have had to keep her alive but since all the children agreed that they wanted to honor her living will, the doctors would remove the tubes that were sustaining her. She died shortly after this procedure. Her children were present and accounted for, and they each defined themselves in letting go of their mother. At the same time, they knew they would greatly miss her.

This three-generation family indicates a higher level of differentiation in the face of mortality. Members of each generation chose intentionally to end their lives when facing physical illness, severe pain, and the inability to sustain their lives if they could not manage themselves. The grandfather, the first generation, lived with severe arthritis and made a reciprocal arrangement with his doctor to end his life peacefully with medicine. Penelope, his niece in the second generation, at 80 years intentionally decided to stop eating and drinking and died in 10 days. M, also in the second generation, lived a full life and died of natural causes at age 82. The day he died he seemed to have an intuition of his impending death and accepted it.

Conclusion

I chose death as an arena for describing variation in levels of differentiation in families because death is, perhaps, the most significant stress a family experiences along a continuum from destabilization to stabilization, reflecting variation of the potential "shock wave effect" of a death in the family.

A Clinical Application for Chronic Illness and Death in the Family: Talk to the Person Behind the Dysfunction

Loretta Nowakowski, RN, PhD, was a nurse clinician who worked from a Bowen theory framework and used the theory in treating chronically ill patients and those in the process of dying. The following is some of her thinking and clinical applications drawn from her article, "Disorientation—Signal or Diagnosis" (1978). Disorientation is prominent in organic brain disorders, but is also present in other types of illness. Bowen (1971, personal comment) introduced Nowakowski to one of his principal maxims: "Talk to the person behind his dysfunction."

Nowakowski applied the following when developing a route for dealing with disorientation:

> In order to remain objective in observing disorientation, I told myself I was dealing with an individual who is responsible for his or her situation in life and plays a part in the condition he is exhibiting. By following this maxim I was able to resist being overly helpful or overly sympathetic with the patient. Later as a nursing instructor in an acute care setting, I found that I could talk to a person exhibiting disorientation clearly and substantively.
>
> (Nowakowski, 1978, p. 297)

Nowakowski describes the importance of understanding the disoriented person's relationship system. She suggests evaluating the family system and the health system, determining the amount of anxiety in those systems, and understanding to what degree the health system is adding anxiety that increases the patient's disorientation. An example of this from families or health care professionals is when they are overly helpful, or in Bowen's term, "overfunctioning," as they try to help the patient without assessing what he or she can do for himself or herself.

In summary, Nowakowski wrote what most characterized the disorientation were "1) abdication of decision-making on a significant issue and dissatisfaction with the outcome of that decision made by others; 2) disruption or deprivation of meaningful relationships; and 3) intense fusion in the marital relationship" (1978, p. 300).

Bowen theory concepts, triangles, and the overfunctioning-underfunctioning reciprocity can explain the relationship issues. When family tensions are high, family systems triangles are available to bring in "outsiders" to absorb the anxiety.

According to Nowakowski:

> The overfunctioning of health care professionals contributes to and usually intensifies the underfunctioning of the patient. The triangle can be changed and the anxiety can be reduced in the presence of a significant other who remains objective about the issue and can maintain a one-to-one relationship with the disoriented individual, the health care team, and other members of the family. When the health professional relates to the person behind the disorientation, she becomes significant to disoriented patients because they have usually been deprived of meaningful relationships in their families during the course of their illness.
>
> (1978, p. 300)

Finally, Nowakowski states:

> When disorientation can be seen as a signal of anxiety in the family system and in the health care system, rather than as a diagnosis of an individual patient, new possibilities for the disoriented person can emerge.
>
> (1978, p. 304)

Reflections

In this chapter the author has followed the thread of Bowen theory that is the foundation of his theoretical understanding relating to family reaction to death along the continuum of differentiation. Dealing with mortality for the individual who is dying and his or her family, and the physicians and other health caretakers in our society, will always include a majority of humans whose level of emotional reactivity—particularly when facing the end of life—will be based on lower levels of differentiation of self. There will be positive societal changes in providing better forms of assisted living for elders facing their mortality, and there will be new cures for illnesses. However, there will also be ups and downs in applying Bowen's approach to the "open communication system" between the dying individual, the family, and the health care practitioners because, as Bowen (1978) wrote: "Death is a biological event that terminates a life. No life event can stir more emotionally directed thinking in the individual and more emotional reactiveness in those about him" (pp. 321–322).

The facts of science are objective for the most part. But emotionally subjective responses to death, rather than objective responses to death, are usually predominant. There is no evidence at this time that the majority of the human population will reach a higher level of differentiation any time soon. Thus, Bowen's approach to facing death directly will most likely not include the majority of humans.

NOTE

1 A partial mental construct triangle includes a mix of living and nonliving entities. The use of the term mental construct is meant to connote the fact that one point of the triangle is occupied by an entity that comes out of man's brain, rather than being a living, biological entity. This form of triangle consists of two or more living individuals, occupying two positions, with the third position occupied by a deceased person, idea, religion/philosophy, or fantasy, among other nonliving entities. These triangles might also be described as quasi-triangles (Titelman, 2008, pp. 25–26).

REFERENCES

Bonanno, G. A. (2005). Resilience in the face of potential trauma. *Current Directions in Psychological Science*, *14*(3), 135–138.

Bonanno, G. A., Westphal, M., & Mancini, A. D. (2011). Resilience to loss and potential trauma. *Annual Review of Clinical Psychology*, 7, 511–535.

Bowen, M. (1971). Principles and techniques of multiple family therapy. In J. Bradt & C. Moynihan (Eds.), *Systems therapy*. Washington, DC: Georgetown University.

Bowen, M. (1972). Toward the differentiation of self in one's family of origin. In Francis D. Andres & Joseph P. Lorio (Eds.), *Georgetown family symposia (Vol. I, 1971–1972)*. Washington, DC: Family Section, Department of Psychiatry, Georgetown University Medical Center.

Bowen, M. (1978). *Family therapy in clinical practice.* New York, NY: Jason Aronson.

Bush Signs Schiavo Legislation [Video file]. (2005, March 21). Retrieved from www.nbcnews.com/id/7212079/ns/us_news/t/bush-signs-schiavo- legislation

Kerr, M. E., & Bowen, M. (1988). *Family evaluation: An approach based on Bowen theory.* New York, NY: W. W. Norton.

Nowakowski, L. (1978). Disorientation signal or diagnosis. In *Georgetown family symposia: A collection of selected papers (Vol. III, 1975–1976).* Washington, DC: Georgetown Family Center.

Titelman, P. (2008). *Triangles: Bowen Family Systems Theory.* New York; London: The Haworth Press/Taylor & Francis Group.

Titelman, P. (2014). *Differentiation of self: Bowen family systems theory perspectives.* New York, NY: Taylor & Francis.

Wikipedia. (2017, July 25). *Terri Schiavo case.* Retrieved from https://en.wikipedia.org/wiki/Terri_Schiavo_case.

3

A HISTORICAL BACKGROUND FOR BOWEN'S PERSPECTIVE ON DEATH IN THE FAMILY SYSTEM

Anne S. McKnight

Death has been acknowledged by families and communities and in every culture and society since the origins of hominid evolution. Death as part of the life cycle is the foundation of religious beliefs, rituals, and traditions over eons of time. Scientists have studied the animal recognition of the loss of one of their species in elephants, dolphins, and magpies, leading to the idea that grief has an evolutionary origin. This chapter explores the history of how the human has acknowledged death and handled the emotions around the loss of a loved one. It also explores how the philosophy and research on the reaction to death have changed over time in modern Western culture. The history of the reaction to death lends a broad perspective to Murray Bowen's concept of the family reaction to death as an indicator of the shifts in the emotional equilibrium of a family system, which will be explored in other chapters of this book.

The Universality of Grief Practices

The recognition of death through ceremonies, rituals, and monuments has been part of the life cycle of *Homo sapiens* from their earliest origins. In discovering remains of four Cro-Magnon individuals who were believed to have been buried 32,000 years ago, Smithsonian researchers noted:

> The condition and place of ornaments, including pieces of shell and animal teeth fashioned into what appear to be pendants or necklaces, led researchers to believe that the

> skeletons have been intentionally buried within the shelter in a single grave.
>
> (Smithsonian Museum of Natural History, August 5, 2016)

In Qafzeh, Israel, 15 individuals buried 100,000 years ago in a cave were covered with red ochre. A Neanderthal boy was found in a grave covered by a slab of stone, while remains of flowers placed around the body were found in others. A Sunghir man and woman, buried in 24,000 B.C., were discovered carefully placed head to head surrounded by artifacts (Smithsonian Museum of Natural History, March 25, 2016). Of course, the tombs and pyramids of the Egyptians filled with objects, animals, and humans that would be important in the afterlife, speak to the importance of rituals in the death of an important person. No less grand was the Mausoleum of the Emperor Qin Shih Huang (259–210 B.C.) in which an entire city was replicated for his use after death. The Terracotta Warriors and Horses are well-known artifacts from that tomb. The magnitude of the tomb of a deceased mirrored the importance of his life. In the earliest history of humankind, gestures such as these signify the emotion that accompanies the departure of a member of a social group and are testimony to the impact of death on the living.

Human practices to acknowledge the dead through ceremonies and gatherings to mourn the loss of a member of the tribe or family are universal. Paul Rosenblatt, an anthropologist, studied the customs of mourning across 264 cultures. Grief is expressed in every culture he studied, although he found a variation in who grieves, how they grieve, and for how long.

> My opinion is that nothing—no feeling, no meaning, or understanding—related to grief is universal across cultures or probably even within a culture. Someone cries in most cultures when someone dies, but not everyone cries, and crying has diverse forms, reason for crying, and meanings from culture to culture. Fear and anger are less common and where there is fear and anger, it varies a lot in meaning, forms, and reasons from culture to culture—and again there seem often, if not always, to be differences within a culture.
>
> (Rosenblatt, Walsh, & Jackson, 1976)

Several influential paradigms about grief have developed in modern times. These include Sigmund Freud's psychoanalytic theories on the work of mourning, the ideas of resilience best embodied by George Bonanno, and scientists who research the evolutionary origins of grief in animals. These ideas are a historical backdrop for the examination of Murray Bowen's systems concept of the family reaction to death that is explored in other chapters of this book.

Psychoanalytic Theories of Grief and Grief Work

Sigmund Freud: The Work of Mourning

In our Western culture, views about grief and how to grieve were profoundly affected in the early twentieth century by the writings of Sigmund Freud. Freud created the foundation for the predominant paradigm in the Western world for understanding grief by proposing that an individual could only overcome feelings of sadness over the death of a loved one by carrying out "grief work."

When his father, Jacob, died in 1896, Freud began a self-analysis of his grief. In 1917, he wrote "Mourning and Melancholia," in which he compared grief and depression. Freud presented the view that grief was comparable to depression, both involving suffering with a longing for something that is lost. In a letter to Ludwig Binswanger, who had lost a son, Freud wrote:

> We find a place for what we lose. Although we know that after such a loss the acute stage of mourning will subside, we also know that we shall remain inconsolable and will never find a substitute. No matter what may fill the gap, even if it be filled completely, it nevertheless remains something else. And actually this is how it should be. It is the only way of perpetuating that love which we do not want to relinquish.
>
> (Freud, 1917, pp. 150–172)

He concluded that suffering was a natural part of the grieving process, necessitating "the work of mourning" to get relief. This effort required reclaiming the psychological energy, the constant longing for someone no longer there, that was invested in the deceased. The inhibition and loss of interest characteristic of grief are fully accounted for by the work of mourning in which the ego is absorbed. The work entails the ego detaching itself from the deceased so that it is free to attach to someone else (Gay, 1989, p. 587). This process included engaging in a review of "each single one of the memories and hopes which bound the libido (life energy) to the object (the deceased)." This review, done "bit by bit" and "extraordinarily painful," was the only way to break the bond with the deceased, reclaim the libido, and move forward (Freud 1917, pp. 150–172).

Freud believed that individuals respond to the loss of a loved one over the course of weeks and months by moving through a succession of phases. The phases included a phase of numbing, interspersed with outbursts of extreme distress, a phase of yearning for the lost figure, a phase of disorganization and despair, and a phase of greater or lesser degrees of reorganization (Gay, 1989, p. 587). For some individuals, mourning becomes "disordered" so that anger and self-reproach are dominant and sorrow absent. Those with disordered mourning tend to include people whose attachment has been insecure and anxious, as well as those disposed to compulsive caregiving (Gay, 1989, p. 212). Disordered variants of mourning lead to many forms of physical and mental ill health, and impair a person's capacity to maintain love relationships (Gay, 1989, p. 137).

Freud proposed that adults who show a prolonged absence of conscious grieving were commonly self-sufficient people, proud of their independence and self-control. After a loss, they took pride in carrying on as though nothing had happened. They were busy and efficient, and may appear to be coping splendidly. But a sensitive observer, he states, notes that they are tense and often short-tempered and susceptible to physical symptoms such as headaches, palpitations, and pain (Gay, 1989, p. 153). That is, the appearance of coping with a death was deceiving—it masked the inability of the individual to adequately grieve. If the work of mourning was not adequately completed, the unresolved attachment to the deceased would be an obstacle in the future life of the bereaved. This became a foundational concept of grief work to present times.

John Bowlby: Attachment and Loss

John Bowlby (1907–1990), an English psychiatrist, psychologist, and psychoanalyst notable for his interest in child development and his work on attachment theory, contributed a body of thinking to Freud's views on grief work. His ideas about grief came from observations of attachment patterns in children and their caregivers. Bowlby believed that when a mother was separated from her children when she gave birth, the infant's reactions progressed through a series of stages. The mourning responses that are commonly seen in infancy and early childhood bear many of the features that are the hallmark of pathological mourning in adulthood. He identified four stages: the unconscious yearning for the lost person; the unconscious reproach toward the lost person and toward oneself; the compulsive caring for others; and the disbelief that the loss is permanent, also thought of as denial. He modified these stages of the infant's responses to separation and presumed they were similar for bereaved adults (Bowlby, 1980 p. 504). These stages in grief included protest, anger, sadness, despair, withdrawal, and disorganization. This approach laid the basis for future thinking about the stages of grief. In his book, *Attachment and Loss*, Bowlby elaborates on Freud's idea of disordered mourning. This process is marked by a prolonged absence of grieving despite "tell-tale signs that the bereaved person has in fact been affected and that his mental equilibrium is disturbed." He lists among the signs of difficult adjustment positive emotions of pride, cheerfulness, optimism, and the appearance of being in good spirits (Bowlby, 1980, p. 153). The idea that people are resilient in the face of death is not seen as credible, but is rather a pathological denial of grief. Unless people reflect the appropriate stages of the grieving process, they cannot truly recover from loss in spite of an appearance to the contrary.

Elizabeth Kubler-Ross and David Kessler: The Stages of Grief

Elizabeth Kubler-Ross and David Kessler, the most well-known theorists in the field of grief and loss in the twentieth century, formulated the current predominant paradigm for grief. Kubler-Ross's ideas about the stages of grief were not derived from work with bereaved people. She devoted her life to helping terminally ill patients and observed the stages they went through in facing death. She then presumed that these stages applied to those who were grieving over the deaths of loved ones.

Kubler-Ross retained Freud's view of grief as a pathology comparable to depression. "Grief work," her term for the work of mourning, involved processing emotions through the identified stages of grief to free the person from clinging to the loss of the deceased:

> The five stages—denial, anger, bargaining, depression, and acceptance—are a part of the framework that makes up our learning to live with the one we lost . . . Our hope is that with these stages comes the knowledge of grief's terrain, making us better equipped to cope with life and loss.
>
> (Kubler-Ross & Kessler, 2005, p. 7)

Individuals process these stages in different orders and could revisit a previous stage before proceeding on to acceptance. The goal of therapy was to express the suppressed feelings of loss that prevented the individual from engaging in the "grief work." If a person did not "process the death" and "work through the stages," they were considered "not in touch with their grief." This idea extends Freud's view that focusing on the loss of the loved one contributes to a necessary catharsis of the feelings of grief (Kubler-Ross, 1973). "Telling your story often and in detail is primal to the grieving process," she maintains (Kubler-Ross & Kessler, 2005, p. 63). At present, the necessity of processing grief through stages of grief work not only dominates the professional world of therapy, but also is widely accepted in the population as a whole.

American Medical Association: Diagnosis and Medication of Grief

The medical world has increasingly embraced the construct of grief as a pathology. In the *DSM-3*, the Diagnostic Manual of the American Psychiatric Association published in 1980, grief first appeared as "Uncomplicated Bereavement" and was defined as a "normal reaction to the death of a loved one" that occurs within the first two or three months. It was listed as a V code, or nonpsychiatric problem. In the intervening years, a decades-long campaign was carried out, led by Holly Prigerson, to create a full-fledged entry for "complicated grief" in the *DSM-5*. She concluded that complicated grief was a diagnosable symptom in 10–15% of the population (Maciejewski & Prigerson, 2017, pp. 189–191). Complicated grief (originally raised by Freud as disordered grief) is influenced by dependency on the deceased, rumination, lack of protective resources, lack of social skills, previous loss, isolation, anxiety, depression, and adjustment problems before death. Treatment involves "revisiting" the death repeatedly in addition to practical advice on reengaging with the world (Konigsberg, 2011, p. 136).

In contrast to the *DSM-3*, in the newly published *DSM-5* bereavement is included in the diagnosis for major depressive disorder. Feelings of sadness, loss, sleeplessness, crying, inability to concentrate, tiredness, and loss of appetite that lasted *more than two weeks* are now diagnosed as depression, rather than a normal grief reaction. Grief is presented as a diagnosable condition treatable with medication (American Psychiatric Association, 2013). *The Lancet*, the English medical journal, disagreed with the new categorization of grief: "Medicating grief so that treatment is legitimized routinely with antidepressants is not only dangerously simplistic, but also flawed. Building a life without the loved person who died cannot be expected to be quick, easy, or straightforward" (The Lancet, 2012, p. 589).

Freud's conception of grief and its treatment has had a major impact on psychiatry, mental health, and the field of grief therapy over the last century. His ideas on "the work of mourning" and the similarity of grief to depression as a pathology have evolved and been reinterpreted by other theorists to include the ideas of disordered mourning, complicated grief, and the stages of grief work elaborated by Kubler-Ross. The view of grief as a pathology, with the need for diagnosis, treatment, and medication, has been codified by psychiatry in the *DSM-4*.

Grief in the Natural World

The perspective of grief as a pathology is being challenged through observations in animal behavior and human research. The roots of thinking about grief from an evolutionary framework surfaced as early as the work of Charles Darwin.

Darwin, one of the first to initiate the scientific study of human behavior, observed that the expression of emotion was visible and observable in the human. He believed that the universality of emotional expression in animals and humans provided a thread of continuity in the evolution of species. Although he did not examine grief among animals, he observed the universality of the reaction to death in humans: "The expression of grief, due to the contraction of the grief-muscles, is by no means confined to Europeans, but appears to be common to all races of mankind" (Darwin, 1899, p. 194). The observation of the universality of grief serves to lay the basis for its function in the natural life cycle of the human.

Many animal behavior scientists have recorded observable grief reactions in animals. In a longitudinal study of elephant families, Cynthia Moss described a troop surrounding a dying matriarch:

> They stood around Tina's carcass, touching it gently . . . By nightfall they had nearly covered her with branches and earth. Then they stood vigil over her for most of the night and only as dawn was approaching did they reluctantly begin to walk away.
>
> (Moss, 1988, p. 34)

She goes on to depict elephant mothers responding to a dying infant: "[They] became frantic and knelt down and tried to lift her up . . . Her family tried everything to rouse her, kicking and tusking her" (Moss, 1988, p. 272). When 19 groups of wild elephants were studied, researchers found that the animals could distinguish skulls of their own species, spending twice the time examining elephant remains than those of buffalo or rhino (McComb, Baker, & Moss, 2006, pp. 26–28).

Geza Teleki writes about the response of a chimpanzee troop to an accidental death of a member in Gombe. An adult male, Rix, fell into a gully and broke his neck. "The reaction was immediate pandemonium—apes screaming, charging, displaying, copulating, throwing stones, barking, and whimpering. They stayed close to the body, then drifted away" (Teleki, 1973, pp. 81–94). Frans de Waal describes the death of Luit, in his research colony, after a fight for dominance:

> By the time of death the rest of the colony had entered the sleeping quarters. They were completely silent during the time that Luit's body was lying in his cage. The following morning, even at feeding time, hardly any sounds were heard.

> Vocal activity resumed only after the corpse had been carried out of the building.
>
> (de Waal, 1989, p. 69)

In *How Animals Grieve* (2013) Barbara King cites many examples of animal grief. The bottlenose dolphin mother tried to revive her calf over and over for several days by lifting the body, then submerging it (King, p. 97). Maternal corpse carrying is also described in the gelada monkey in Guassa, Ethiopia. Over a period of three years, Peter Fashing and colleagues observed 14 mothers carrying dead infants for periods of one to four days (King, p. 68). Christophe Boesch and Hedwig Boesch-Achermann describe an incident in which a female chimpanzee was killed by a leopard. These researchers found 12 chimpanzees surrounding the body, who groomed the body and played gently around it (King, p. 84).

Marc Bekoff observed the reactions of magpies to the corpse of a magpie lying on the side of the road:

> One approached the corpse, gently pecked at it—just as an elephant noses the carcass of another elephant—and stepped back . . . Next, one of the magpies flew off, brought back some grass, and laid it on the corpse. Another magpie did the same. Then all four magpies stood vigil for a few seconds and one by one flew off.
>
> (Bekoff, 2007, p. 1)

In another situation, when a fox was killed by a mountain lion, a female fox circled the carcass, covering it with dirt with her back legs. The next day Bekoff returned to find it completely buried (Bekoff, 2007, p. 64).

Bekoff speculates on the evolutionary value of grief among animal species:

> Grief itself is something of a mystery, for there doesn't seem to be any obvious adaptive value to it in an evolutionary sense. It does not seem to increase an individual's reproductive success. Some theorize that perhaps mourning strengthens social bonds among the survivors who band together to pay their last

> respects. This may enhance group cohesion at a time when it's likely to be weakened. Whatever its value is, grief is the price of commitment, that wellspring of both happiness and sorrow.
>
> (Bekoff, 2007, p. 63)

Jaak Panksepp: The Neurochemistry of Grief

Jaak Panksepp, a scientist who has studied the neurochemistry of affection bonds in humans and animals, elaborates on the evolutionary importance of the grief response. He views the neurobiology of grief as related to the disruption of feelings of safety and comfort in a social group. He describes the triggering of grief in the following way:

> We simply feel normal and comfortable when we are in the midst of friendly company, and that same feeling becomes warmer when we are among those we love deeply . . . We often take these feelings, like air itself, for granted. But we should not, for when this feeling of normalcy is suddenly disrupted by the undesired loss of a lover or the unexpected death of a loved one, we find ourselves plunged into one of the deepest and most troubling emotional pains of which we, as social creatures, are capable. In everyday language, this feeling is called sorrow or grief, and it can verge on panic in its most intense and precipitous forms.
>
> (Panksepp, 1998, p. 261)

In an evolutionary sense, this psychic pain informs the individual of the importance of the loss of the loved one—usually those with whom one has invested great genetic effort, such as children, or those who helped one thrive, such as parents, friends, or relatives. Panksepp believes that this type of psychic pain emerged from a brain emotional system that evolved early in the mammalian evolutionary line to inform individuals about the status of their social environment.

The neural circuit, which Panksepp named the panic response, is one of the major forces that guide the construction of social bonds. When this circuit is aroused, animals seek reunion with others that help to create a feeling of a "secure neurochemical base" within the brain. He finds there is variation in the panic response in how people react to loss. He points out that the capacity to re-engage the safe, secure neurochemistry varies among individuals, with those most dependent on the one who died being the most susceptible to disorders that emerge from feelings of social loss (Panksepp, 1998, p. 263). Panksepp's ideas are consistent with human practices across cultures. Human reactions of grief and mourning lead to participation in a social acknowledgement of death through rituals, celebrations, or funerals. A death creates a void that draws humans together to reconnect with important others of their social group, thus restoring some feelings of safety and connection.

George Bonanno: A Science of Bereavement

In keeping with evolutionary views of the grief process, Bonanno developed a science of bereavement by introducing rigorous methods of research with populations of bereaved adults. By interviewing large samples of individuals who had lost a loved one, he discovered that a natural resilience was a major component of grief and trauma reactions in people who face the loss of loved ones. The idea that individuals are resilient in coping with death challenges the conceptual framework of the Kubler-Ross model that grief must be processed through stages in order to prevent future difficulties for the individual. Bonanno found through his research that the focus on having people talk or cry about a loss of a loved one can actually intensify the feelings of grief. He proposed that the focus of therapy should be supporting the natural resilience in the individual.

Bonanno's interest in resilience in bereavement is linked to the research on resilience as a general human trait. In studying resilience in children who grow up with maltreatment and abuse, researchers have discovered that some children cope extremely well with adversity. Durable children can be resilient to deaths of a parent, natural disasters, and abuse. Only a small percentage of children exposed to trauma have a diagnostic trauma reaction. This resilience in children overcoming childhood difficulties is replicated in the resilience of adults (Bonanno, 2009, p. 96). Bonanno found through his research that many traumatic events are simply forgotten over time. His research team studied a survey of the mental health of the population of New York after the 9/11 attacks. They found that a large majority of residents had no trauma symptoms or psychological problems from the event six months after the attacks. An exception to this was those who had witnessed the attack firsthand and lost a loved one. For them, grief was more profound. Yet only a third of them met the criteria for post-traumatic stress disorder (PTSD), whereas two-thirds did not (Bonanno, 2009). In a survey of 55 widows one month after the death of a spouse, Toni Biscotti found that those with the lowest amount of stress had dispositional resilience defined by three characteristics: they were connected to other people, they felt their grief was manageable, and they embraced and learned from new experiences (Konigsberg, 2011, p. 160).

What influences resilience in the face of death? Bonanno found that resilient people consistently fare better when they have the following characteristics:

- They have people to talk to about the deceased.
- They possess power in positive memories about the deceased and positive emotions.
- They have the ability to adjust to shifting demands by being optimistic and exerting control over outcomes.
- They have flexibility in expressing sadness and grief.
- They are willing to accept that death opens new possibilities in life.

According to Bonanno, grief is a stress reaction in the normal population. It is experienced in waves in which an individual has periods of loss-oriented thinking, alternating with periods that are restoration oriented. Reflective of Panksepp's theories of the neurochemistry of grief, he believes sadness is wired into the human brain and is "functional" in helping the bereaved take stock of his or her loss and reflect on its impact on their lives. Expressions of sadness engage sympathy and support from those around them, engaging social bonds. For the most part, people have a natural resilience that allows them to go forward in life while mourning the death of a loved one (Bonanno, 2009, p. 96).

For some who are dependent on a loved one, however, grief becomes more debilitating. Dr. Bonanno found that 10–15% of the population he studied had difficulty overcoming grief. Those people overwhelmed by grief were characterized as excessively dependent, submissive, or clingy to the one who had died. These individuals had an "exaggerated need for care, nurturance, and protection even when one is capable of functioning independently to meet normal everyday challenges" (Bonanno, 2009, p. 102). Their grief reactions were debilitating as they withdrew from life and were endlessly preoccupied with the deceased person. He summarizes these individuals:

> When grief persists for longer periods of time, when it drags on for months and then years, the image of the deceased becomes elusive, fragmentary, and increasingly disturbing. Relentless suffering and yearning color everything. What was once a feeling of safety or happiness becomes mixed up with worry and fear and dread.
>
> (Bonanno, 2009, p. 100)

Murray Bowen: The Family as an Emotional Unit

Murray Bowen's research on the family and on the human's reactions to death is based in an evolutionary framework of the function of grief of the animal behaviorists. However, family systems theory offers a broader view of grief in the family system and the impact of death on a family over generations. His view that human families vary in the ability to manage emotion, including around death, is based on the level of maturity of the family members in adapting to the stressors they face. The view of the family as an emotional unit sets the structure for seeing the capacity of the family to handle the loss of a family member within a larger context of the management of anxiety in the system. Families whose members have a greater capacity to manage their emotions in the face of loss or stress have more ability to communicate thoughts and feelings around the death—to maintain an open system—as well as to become a resource to one another. These families are less dependent on one another and more capable of rebounding from the death of a loved one. They are less susceptible to the shock wave of emotion that can create ripples of symptoms across generations.

The capacity to conceptualize grief within the family system can be of use to both those who are bereaved and those professionals who aid the grieving. It provides the opportunity to step back from focusing on the emotionality of grief in an individual to examine the bigger picture of how the family adapts to a death and moves forward in the cycle of life (Bowen, 1978).

Summary

A conceptual framework for mourning and bereavement is significant in human history. In the twentieth century, Freud's ideas on the work of mourning laid a foundation for others, including Bowlby and Kubler-Ross, to formulate the stages of grief and the necessity for grief work as the predominant view in the mental health field in the modern age. This focus on the pathology of grief has led to diagnosis and medication of this natural part of human life.

Since Darwin, however, the study of the universality of grief in both animal species and humans has been researched through an evolutionary lens. Rather than focusing on grief as a pathology to be treated, researchers have examined the evolutionary function of grief as a mechanism to draw the mourners into community (Bekoff, 2007) and to reset the neurochemical basis for feelings of connection and safety through social affectional bonds (Panksepp, 1998). Bonanno's research, published in 2009, proposes that a natural resilience is a part of the human capacity to manage the death of a loved one, although people vary in the ability to recover from loss and trauma.

Bowen departs from all the previously discussed theorists by establishing a wider lens for viewing the impact of a death. He views the family as an emotional unit composed of interdependent family members adapting to their environment. The influence of a death is not simply on an individual who is grieving, but on the entire family system, including succeeding generations over time. A person's position in a family affects how their death impacts the relationship system. Bowen's concept of differentiation of self addresses the variability of grief among individuals and families, as does Bonanno's concept of resilience (Bowen, 1978).

REFERENCES

American Psychiatric Association (1980). *Diagnostic and statistical manual of mental disorders* (3rd ed.). Washington, DC: American Psychiatric Association.

American Psychiatric Association (2013). *Diagnostic and statistical manual of mental disorders* (5th ed.). Washington, DC: American Psychiatric Association.
Bekoff, M. (2007). *The emotional lives of animals.* Novato, CA: New World Library.
Bonanno, G. (2009). *The other side of sadness.* New York, NY: Basic Books.
Bowen, M. (1978). *Family therapy in clinical practice.* New York, NY: Jason Aronson.
Bowlby, J. (1980). *Attachment and loss, vol. III, sadness and depression.* New York, NY: Basic Books.
Darwin, C. (1899). *The expression of emotions in man and animals.* New York, NY: D. Appleton.
De Waal, F. (1989). *Chimpanzee politics.* New York, NY: Harper & Row.
[Editorial] (2012, February 18). *The Lancet, 379*(9816), 589. London.
Freud, S. (1917). Mourning and melancholia. In J. Strachey (Ed.), *The standard edition of the complete psychological works of Sigmund Freud*, vol. 14 (pp. 152–170). London: Hogarth Press.
Gay, P. (Ed.). (1989). *The Freud reader.* New York, NY: W. W. Norton.
King, B. (2013). *How animals grieve.* Chicago: University of Chicago Press.
Konigsberg, R. (2011). *The truth about grief.* New York, NY: Simon & Shuster.
Kubler-Ross, E. (1973). *On death and dying.* New York, NY: Routledge.
Kubler-Ross, E., & Kessler, D. (2005). *On grief and grieving: Finding the meaning of grief through the five stages of loss.* New York, NY: Scribner.
Maciejewski, P., & Prigerson, H. (2017, October). Prolonged, but not complicated grief, is a mental Disorder. *The British Journal of Psychiatry, 211*(4), 189–191.
McComb, K., Baker, L., & Moss, C. (2006). African elephants show high levels of interest in the skulls and ivory of their own species. *Biology Letters The Royal Society, 2*, 26–28.
Moss, C. (1988). *Elephant memories: Thirteen years in the life of an elephant family.* New York, NY: Fawcett Columbine.
Panksepp, J. (1998). *Affective neuroscience: The foundations of human and animals emotions.* New York, NY: Oxford University Press.
Rosenblatt, P., Walsh, R., & Jackson, D. (1976). *Grief and mourning in cross-cultural perspec*tive. New Haven, CT: Human Relations Area Files.
Teleki, G. (1973). Group response to the accidental death of a chimpanzee in Gombe park, Tanzania. *Folio Primatologica, 20*, 81–94.
"What Does It Mean to Be Human? Cro-Magnon-1". (2016, August 5). *Smithsonian Museum of Natural History.* Retrieved from http://humanorigins.si.edu/evidence/human-fossils/fossils/cro-magnon-1
"What Does It Mean to Be Human? Social Life". (2016, March 25). *Smithsonian Museum of Natural History.* Retrieved from http://humanorigins.si.edu/human-characteristics/social-life

4

TOWARD AN OBJECTIVE VIEW OF MORTALITY

Biology, History, and the Emotional System

Stephanie J. Ferrera

> *All of the life of the earth dies, all of the time, in the same volume as the new life that dazzles us each morning each spring.*
>
> (Thomas, 1974, p. 115)

All lives come to an end. And life goes on. The connection between these two facts, captured by Lewis Thomas in one elegant sentence, is rooted in biology. Death and the continuation of life in new generations have always been part of the human experience, but as pointed out by Ernst Mayr (1997), this could not be understood scientifically until Charles Darwin came forward with the theory of evolution through natural selection. He credits Darwin's follower, nineteenth-century biologist August Weismann, with demonstrating that "a rapid sequence of generations is necessary to provide the number of new genotypes required to cope permanently with a changing environment" (pp. 1–2). Each new generation brings new characteristics, mostly similar yet slightly different from the parent generation; these play out in the struggle for existence, "leading to the preservation of each profitable deviation of structure or instinct" (Darwin, 1859/1979, p. 435). Variation is the *sine qua non* of evolutionary change. Without it, the species does not evolve and therefore does not survive.

Sherwin Nuland (1994) writes of death as essential to the balance, or economy, of nature. A doctor dedicated to saving lives, he asserts that death is natural, not pathological:

> Mankind, for all its unique gifts, is just as much a part of the ecosystem as is any other zoologic or botanical form, and

> nature does not distinguish . . . We die so that the world may continue to live. The tragedy of a single individual becomes, in the balance of natural things, the triumph of ongoing life.
> (p. 267)

Becoming Aware of Death

> *We behold the face of nature bright with gladness, we often see superabundance of food; we do not see, or we forget, that the birds which are idly singing round us mostly live on insects or seeds, and are thus constantly destroying life, or we forget how largely these songsters, or their eggs, or their nestlings, are destroyed by birds and beasts of prey.*
> —Charles Darwin (1859/1979, p. 116)

It is easy, Darwin thought (1859/1979), to admit "the truth of the universal struggle for life" (p. 115) but difficult to bear in mind that death is inherent in that struggle. Thomas (1974) suggests that although dying surrounds us, it goes mostly unnoticed. Insects by the ton are steadily being eaten or dropping in their tracks, invisibly. To see a dead animal in the open is a rare and startling experience. "It is in the nature of animals to die alone, off somewhere, hidden" (p. 113). Able to forget about death much of the time, we know it "as a kind of abstraction" (p. 113).

The tendency of nature to keep death out of sight fits with the human preference to keep it out of mind. Given the nature of human attachment, separation from a loved one and the end of one's own life are profoundly painful subjects to think about often or closely. The emotional reactivity that makes death a difficult subject to think about also makes it difficult to talk about. Murray Bowen (1978) wrote: "Chief among all taboo subjects is death" (p. 322). Sensitive to the anxiety in self and others around death, one treads lightly. We see this in the language used to soften the reality: People do not die, they "pass away" and go on to "a better place."

Our ancestors did not have the luxury of keeping death at a distance. Life for them often ended early, suddenly, and violently. According to W. M. Spellman (2014), the norm was early death from disease, famine, natural disaster, or sudden trauma at the hands of predators.

Thousands of years of scientific and economic progress have brought us to the other end of the spectrum: "Today in the developed West death and dying are often kept tidily out of sight, relegated to hospitals, skilled care facilities or nursing homes . . . Death today is commonly at a distinct remove from life, very nearly clandestine, almost always unwelcome" (p. 7).

Modern medical education plays its part in looking away from the reality of death. Atul Gawande (2014) opens his book, *Being Mortal*, stating: "I learned about a lot of things in medical school, but mortality wasn't one of them . . . Our textbooks had almost nothing on aging or frailty or dying" (p. 1).

The difficulties we have in looking squarely at death arise from the nature of emotional attachment and separation. We are ever aware at an instinctual level of how life would change if we were to lose a member of that inner circle, those who are central to our well-being, our very life. For families, the loss of a person who has been pivotal to the functioning and emotional equilibrium of a family leaves a void to be filled. With the absence of such a person, we become aware of the degree to which we had oriented our lives around him or her and had come to count on them for resources, energy, security, comfort, guidance, and so much else. The whole system of relationships begins to shift and change. There are certain deaths that will disturb the functioning and stability of a family for months or years. Grieving families are vulnerable to increased anxiety that can trigger further losses (Bowen, 1978). At this crucial time, the attempt to balance intense subjectivity with a bit of objectivity is a step toward resolving loss and moving forward.

Objectivity and Subjectivity

Why is it important to become objective about life and death? What is gained in the effort to think objectively about one's own life, one's place in the world, one's death? Michael E. Kerr's (1988) distinction between objectivity and subjectivity provides a starting point for reflections on these questions.

> Objective means that what is being defined belongs to the object of perception or thought and is not affected by

> personal feelings or prejudice. Subjective means that what is being defined belongs to the thinking subject rather than to the object of thought and that it relies on one's personal feelings or opinions.
>
> (Kerr & Bowen, 1988, p. 18)

Paul MacLean (1970) explained the influence of emotion and subjectivity on scientific work as a natural consequence of the way the brain evolved:

> No measurement or computation obtained by the hardware of the exact sciences enters our comprehension without undergoing subjective transformation by the software of the brain . . . primitive systems of the brain have the capacity to generate affective feelings of what is real, true, and important and thereby to influence scientific attitudes.
>
> (p. 337)

Bowen (1982) saw subjectivity as the "major barrier" to the pursuit of a science of human behavior. His writings on the years of work that went into the development of family systems theory, from his first inklings of the disparity between Freudian theory and science to his concept of the family as an emotional unit, are a case study in managing subjectivity and maintaining a focus on functional facts.

Objective thought is a strict discipline. It calls for reflection on one's own inner process, identifying assumptions and biases, questioning oneself rigorously, seeing the gaps in one's data, seeking more facts and a broader perspective, and most importantly, recognizing the influence of others on one's thinking. Consider the difficulties encountered in trying to keep personal feelings and opinions separated from facts in one's thought process. Even for a scientist trained to view data objectively, there are unrecognized biases, what Mayr (1982) calls "the silent assumptions that are taken so completely for granted that they are never mentioned" (p. 835). There is also the issue of the emotional attachment to ideas and the comfort of togetherness with a community of people who think alike. MacLean (1970) observed that scientists become emotionally invested in theories and their founders: "important theories, marked for death by the discovery of contradictory evidence, seldom die before their authors" (p. 337).

The discipline of objectivity is most valuable, but also most difficult, in arenas in which one has significant personal investment. Michael Kerr (1988) writes: "The closer we get to ourselves, the greater the pressure to see what we want to see, or, at least to see what we have always seen" (Kerr & Bowen, 1988, p. 18). When close-to-home concerns are at play, sensitivity to others and scrutiny of their behavior increase; there is increased likelihood of listening selectively and missing important facts. Subjective interpretations of behavior are daunting barriers to overcome. Attributing a motive or meaning to another person's behavior (for example, saying "I know why you did that,") is a boundary violation likely to trigger a reaction and increase tension.

Family members experience events somewhat differently, especially those, like illness and death, that are laden with emotion. Each member of a family or group will have his or her own perceptions and biases and will remember the event differently, and most will develop narratives to explain events and outcomes. The part that self has played is often the hardest to see. A narrative becomes self-serving when it shields one from seeing one's own part, whether it be a greater or lesser part, in the total process. A narrative may also place blame on oneself and miss seeing the realistic limitations on what one could do. In either case, blame of others or of self, one is tied to a defensive posture that can perpetuate anxiety and all of anxiety's impacts on relationships. Kerr (1988) states: "Anxiety can intensify the feeling process to the point that the capacity for objective thinking is completely obliterated" (Kerr & Bowen, 1988, p. 125n).

In moving toward objectivity, one begins to replace blame and guilt with a sense of responsibility as a guide to action. A memorable moment in my early training in Bowen theory was the coaching I received from Kathleen Kerr as I was dealing with a challenging event. I have saved the letter in which she wrote: "I think it is worthwhile to look at the process and to see what part of the responsibility you own and try to face that square, neither denying any part, nor accepting it all" (K. Kerr, 1979, personal correspondence).

The Perspective of History

Before considering how earlier generations of humans thought about death and dealt with its sorrows, it is worth thinking about how they experienced death. In *A Brief History of Death*, W. M. Spellman (2014) offers this overview:

> Prior to the industrial revolution the earth could be seen as an especially unfriendly host, replete with seasonal terrors, inexplicable natural disasters, and mysterious illnesses . . . The sometimes hostile ecosystem was made more dangerous by an even harsher social environment marked by the propensity of the species to do harm against its own kind.
>
> (p. 132)

In Spellman's accounts, one is struck by the close association between death and violence. History is marked by episodes of massive casualties driven by four main causes: natural disaster, disease, famine, and death at the hands of other humans.

Life was transformed "once humans stopped chasing after their dinner and began growing it around 12,000 BCE" (Spellman, 2014, p. 134). After millennia of life as hunter-gatherers, humans developed the ability to domesticate plants and animals. Agriculture arose independently in many parts of the world, and with it came more abundant food supplies and rapid population growth, followed by the invention of the territorial state, organized armies, the development of trade and mobility, urbanization, and rampant disease. Humans now acquired diseases from animals, insects, worms, and parasites and carried these diseases to other populations as they pursued commerce and conquests. The bubonic plague of the mid-fourteenth century claimed an estimated one-third of Europe's population. Spellman (2014) puts a human face on this catastrophe:

> So powerful was the ripsaw of plague in Europe that survivors could not bury the dead fast enough . . . Neighbours avoided neighbours, parents abandoned children, spouses departed their partners with no thought of prayers, much less physical comfort, for the dying.
>
> (p. 138)

The sixteenth century saw European explorers arriving in the Americas, bringing new plants and animals, and pathogens against which the indigenous population had no immunity. The result was "an unprecedented demographic disaster" (Spellman, p. 139) with populations falling in the invaded areas, as much as 90% in Meso-America and Peru. Virulent epidemics struck with regularity well into the twentieth century. The influenza pandemic of 1918–1919 killed at least 50 million people, more than the military dead of World War I. Spellman describes the response as "unprecedented": Rather than turning to the religious explanations that had prevailed over centuries, governments and the public looked to scientific medicine. With science, humans have begun to conquer infectious disease by understanding its mechanisms and developing vaccines and antitoxins. Victories have been won. Smallpox was eradicated in 1980. We have come to understand the human interface with microorganisms as a co-evolutionary "arms race." While gaining some control over disease, we find ourselves facing "new and emerging infections that guarantee an ongoing struggle in an increasingly interconnected world" (Spellman, p. 141).

A most sobering set of facts in Spellman's history of death is his account of infant mortality and infanticide. "Death was most commonly associated with the very young, not, as is the case today, with the very old" (p. 146). In agricultural societies before the past two centuries, an estimated one-third to half of children died before the age of two, due primarily to malnutrition and disease. How, we may ask, did families endure the sorrow of such losses? Spellman's answer is that adults adopted a posture of resignation, sometimes not naming a baby or investing emotionally until there was a reasonable expectation that he or she would survive infancy.

Infanticide, the willful killing of infants, has been practiced in human culture from the hunter-gatherers to agrarian societies and, though now widely condemned, into modern times. Abandonment and exposure to the elements were most often the means and most often carried out by the mother. Female infants were more likely to be killed than males. Fathers had legal rights over children and over the decision whether or not to admit a newborn to the family. Infanticide, which seems to go against basic human instincts, needs to be understood in the context of biological, social, and economic realities. Spellman (2014) explains:

> Following—ironically perhaps—the modern notion that it is better to die than to suffer, the act was most often a method of family planning or birth control, where a decision was made that food and other essential resources were inadequate to sustain an expanding population.
>
> (p. 149)

The violence done to humans by one another, directly or indirectly, must be considered the most problematic of the causes of death. Violence is familiar to us today, as it has been through much of history, in the forms of famine, warfare, genocide, and terrorism. I begin the list with famine because, though food crises are tied to environmental factors, famine has on occasion been used as a weapon of state terror, as it was in the regime of Stalin (1929–1933) when approximately 14 million people, almost all unarmed civilians, perished.

Karen Armstrong (2014) speaks to the biological and historical roots of human violence:

> Much of what we now call "religion" was originally rooted in an acknowledgement of the tragic fact that life depended on the destruction of other creatures; rituals were addressed to helping human beings face up to this insoluble dilemma. Despite their real respect, reverence, and even affection for their prey, however, ancient huntsmen remained dedicated killers. Millennia of fighting large, aggressive animals meant that these hunting parties became tightly bonded teams that were the seeds of our modern armies, ready to risk everything for the common good and to protect their fellows in moments of danger.
>
> (p. 9)

The "insoluble dilemma" is at the core of human nature, rooted in the reality that we are part and parcel of nature. With remarkable clarity, Armstrong puts forward the contradictions, ambivalences, and perpetual tensions that inhabit our minds and complicate our relationships. Reverence for nature vies with exploitation of nature; empathy and altruism vie with mistrust and hostility; reason contends with instinct.

Armstrong draws an important distinction between the organized violence of warfare and another, more covert type of aggression: structural or institutional violence. Hunter-gatherers lived near subsistence level and developed relatively egalitarian communities. Sharing resources was essential; accumulating wealth was not an option. With agriculture, a new way of life, an economy of surplus, emerged. Armstrong (2014) explains: "In societies that produce more than they need, it is possible for a small group to exploit this surplus for its own enrichment, gain a monopoly of violence, and dominate the rest of the population" (p. 14).

Structural violence becomes woven into our social systems through institutions and ideologies that support the concentration of resources and privilege in the hands of some at the expense of others. Melvin Konner (2015) describes the social, economic, and political developments that led to societies becoming patriarchal as well as hierarchical. As societies became more stratified, a minority, primarily high-ranking men, gained control over territory and resources and thereby gained a large measure of control over the lives of the majority. They became, Konner writes, "hugely over-represented in positions of power" (p. 7). A prime example of structural violence is slavery, which was universal in the ancient world and continues today in the forms of sexual slavery and labor slavery. Structural violence includes suppression of dissent, confiscation of property, and displacement of people; it goes further with the discriminatory policies and practices that target certain individuals and groups; the barriers to equal access embedded in political and economic structures such as elections, finance, education, housing, law enforcement, and the law itself.

It is not easy to calculate the number of illnesses and shortened lives that result from structural violence. Embedded in the institutions of society, this violence is covert; because it is systemic, it is difficult to locate particular individuals or groups that are responsible.

Evolving Beliefs About Life and Death

> *With his intellect, man has devised philosophies and beliefs about the meaning of life and death that tend to deny his place in nature's plan.*
>
> (Bowen, 1978, p. 321)

The natural world in which humans evolved has to a great extent been a world of trials and tribulations for our species, a world of forces and dangers that were beyond human understanding or control. Until the rise of the natural sciences in the Enlightenment period of the seventeenth and eighteenth centuries, the dearth of scientific facts left people to their subjectivity—imagination, speculation, magical thinking, philosophical constructions, and religions—to create systems of belief about life and death that provided meaning and guidance through life. Spellman (2014) proposes that, across centuries and cultures, humans have approached mortality and the possibility of an afterlife from three basic standpoints. One is the naturalist position, held mainly by scientists, who see no empirical evidence of any continuity of life beyond biological death. Death is "the end of life, plain and simple" (p. 9). The meaning of life is to be found in the joys and challenges of this world. The second perspective is that of the agnostic who sees no evidence for belief in an afterlife but does not rule out the possibility. The final reality remains a mystery beyond our power to know.

The third view, the transcendental position, holds that there is something larger than this life, something beyond the grave, and that supernatural beings more powerful than limited human beings govern the world. Transcendental thinking in its many variations has held the strongest influence in shaping human beliefs about life and death. Although there is no empirical evidence to support the existence of supernatural gods or one God, an immortal soul, or an afterlife, there is abundant evidence that these beliefs have met important needs for humans and served essential purposes. This evidence is seen not in the content of the beliefs but in the actions that they inspire: from the building of great cathedrals, mosques, and temples, to the billions who gather to worship, to the millions of pilgrims to holy sites, to the pervasive presence of religious traditions in literature and the arts, to elaborate and costly burial rituals, to the reliance on the supernatural for moral guidance. Religion has addressed the most compelling human needs: the need to find purpose and meaning in life, and the need to do so in a community of like-minded others. Spellman (2014) speaks to the functions of transcendental beliefs:

> Especially in the world's great religious traditions, death as but a stage in life served the cause of justice in an all-too-cruel world, offered reward or reunion with creator god after the trials of the earthly tenure, and even assured perfection that was withheld from those still in the flesh.
>
> (p. 11)

He goes on to describe the God-centered view of the world that prevailed from the time of Aristotle to the mid-sixteenth century:

> For upwards of 2000 years most thinkers understood this universe as limited in scale, hierarchical in nature and monarchical in governance. Animated by angels, spirits, and the workings of divine grace, God's creation was alive with energy and activity. The sun, moon, and planets all revolved around the earth, the definite centre of the cosmos, in perfect concentric circles, their movement regularly influencing daily lives. In the end, the whole of creation was micro-managed by a prime mover who was constantly and intimately involved in his handiwork, solicitous of human welfare and quick to punish those who rejected his sovereignty.
>
> (p. 69)

Shortly before his death in 1543, Nicolaus Copernicus published a model of the universe that placed the sun, not the earth, at the center. Galileo Galilei later championed this model at expense of being imprisoned for his view. In the new intellectual environment of the Enlightenment of the seventeenth and eighteenth centuries, the empirical perspective began to gain ground. A picture of nature emerged which called into serious question the need for nonmaterial explanations. A monumental step forward (though some would say "backward") was the publication of Charles Darwin's *On the Origin of Species by Means of Natural Selection* in 1859, followed by *The Descent of Man* in 1871. What could be more disturbing to the view of the human as the pinnacle of creation, holding dominion over the earth and its bounty, than Darwin's proposition that *Homo sapiens* is kin to other species by common descent and subject to the same forces of natural selection? Spellman (2014) captures the shock felt by the religious establishment and laypeople alike: "Gone was the great chain of being and its static hierarchy of life forms from lowest to highest; in its place were species transformed slowly over great sweeps of time, the result of mere accident and impersonal forces" (p. 78).

Edward O. Wilson (1998) defines the transcendental and empirical positions as fundamentally different ways of thinking about moral values. "Either ethical precepts, such as justice and human rights, are independent of human experience or else they are human inventions . . . The choice between the assumptions makes all the difference in the way we view ourselves as a species" (p. 238). Transcendentalism is the province of theologians and philosophers. "They seek the grail of natural law, which comprises freestanding principles of moral conduct immune to doubt and compromise" (p. 239). The doctrine of natural rights follows from natural law and is considered to be self-evident. In contrast, empiricists, himself included, look to objective knowledge as the basis of discerning moral codes. Knowledge of how the brain works, how the mind develops, and how biological and cultural evolution have shaped moral sentiments is the foundation needed for more accurate, science-based ethical decision-making.

Following "the Copernican and Darwinian dethronement of the species" (Spellman, p. 206), and through the scientific revolution of the past several centuries, empiricism has gained ground. The science and technology of medicine together with advances in public health have dramatically changed the way death is experienced. Death for most comes at the end of a long life, in contrast with the sudden, premature, and violent death that was the norm for 99% of human history (Spellman, 2014). In the past century, dying has become more a process over time, involving a series of losses and raising a host of new questions: how to maintain quality of life as physical health and/or cognitive capacity decline; how to deal with the complexities of medical interventions; how to create resources for care and allocate resources wisely. As death approaches for oneself or a loved one, these become very personal, moral questions.

Though we now have much greater empirical knowledge than early humans, transcendental thinking still holds strong appeal. Wilson (1998) writes: "Transcendentalism, especially when reinforced by religious faith, is psychically full and rich; it feels somehow *right* . . . even as empiricism is winning the mind, transcendentalism continues to win the heart" (pp. 261–262). For some, the two paths to truth are held in separate categories: science and reason for those things that can be explained; faith for those things that cannot. A great many people turn to religious beliefs and the community of believers for comfort, especially at times of illness, dying, and death.

Humans have always been a transcendental species in the larger sense of the word. We have a great gift: the capacity to transcend fear, adversity, suffering, and loss by coming together in community, putting differences aside, joining collective intelligence and collective passion in pursuit of a common cause. Each time we set a mission, in our personal lives and as a society, each time we overcome obstacles and our own limitations, each time we reach a new level of knowledge, or solve an intractable problem, or resolve an impasse in a relationship, or achieve as a team what no one person alone could achieve, we feel the power of community at its best, a transcendent spiritual experience. At such times, we find ourselves without words. We turn to the poets, the artists, the musicians.

Mortality and Morality

What teaches us more about our common humanity than the experience of losing someone dear to us or facing our own frailty and dying? Once we know death, both intellectually and emotionally from direct encounter, it can never go back to being "a kind of abstraction." We know that the deaths of those far removed from us are as real in human suffering as those close to us. In this way, being mortal and being moral are wedded in our thinking and in our emotions.

As numbered days grow fewer, one sorts out what is important from what is not. The legacy one will leave for the future is in the important category. Years of lived experience bring a perspective, and possibly greater objectivity about one's place in the universe, one's place in human history, and in the personal inner circle of loved ones. What is important now is the younger generations. With them in mind,

I bring up three large areas of concern for the twenty-first century, all well known and observable in daily news reports.

First is the age-old "insoluble dilemma" of violence against one another. Although the accelerated growth of knowledge in the last three centuries has brought us remarkable success in shaping the environment to meet human needs, in overcoming famine and disease, reducing child mortality, alleviating poverty, and extending the life span, it has not brought the gains in wisdom and maturity we need to settle our tribal differences without violence. Spellman (2014) writes:

> The very human ingenuity and technical prowess responsible for improving the quality of life over the past 100 years has also allowed us to kill one another more effectively, on a sweeping scale, and at greater distances . . . Although an appalling constant in the human experience, organized warfare was not a major cause of death in terms of total population until the advent of mechanized combat in the mid-nineteenth century.
>
> (p. 154–155)

It should be noted that an increasingly high percentage of the casualties of war are the injuries and deaths of noncombatants, including, of course, children.

The second concern is social and economic inequality and its multiple effects. Statistics abound, underscored by popular uprisings in the United States and around the world, showing that distribution of resources has become increasingly unequal, the gulf between rich and poor wider. One way that this plays out on the ground in regard to health care is illustrated in the experience of Sunita Puri, a physician of palliative medicine in California. In an essay titled "Unequal Lives, Unequal Deaths," Dr. Puri (2016) describes her work with families in the poorest neighborhoods of Los Angeles. "In these neighborhoods, people die an average of 10 years earlier than those who live less than ten miles away." Her work includes explaining to overstressed caregivers the rules of what the health care system will pay for, and she wonders why our health care system will pay for last-ditch-effort interventions for a dying patient but not for one trained caregiver to help a family provide comfort at home. She offers this perspective:

> "Death may be humanity's great equalizer, but the inequalities suffered in life—leading to a shorter life expectancy—become inequalities in the experience of dying as well."
>
> (http://opinionator.blogs.nytimes.com/2016/01/20/dying-at-home-when-youre-poor/)

There is the obvious problem of doing too little for ill and dying patients, but there is also the danger of doing too much. With the great advances in the science of medicine, the art and practice of medicine has become divided into narrow specializations; focus goes to symptoms and failing organs; patients may be viewed more as candidates for interventions than as whole persons. Katy Butler cared for her parents at the end of their lives and later wrote about the close-up experience of medical decision making from the perspective of the patient and the family. Following a stroke, her father's life was extended with technology, resulting in prolonged suffering and a diminished life for him along with severe pressure on her mother to meet the demands of his care. Butler (2014) offers this brave proposal:

> I think the whole family should be regarded as the patient . . . What have we accomplished if we've just shifted the illness from one member of a family to another? If you're a doctor, I think you have to look at whether you're adding suffering to the family as a whole when you extend the life of an individual.
>
> (Mowe, 2014, p. 7)

Atul Gawande (2014) is one of many in the medical field who are looking closely at the cost–benefit balances involved in decision making at the end of life. He advocates for the new specializations of geriatrics and palliative medicine. He writes:

> The battle of being mortal is the battle to maintain the integrity of one's life—to avoid becoming so diminished or subjugated that who you are becomes disconnected from who you were or who you want to be. Sickness and old age make the

> struggle hard enough. The professionals and institutions we turn to should not make it worse. But we have at last entered an era in which an increasing number of them believe their job is not to confine people's choices, in the name of safety, but to expand them, in the name of living a worthwhile life.
> (p. 141)

The third area of concern encompasses all of the issues that are now called "environmental." Wilson (1998) wrote almost 20 years ago: "Humankind is like a household living giddily off vanishing capital" (p. 286). He alerted us to the precarious position we are in, facing an environmental bottleneck or worse, in the twenty-first century.

Joining the voices of the scientists, now comes the voice of Pope Francis. He, of course, comes from the transcendental tradition, but has proven himself a keen student of the empirical research on our relationship to the planet. His thinking, in fact, is an example of how transcendental and empirical avenues can combine in a powerful way and lead to agreement on solutions when applied to the practical realities of life.

The Pope begins the encyclical letter *Laudato Si'* (2015) recalling the devotion of Saint Francis of Assisi to "our Sister, Mother Earth" (p. 7). Under the heading, "The Human Roots of the Ecological Crisis," he names the developments that have brought us to this point. They include the creation of immense technological power and economic resources without sufficient wisdom and responsibility to control them or use them wisely; interventions in nature that lack the ancient attunement and respect for nature; the illusion of unlimited growth based on an infinite quantity of resources which can be renewed quickly; lifestyles conditioned by dependence on technology; wasteful consumerism that stands in unacceptable contrast with dehumanizing deprivation; the overwhelming of the real economy by finance and the profit motive; fragmentation of knowledge and loss of appreciation for the whole and for the relationship between things.

As I read the encyclical, the words "down to earth" come to mind. The Pope has shown himself to be refreshingly down to earth in his personal style. In *Laudato Si'*, Francis is calling us down to earth, as in these passages:

> Nobody is suggesting a return to the Stone Age, but we do need to slow down and look at reality in a different way, to

> appropriate the positive and sustainable progress which has been made, but also to recover the values and the great goals swept away by our unrestrained delusions of grandeur . . . our "dominion" over the universe should be understood more properly in the sense of responsible stewardship.
>
> (pp. 78–79)

> If the present ecological crisis is one small sign of the ethical, cultural and spiritual crisis of modernity, we cannot presume to heal our relationship with nature and the environment without healing all fundamental human relationships.
>
> (p. 80)

The Emotional System

Murray Bowen introduced a new way of understanding how we have arrived at the levels of violence, inequality, and environmental degradation that concern us today. In Bowen's natural systems theory, these extremes are seen as part of a broad continuum of human behavior that encompasses calm, thoughtful, responsible functioning at one end and anxiety-driven, reactive, out-of-control functioning at the other.

Bowen believed that humans had the faculties in our brains that could, with disciplined effort, permit us to think scientifically and objectively about ourselves. Not everyone thought this was possible. He designed and led an empirical study of the human family, arguably nature's most complex system. The result was the concept of the family as an emotional system in which individual development is significantly shaped by the system as a whole.

Over the years of research and development of family systems theory, Bowen kept notes on indicators of emotional process in the larger society. In 1972, in response to an invitation from the new Environmental Protection Agency to write a paper on man's reaction to crisis, he began to organize these data into a conceptual framework and later added the concept, emotional process in society, to the theory. Seeing the same emotional process in society as in the family, he identified the common elements: chronic anxiety, the balance between thinking and emotion, and the balance between the pressure for togetherness and the force for individual autonomy.

In the family and in the society, an anxiety-driven process leads to emotional and social regression:

> When a family is subjected to chronic, sustained anxiety, the family begins to lose contact with its intellectually determined principles, to resort more and more to emotionally determined decisions to allay the anxiety of the moment . . . The societal concept postulates that the same process is evolving in society.
> (Bowen, 1978, p. 386)

Regression deepens as togetherness pressures intensity and individuality is reciprocally constrained. The endpoint is reached "when viable members desert the group and there is overwhelming reactivity, violence, and chaos" (278).

Bowen saw the same human phenomena that environmental leaders and the Pope see: the pressure of exponential population growth and unsustainable lifestyles on the earth's resources, the resort to short-term solutions that exacerbate problems, and the difficulty of getting cooperation between societies. He believed that the origin of the anxiety that drives regression is in the disharmony between man and nature more than the disharmony between man and his fellow man.

Bowen did more than name and describe the end results of family and societal regressions; he developed an original body of knowledge to explain regression as a product of instinctually driven human emotional systems. He identified the relationship patterns that operate automatically, out of awareness, when fear and contagious anxiety are on the rise. Distancing, conflict, dominant-adaptive reciprocal functioning, triangling, the projection process, and emotional cutoff work in combination to produce insider–outsider polarities and the host of "-isms" that divide us and fuel chronic anxiety. The phenomenon of the "emotional shock wave" that Bowen observed in families is undoubtedly part of the emotional process in societies. It is not hard to see how the massive losses suffered in human conflicts could propel further conflict and loss.

Bowen saw a pathway out of regression that operates in both families and societies. That pathway is leadership through differentiation of self. Those individuals who are able to observe systemic regression, recognize and change their own participation in it, and find more responsible avenues for action become the leaders who gradually move the larger system to a new norm of higher functioning. Bowen (1978) described this remarkable process:

> A shift toward individuality on a family level can be illustrated by a single, responsible family member who proceeds on an individually determined course . . . When one family member successfully makes such an individuality move, then another, and another will do the same. In a small or large social system, the move toward individuality is initiated by a single, strong leader with the courage of his conviction who can assemble a team, and who has clearly defined principles on which he can base his decisions when the emotional opposition becomes intense.
>
> (pp. 278–279)

Increasing regression means increasing pressure to think and act with the group, more difficulty developing an independent view, more risks and costs in expressing or taking action on a different view. At the extreme, it becomes life threatening to challenge the status quo. Nevertheless, there have always been people who recognized regression and had the motivation and courage to speak and act for more responsible courses of action.

Taking a Position for Self on Mortality

> *Each individual has to define his own place in the total scheme and accept the fact that he will die and be replaced by succeeding generations. His difficulty in finding a life plan for himself is complicated by the fact that his life is intimately interwoven with the lives about him.*
>
> (Murray Bowen, 1978, p. 321)

There is something very personal and solitary about dying. As social as we are, there are things in life that one must do alone. Leaving this world is one of those things; defining a position for self on how one hopes to leave this world is another. Both are done in intimate contact with important others who have an influence and an investment in the outcome.

Biology tells us that humans are the only species with the ability to anticipate and plan for the future; history tells us that only a small percentage of people have had the opportunity of time and thinking space to do so. One is fortunate indeed to live long enough to have a perspective on one's "place in the total scheme," to develop beliefs and principles that hold solid, and to meet death with a degree of peace within self and with those important to self.

My own movement toward objectivity, and effort toward differentiation of self, led me to cross the bridge from transcendental beliefs to empiricism and a nature-based spirituality. With my introduction to the thinking of Murray Bowen in the 1970s, I became interested in learning science, biology in particular. Eyes that had searched the great beyond for guidance began to focus on the earth and its wonders.

At the bicentennial celebration of the founding of Georgetown University in 1989, Edward O. Wilson made this comment: "Humanity, I would suggest, is exalted not because we've risen so far above other living creatures but because understanding them very well elevates our very concept of life" (Papero, 1989).

Life itself—its origins, its evolution, its amazing adaptability and tenacity, its vast diversity, its complex relationships, its beauty and its mystery, and its hardships and struggle as well—life itself holds the meaning and purpose for which we search. The brain that allows us to discover, within limits, who we are and where we came from, and to make enlightened choices, within limits, about where we are going—this brain is a product of natural processes. To be attuned to nature, to be touched by its beauty and nourished by its bounty, to know oneself as part of it and live responsibly within it, are spiritual pursuits. The mind and spirit are elevated as one opens oneself to the natural world. No wonder Darwin saw "grandeur in this view of life." (Darwin, 1859/1979, p. 459).

REFERENCES

Armstrong, K. (2014). *Fields of blood: Religion and the history of violence.* New York, NY: Alfred A. Knopf.

Bowen, M. (1978). *Family therapy in clinical practice.* New York, NY: Jason Aronson.

Bowen, M. (1982/1997). Subjectivity, *homo sapiens*, and science. In Sagar R. Ruth (Ed.), *Bowen theory and practice.* Washington, DC: Georgetown Family Center.

Darwin, C. (1859/1979). *The origin of species.* New York, NY: Avenel Books.
Gawande, A. (2014). *Being mortal.* New York, NY: Henry Holt.
Kerr, M. E., & Bowen, M. (1988). *Family evaluation.* New York, NY: W. W. Norton.
Konner, M. (2015). *Women after all.* New York, NY: W. W. Norton.
MacLean, P. D. (1970). The triune brain, emotion, and scientific bias. In F. O. Schmitt (Ed.), *The neurosciences: Second study program.* New York, NY: The Rockefeller University Press.
Mayr, E. (1982). *The growth of biological thought.* Cambridge, MA: The Belknap Press of Harvard University Press.
Mayr, E. (1997). *This is biology.* Cambridge, MA: The Belknap Press of Harvard University Press.
Mowe, S. (2014, April). The long goodbye: Katy Butler on how modern medicine decreases our chance of a good death. *The Sun*, pp. 4–12.
Nuland, S. B. (1994). *How we die.* New York, NY: Alfred A. Knopf.
Papero, D. V. (1989). E. O. Wilson speaks at Georgetown bicentennial. *Family Center Report, 10*(3). Washington, DC: Georgetown Family Center.
Pope, F. (2015). *Laudato si': On care for our common home.* Huntington, IN: Our Sunday Visitor Publishing Division.
Puri, S. (2016). *Unequal lives, unequal deaths.* Retrieved from http://opinionator.blogs.nytimes.com/2016/01/20/dying-at-home-when-youre-poor/
Spellman, W. M. (2014). *A brief history of death.* London: Reaktion Books.
Thomas, L. (1974). *Death in the open: Lives of a cell* (pp. 113–116). Toronto: Bantam Books.
Wilson, E. O. (1998). *Consilience: The unity of knowledge.* New York, NY: Alfred A. Knopf.

II

DEATH IN THE THERAPIST'S OWN FAMILY

5

EMOTIONAL SHOCK WAVE AND DIFFERENTIATION OF SELF

Sydney K. Reed

In 1989 I interviewed Dr. Bowen regarding his thoughts about family reaction to death, asking him if there was a way to prepare oneself and one's family to be able to avoid an "emotional shock wave." In this interview he makes the connection between emotional shock wave and differentiation of self.

Mrs. Reed: *Dr. Bowen, I have been interested in your theory since 1972 when I first read your anonymous article* (Framo, 1972). *It happened to be the summer when my grandmother died. The concepts were useful for my understanding of what I saw happening in my family. In 1975 I visited Georgetown for the first time. You were speaking about the death of your father. At the same meeting several others spoke about deaths in their families. The emotional climate at the meeting was calm and thoughtful. The week before I had attended a meeting in Chicago on the topic of death and I would have described the climate as uptight and anxious. It was clear to me that there was something different at Georgetown. My head and my physiology responded differently. Would you speak to the concept of emotional shock wave?*

Dr. Bowen: *I ran into families in which shock wave was prominent. They were mostly poorly differentiated families. In that chapter ["Family Reaction to Death"] I was trying to define the notion of shock wave. That would be when the whole family is influenced by the emotional system. Then you can have a shock wave. If a shock wave exists in your family, you've got a lot to work on. What you are trying to do is get to "easy come, easy*

> *go." Not so dependent on a single emotional figure. That's what differentiation is all about.*
>
> (Reed, 1989)

My interest in family reaction to death stemmed from the coincidence of learning about Bowen theory the summer my maternal grandmother died. That summer I also made the decision to go to social work school to become a family therapist. This chapter is my attempt to describe the emotional shock wave that I believe began in my family in 1972 when my grandmother died.

Important Concepts in Bowen Family Systems Theory

The foundational principle of Bowen family systems theory is that the family, not the individual, is the emotional unit. As individuals respond to events in their lives and to other family members, they face the challenge of sorting out their own emotional responses from that of others with whom they are tightly connected. The pull for togetherness is such that an individual will often move in the direction of going along with the group in order to belong, or they will do the opposite and move away from the group in order to protect themselves from being absorbed by the emotional process of the group. Differentiation of self, the most important concept of Bowen family systems theory, represents a third path. The concept of differentiation of self is fundamental to all of the other seven concepts. Differentiation of self allows one to define one's own emotional responses and set one's own course in life while staying emotionally connected with one's family and other important people in one's life (Bowen, 1978, pp. 468–478). Human reactivity is such that maintaining a self in an important relationship, particularly at a time of stress or heightened anxiety, can be difficult. As tension and anxiety rise, there are automatic responses that individuals will use to protect themselves and make themselves more comfortable. Individuals can move away from anxiety-producing relationships toward less intense relationships. As the emotional tension from the first relationship is transferred to another relationship, a "triangle" is created. This transfer of emotional energy from one relationship to another as anxiety and discomfort arise and spread through a family or a collection of individuals creates "interlocking triangles" (Bowen, 1978, pp. 478–780).

Bowen observed an intense emotional process, driven by high anxiety, operating via interlocking triangles after a death in the family. This is particularly common in families with a lower level of differentiation. This phenomenon occurred frequently enough that it led him to develop the idea of the emotional shock wave. He saw that emotional reactivity to the original event would travel through relationship triangles that were often hidden or "underground." Symptoms might then develop in individuals far removed from the key events and/or relationships of the nodal event. Dr. Bowen used the example of a pebble being tossed into a pond resulting in concentric ripples that move out from the original pebble drop. In a family, individuals in the outer ring may not be aware of the original source of the anxiety as it moves through interlocking triangle relationships and now touches them (Bowen, 1978, pp. 324–326).

Optimum functioning is seen as the closest each individual can get to achieving a workable balance between operating for and investing in self and operating for and investing in the welfare of the family. This balance can be reached by recognizing and managing two separate but interrelated processes within self: 1) the tendency to react automatically out of the emotional part of the brain and 2) the ability to act for self by looking at functional facts, defining one's own life principles, and managing self in a thoughtful manner. Both of these processes are needed to define a self (p. 541).

The ability to define a self in one's family is one of life's greatest challenges. Being present and accounted for is the ongoing process of working to be responsible for yourself and to be responsible to one's family.

The Importance of Being Present for Deaths in the Family

This chapter describes two nodal events in my family, the death of each of my grandmothers. It describes the emotional process in me and in my family as two examples of an individual's experience with death in the context of the extended family. I was very new to Bowen theory at the time of the first death, 1972, with a limited understanding of the family as an emotional unit and the importance of being present at significant events in the life of one's family. The funeral of my maternal grandmother, Grandma Strecker, in 1972, for which I was not present, was followed by an emotional shock wave. I eventually understood the emotional shock wave three years later at the time of the death and funeral of my paternal grandmother, Grandma Zeiler, for which I was present. In contrast to my absence at the funeral in 1972, my thoughtful presence during the days after my paternal grandmother's death in 1975 allowed me to be present and accounted for in my extended family. My reconnection with relatives in Montana on both sides of my family provided an opportunity to work on differentiation of self. The shifts in the triangles and the new sense of self gained in these relationships enabled me to formulate an I-position, when previously I had been unable to do this. The shifts in all the triangles involving my mother were the most important, particularly the primary triangle with my father. As I deepened relationships with my aunts, uncles, my sister, and my father, the intensity of the attachment with my mother was modified and lowered. These triangles will be described later in the chapter.

At this time there was an unresolved issue in my marriage. The issue revolved around my belief that I needed more than one child to satisfy my idea of family. My husband was ambivalent about adding a second child to our family. The opportunity to be with my family and the experience of being one of 200 people present at my grandmother's funeral, all related to my paternal grandmother and to each other, provided an existential reality to the meaning of family.

I had lived in another part of the country since I was 18 and had lost touch with the experience of being part of a large extended family. The multitude of triangles in these large extended families, in which I was one of 64 first cousins, had the capacity to absorb and lower anxiety under the right conditions. Under situations of higher anxiety, as in a death in the family, the triangles were more likely to intensify and provide the conditions for an emotional shock wave. In 1975, with a deeper understanding of the family as an emotional unit, I was able to observe emotional process in the family and in myself through the lens of Bowen theory. This enabled me to have a calmer and more productive presence. The experience of the diversity and the resources in my extended family also helped me to clarify my own beliefs and values about what constitutes a family.

The Importance of Being Present for Deaths in the Family

Murray Bowen suggested that being "present and accounted for" in one's nuclear and extended family allows one to make choices to function in a manner that could be a benefit to the family as a whole as well as to self. He particularly urged individuals to be present for nodal events in the family at times of major life transitions and celebrations. At these times families can frequently function a bit more openly than usual. "Being present and accounted for" can be defined as the presence of a thoughtful person making an effort to connect with family members while managing self, responsibly and respectfully, at a time of heightened anxiety. Family members who can be present and accounted for can contribute to the family system remaining relatively open. In addition, a calm and thoughtful presence of a family member who makes a connection with most, or all, members of the family can help dampen anxiety and reactivity that often accompany an intense emotional experience. In a system that is open in this way, one has a better opportunity to make meaningful emotional contact with family members. This openness offers opportunities to strengthen existing relationships and provides a platform for creating new "one to one" relationships with more distant relatives.

The Death of My Maternal Grandmother in 1972

The emotional shock wave I experienced occurred after the death of my maternal grandmother, Grandma Strecker, in July 1972. My husband and I had made plans to travel from Chicago to my parents' home in Montana in August 1972. Consequently, I was not present in July for my maternal grandmother's funeral in Montana. This shock wave, which began in my mother's family of origin, subsequently affected the functioning of my sister and myself via the triangle with our mother. In addition to the illness and the loss of her mother, my mother was reacting to the conflict that developed in her family in response to the will left by my grandparents. The will, which was common among German immigrant families at the time, left all the farmland to the men in the family, and the contents of the house and whatever savings there were to the women. This farmland was now part of the city of Billings, the largest city in Montana, and worth a lot of money as land for residential housing development. There was difference of opinion about how the estate should be distributed. Arguments were made about why the brothers deserved the money while their sisters did not. My mother never told me a word about this conflict. I found out about the conflict by chance in 1975 when I was in Montana for my first trip home to do "family work" as part of my effort to work toward differentiation of self.

Both sets of grandparents, the Streckers and the Zeilers, had settled in Montana when they emigrated from Russia at the turn of the century, and most of my extended family lived there. Over the phone in July, and on my visit home in August, my mother said very little about the death and funeral of her mother, Grandma Strecker. As part of my family's vacation, I traveled to Glacier Park in northern Montana with my husband, my four-year-old child, and my unmarried sister, Jacque. On this trip my sister informed me that she was pregnant and planned to have the baby and swore me to secrecy.

Looking back at this time, I cannot explain why I agreed to keep the secret except to say I was caught up in the emotional triangle consisting of my mother, my sister, and myself. The triangle usually functioned with each of us sisters in a close leg of the triangle with our mother and the distance leg of the triangle between us. This move to swear me to secrecy increased the connection with my sister and created a certain amount of tension in the relationship with my mother. As the oldest child of three, I had assumed responsibility for my younger siblings most of my life. My sister is six years younger than I. When I was six and she was an infant, my mother asked me to take care of her one morning. I thought if I put her in a barrel in the yard, my brother and I could continue playing ball. I fell and my sister's nose was cut. There was a lot of blood, and I was terrified. She has a slight scar to this day. I suspect this incident and my heightened responsiveness to the anxiety in my mother contributed to the overfunctioning care-giving position I have assumed with my siblings. I felt responsible for helping my sister through this pregnancy.

My father and my brother, with whom I had more distant relationships, were outside of this triangle. They had a closer relationship to each other as a result of my brother working in my dad's market after school and on weekends. My mother was the active, hands-on parent, whereas my father's role was mainly breadwinning. I was quite distant from him, but I thought that was normal for most families at that time.

My sister was two years old when my parents moved from Billings, Montana, to a small town, Hardin, 50 miles away. My father was busy with his new business, a small meat market and grocery shop. There were no relatives in the town. This was quite a change from the large extended families on both sides that had surrounded my mother during the childhoods of my brother and myself. My sister was very shy and closely connected to my parents growing up. She was an excellent student in high school, a cheerleader, and president of the student council. She had only one serious boyfriend who went to a Catholic boarding school in another state but returned to our small town in the summer. From 1966 to 1968 she attended Mills College, a girls' school in California. Her boyfriend was also at school in California. After two years at Mills College, she returned home and went to a Montana University closer to home. After one semester in 1968, she dropped out of that program. At Christmas time in 1968, my husband, son, and I had returned to Montana for a visit. Hoping to help my sister move along in life, we offered to have her return with us to Oberlin, Ohio, where we were working and going to school. I offer this as an example of the rescuing posture I took with my sister after she left home. Looking back at this time, I realize that it would be a continuation of my role as big sister, helping to calm down the anxiety in my mother.

My sister lived and worked in Oberlin for six months, but returned to California to live with her longtime boyfriend when my husband and I left Oberlin for the summer. They lived together beginning in 1969. I was frequently triangled in by my mother to "do something" about my sister. They married in January 1973. Their first child, a healthy daughter, was born in February 1973. My sister had become pregnant nine months earlier when our grandmother was hospitalized with a stroke in June 1972. This was the pregnancy to which I had sworn secrecy. My sister told our mother about the pregnancy around Christmas. Our mother did not attend my sister's wedding in early February 1973 but was there in California a few weeks later to help her daughter after the birth of her child. I was not able to attend the wedding due to financial concerns. Only the groom's mother and his older sister attended the wedding. Sometime later my mother expressed her anger at me for having kept my sister's pregnancy a secret.

My Emotional Response to the Hidden Triangles

When I returned to my home in Evanston, Illinois, in fall of 1972, I was quite depressed and had a hard time managing my life. I had just started graduate school and had a four-year-old son and a husband in graduate school. I accepted a fieldwork assignment at a child guidance clinic on the condition that they would allow me to see families in the evening. This meant I was essentially unsupervised in providing family treatment. This was my preference, because I believed using Bowen theory to inform my work was more useful than the child-focused model being used at the clinic. The two previous years I had been part of an inpatient treatment team at the state mental hospital. None of us had formal training in family therapy, but our monthly consultant was Dr. Carl Whitaker, who practiced a form of family therapy that involved becoming part of the family emotional system and then challenging its members to change. Dr. Whitaker suggested I study Bowen's writings. In graduate school I asked a professor to do a reading course with me on Bowen theory. This was the beginning of my study of Bowen family systems theory. The theory gave real meaning to the clinical work I had done in the hospital. It also gave intellectual meaning to Dr. Whitaker's clinical work although the clinical methods were quite different. Since I was at odds with the general philosophy of the agency, the supervision I had in individual and group treatment was not the most comfortable for my supervisors or me. It was an extremely challenging time.

I felt compelled to make sure that my sister was managing her pregnancy in a responsible manner, which in fact she was not doing to my satisfaction. In October 1972, three months after my grandmother's death, I terminated an unplanned pregnancy, the result of a defective intrauterine device (IUD).

I had some theoretical sense that my inability to cope well with these events could be related to my mother's reaction to her mother's death and the secret of my sister's pregnancy, but I had no real data to support that idea. Even though I talked to my mother every week on the phone and saw my parents twice a year, anxiety manifested as distance, both emotional and geographical, and created tension in our relationships. At this time, I had just been introduced to Bowen's "anonymous paper" and had limited understanding of Bowen theory and the importance of "being present and accounted for" at significant family nodal events. I did not have the theory or the information that I would have needed to recognize the emotional process around the death of my grandmother and the subsequent life difficulties of my mother, my sister, and myself.

Triangles in the Maternal Side of My Family

Three years later in 1975 I had begun a serious study of my family using Bowen theory as the lens to gain a new and more complete understanding of the emotional process. I embarked on an assignment given to me in a coaching session with Dr. Bowen, namely to get a relationship with my mother's brothers' wives in Montana. I didn't understand the assignment, nor did I question it. I trusted that Dr. Bowen knew it would be useful. I assumed the assignment represented an opportunity to be in relationship with my aunts and uncles as an adult.

My mother was the only daughter of the five daughters of her sibling group of 14 who lived in Montana. She was a close member of the interlocking network of sisters-in-law in the area. This visit was my first trip home without my husband and child since I had married nine years earlier. Telling my mother that I would be spending half my limited vacation time with relatives in another town was my initial difficult task. I was able to complete visits with 3 of the 13 families of my mother's siblings after choosing those families I thought would be easiest (Figure 5.1).

These visits forced me to give up long-held assumptions about what others thought of me and were the beginning of more meaningful relationships with these relatives. I had considerable dread at the thought of seeing one particular uncle, Jake, who had teased me as a teenager about how I looked: skinny. That painful memory was something that I had carried for 15 years in spite of having little contact with this uncle since I had left home for college in Ohio at 18.

Additionally, this uncle and two of his brothers had challenged my husband-to-be, then-boyfriend, with a common, somewhat crude, "Westerner to Easterner, no college to college, Republican to Democrat" put-down. In fact, my husband was from Massachusetts, was working on a PhD, and was a Democrat. This confrontational

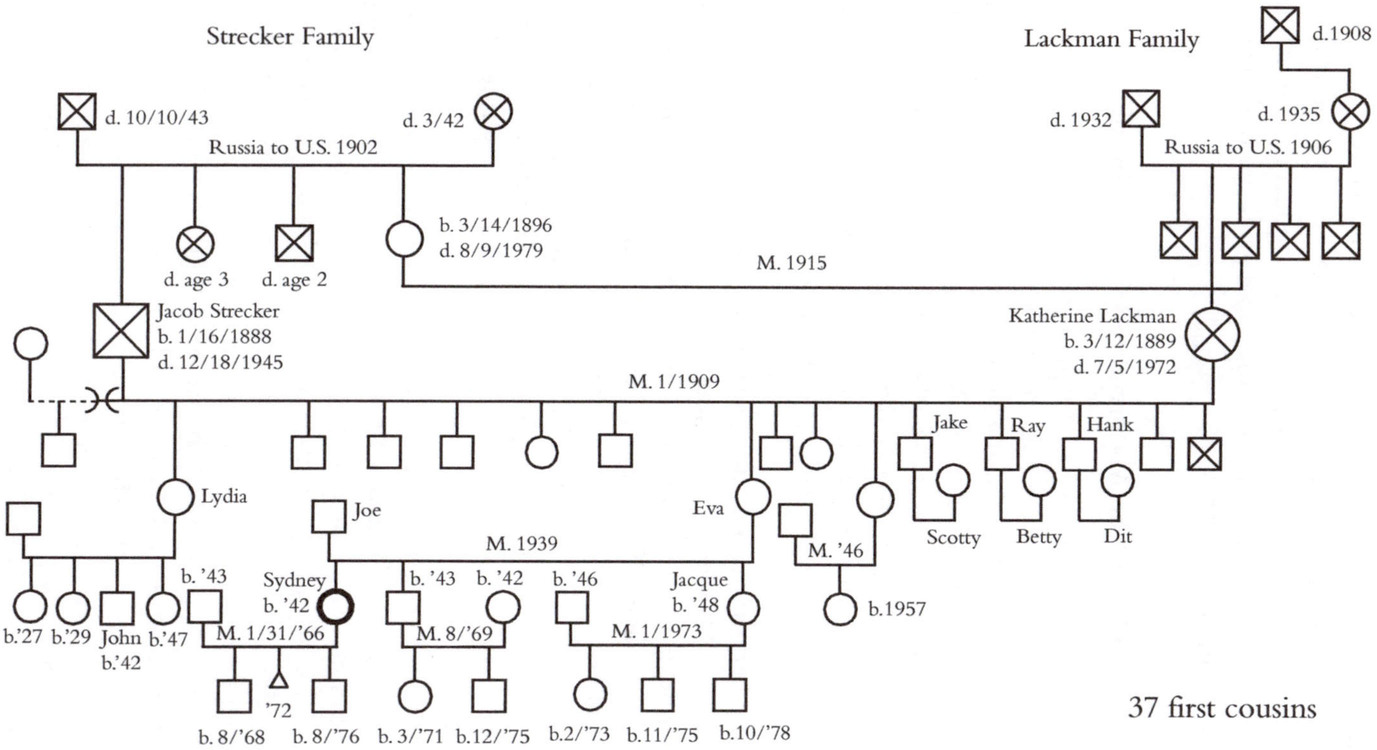

Figure 5.1 Strecker family diagram

encounter occurred before we were married, on a trip to Montana to introduce him to my family. Although my husband-to-be handled himself quite well and remained nonreactive in this confrontation, I was very upset and dismayed by the "testing" and unwelcoming behavior of these uncles. Later experiences with my mother's brothers and my male cousins indicated that "teasing put-downs" were a way the male members of the family often related to each other. However, the memories of 1964 were the ones I had in mind as I faced the prospect of seeing my Uncle Jake. Picking my uncle up from his work, I was surprised by his warm greeting, "You look great. So happy you are having supper with us." I was greatly surprised and relieved. This uncle had always teased me about being "too skinny" and unattractive. There is something profound that happens when the brain can be "rewired" in the actual relationship where the initial neuronal connections were established. Some significant impact on body image occurred in me that day, changes that, I believe, were more powerful and immediate than any changes that could have occurred talking with a therapist about the situation. This speaks to the significance of being present in one-to-one relationships in one's extended family. Six years later at a family reunion this uncle had warm greetings for me and my husband, mixed, of course, with the predicable teasing.

Visiting with Jake's wife, Scotty, earlier in the day, I gathered information that provided a clearer understanding of the triangles and the anxiety in my extended family. Jake, his wife, and two children had lived with his mother, my grandmother, for many years before her death. The large extended family had expressed great appreciation for the fact that Jake and his wife were living with and caring for Grandma Strecker as she aged. Scotty presented a different and somewhat alarming version of the situation. She described being so distressed by the abusive treatment she felt she received from her mother-in-law that she had considered taking her children into her car and driving off the rim rock cliffs that surrounded the city of Billings where they lived. Clearly shocked by this information, I remember this conversation and the circumstances of the luncheon vividly to this day. This represented a side of my grandmother I had never seen or heard of. The story also gave me some sense of the anxiety in the family system with which my mother was in regular contact. What was it like for my mother, the only daughter of her mother living in the area, to manage all of the triangles with her brothers' wives and their mother-in-law? Now I had more information by which to understand the level of anxiety in this family system and new questions to ask my mother. I also had a growing appreciation for my mother's ability to handle these relationships as well as she did. When I asked my mother about the situation at my grandmother's house, she dismissed it as not significant.

The second family I visited was totally different. My mother's brother was working in the fields so I had time alone with my aunt, Betty. However, my aunt was in such pain from a headache that talking was difficult for her. I was confused about how to proceed, finally offering to give my aunt a back and neck massage. This was appreciated by my aunt, but did little to relieve her pain. When my cousins came home from school, my aunt suggested I put on rubber boots and accompany them to the barn yard where I could help them curry and clean their steers for the 4-H fair that was happening the next day. As I timidly brushed the hides of these huge animals that were much bigger than I was, I wondered with amusement if this is what family-of-origin work was about, wading through "cow manure." (Later in my family work, I decided that this experience was, in fact, not atypical of what was required to connect with family. Often the "manure" is more symbolic than it had been on that day.) Over dinner I asked many questions about the family in which my mother had grown up. However, my efforts to learn more about the time of my uncle's and mother's childhood failed. Respectful of my uncle's refusal to talk about his family, eventually, I was able to get the names of the horses and the dogs they had on the farm as he was growing up, the total sum of new information. In later years, more information about the emotional system of the Strecker family helped me understand his reluctance to talk about his family.

The third uncle and aunt I knew somewhat better and have no memory of a significant conversation with them. They lived one block from my paternal grandfather's home and encouraged me to spend time with the Zeiler family who were gathering there to mourn the death of my paternal grandmother, who had died the morning I arrived.

I believe that creating these new and renewed relationships with my mother's brothers' families served to loosen the emotional fusion (emotional overconnectedness) between myself and my mother. In addition, I gained some understanding of the issues with which my mother was dealing; factual information that helped me understand the source of some of the anxiety I experienced coming from my mother. I was somewhat more objective in our phone conversations to comments that in the past would have made me very anxious.

The Strecker Family Emotional System

In 1978 when I was attempting to reconnect with my extended family, I wrote a letter and sent it to my 13 aunts and uncles asking for information about my maternal grandfather who had died when I was three. Most of the aunts and uncles responded. Interestingly, the responses were split between those who had fairly positive things to say about him (he was musical and liked to read) and those who were very negative (he was angry, abusive, and drank too much). The range of differences in the descriptions of their father undoubtedly represented the variation in their experiences, their memories, and the choice of how to describe their father to their niece. I suspected that all of the responses represented part of the truth about who he was. This notion was later confirmed by my mother's more comprehensive view of her father.

Understanding My Father's Individual Behavior in the Context of His Whole Family

On the same day as my arrival for the visits I described earlier in 1975, my paternal grandmother, Grandma Zeiler, died unexpectedly of a sudden heart attack. In between visits to my maternal relatives, I was able to be "present and accounted for" at my paternal grandparents' home as local representatives of my large extended family that included 16 aunts and uncles and 27 cousins gathered together to console and support each other and my grandfather. Careful observation of the emotional process and the resulting relationship patterns at this time of heightened anxiety provided invaluable information about the functioning of this side of my extended family (Figure 5.2). The predictable openness of some relatives at the occasion of a death in the family led to more authentic connections, as once again, childhood assumptions were modified with new information, including

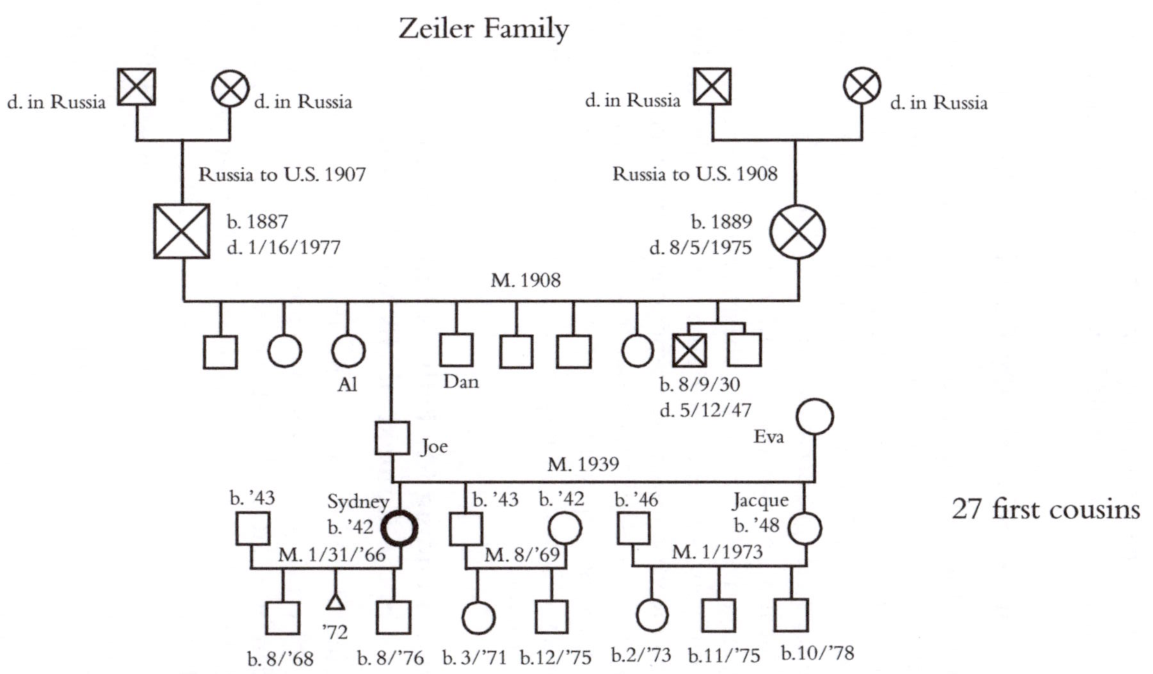

Figure 5.2 Zeiler family diagram

my new assessment of my father. I happened to be present as the six sons carried the coffin to the back of the church. As the lid to the coffin was being sealed, my father was the only son who showed outward, though constrained, signs of emotion. Having viewed my father as a distant and an emotionally inhibited person, seeing him in the company of his even more stoic brothers caused me to reassess my perception of him.

Additionally, a conversation with an aunt, who I considered very judgmental of me, helped me to get a broader view of the critical nature of my father and a better understanding of the family in which he had grown up. The aunt, a mother of three sons, confided while we were washing the dishes after a family gathering in the days before the funeral that she had always thought if she had had a daughter she'd hope she would have been just like me. I was shocked, surprised, and touched by this statement, which was the opposite of what I had always assumed. This positive and loving encounter with my aunt gave me a broader understanding of the importance of seeing the individual in the context of the whole family. My father and my aunt had grown up in a family that was very critical and judgmental. Being present and accounted for had provided opportunities for me to learn the facts by observing the functioning of myself and my family. Emotional patterns revealed in the multigenerational process, the reactivity in the triangles, and the various use of coping mechanisms, once observed in the family, can often be operating in self as well. This experience helped me to be more aware of how critical I can be and how useful this awareness can be in relationships.

The fact that I was present for the funeral of my father's mother provided an opening for a less distant relationship with him. In the triangle with my mother, she and I would have been on the close inside positions with my father on the outside. He was hard working and involved in running his own business. My mother was the active parent, sometimes conveying the message of what she said my father thought about things. Growing up, I never felt I had a personal relationship with him. As I began my family work, I focused on getting a one-to-one relationship with each parent. This effort continued to reshape the triangle that had been opened up by my presence at my father's mother's funeral.

Emotional Process at a Time of Death

By 1975 I had a better understanding of the importance of observing the emotional process in the family as a way to gather knowledge about my own and my family's functioning, and possibly to learn about coping mechanisms that are universal in all families at a time of loss and grief. In my father's family, his brother, Dan, who was thought to be the most distant from his parents, announced that he wanted to buy all the flowers that would be in the church for the funeral. The other eight siblings told him that his idea was ridiculous, and they all wanted to contribute to the flowers. This incident became the topic of conversation over a period of days, a way of triangling that bound the anxiety of the individuals, providing a sense of closeness to those on the togetherness leg of the triangle while the uncle was on the outside. The focus on this uncle may have relieved others from their own feelings of guilt and loss regarding the sudden death of their mother. Regretting one's failure to have done more in a relationship is common after a sudden death. These personal grief reactions quickly become entangled with relationship issues in the family system. Knowledge of triangles is useful when one attempts to disentangle from the emotional process in the family and acknowledge one's own response to the loss. One can then take responsibility for that feeling and determine how best to manage the feeling—what actions seems appropriate to represent one's own feelings without the need to focus on another's feelings.

I was interested in watching my grandfather in the days following his wife's death. There were no signs of overt grief and sadness as I had expected. Instead, he continued to move through his day in a somewhat orderly manner. I noted my surprise when I saw him put "green stamps" into a booklet. "Well," I thought, "I guess one needs to keep on living and doing what needs to be done." Similarly, when my father did not come to his father's home immediately, but rather worked in his business during the day and came with my mother after work, I began to understand the necessity of continuing the tasks that are demanded in one's own life while finding a way to be as present as possible to the rest of the family. Looking back on the occasion, I would have been surprised if my father had not brought German sausages from his meat market to share with the family as they gathered for meals, as this was frequently the way he made contributions to the family indicating his presence. These well-loved sausages were a reminder of their German heritage and a favorite dish at almost every family gathering on both sides of my family. Through careful observation I got a broad view of the multiple ways individuals express their grief and function at a time of death.

The most significant experience occurred at the funeral itself. As the family gathered to follow my grandfather and the casket down the aisle of the church, I was one of over 200 descendants of my grandparents. This experience was profound for me, a combined emotional and intellectual realization of my family. Having grown up as part of two large extended families, 10 siblings in the Zeiler family of my father and 14 siblings in the Strecker family of my mother, I remembered fun and festive holiday gatherings at my grandparents' homes with large numbers of aunts, uncles, and cousins in attendance. The importance of extended family relationships at a time of death was clearly demonstrated by the supportive actions of family members toward my grandfather and toward each other. This made a significant impression on me.

The Shock Wave of 1972, Finally Understood in 1975

After the funeral events, my parents and I made a long-planned trip to Yellowstone Park to visit my mother's brother, Hank, and his wife, Dit, who lived there. The recent death of my father's mother seemed to activate memories in my mother and uncle of the 1972 death of my maternal grandmother. Still upset after three years, they were tearfully recounting the conflict that had occurred in their family at that time. The surviving 14 adult children argued over the terms of the traditional German will that left all the property to the nine sons. Some of the sons felt that they were entitled to the money, as they had worked the hardest on the farm growing up. Others felt that the money should be shared equally with their five sisters.

Sitting with my parents and my aunt and uncle in Yellowstone Park was the first time I had heard this story. It was then I was able to understand the shame and disappointment that my mother had experienced at the time of my grandmother's death. My mother had always described the relationship among her siblings as very close, and I believe she had been reluctant to share this information. Conflict over a will is not unusual at a time of death. It both represents the emergence of long-standing issues in the family and a way that grief can be covered over. The hidden triangles, now made clear, composed of my mother, her siblings, and her parents, helped explain the emotional shock wave that had occurred in my family, my sister, and me. The anxiety had been transmitted to me and my sister without any factual information that might have allowed me to gain some perspective and helped me manage my own reactivity in a more thoughtful manner. Recent conversations with my sister revealed her knowledge of the conflict at the time and the distress it caused my mother. She never shared this information with me, as the system was quite closed at the time related to the secrets and the geographic distance of the family members. This conflict and my mother's grief contributed to the shock wave.

Historical Context

Shock waves can be better understood by studying the historical context of the family as well as its current situation at the time the shock wave begins. Looking at the multigenerational transmission process provides information about the historic themes, events, and relationships that might generate reactivity. Both of my maternal great-grandparents, the Streckers, were born in Russia, descendants of German immigrants who had settled in the Volga River Valley about 1788. The Streckers had four children, two of whom died at ages three and four. I speculated that the death of two younger siblings might have intensified the relationship of my great-grandparents with my grandfather, who was the oldest child. The Strecker family arrived in the United States in 1902 when my grandfather was 14. Their move was prompted by the changing political situation in Russia. The "Volga" Germans were no longer guaranteed freedom of religion, freedom from conscription, and freedom of language and tradition.

The Family Secret

Eleven years into my family research in 1986, the daughter of my mother's oldest sister was visiting Chicago for a conference. Over dinner, she asked me if I was aware of the family secret. The cousin told me that at some point around when our grandfather was 19 or 20 years old, our grandfather's girlfriend, who was not my grandmother, had become pregnant. The story goes that he had wanted to marry his girlfriend and take care of this child but his parents would not give him permission to do so. Instead, they wanted him to marry the daughter of their best friends from Russia, the Lackmans. The Streckers had sponsored the Lackman family to come to the United States. They arrived in 1906. My grandparents, Jacob Strecker, 20, and Katherine Lackman, 19, were married in January 1909.

Multiple stressors surrounded this marriage: It took place one month after the death of Katherine's maternal grandfather in December 1908 and three years after the Lackman family had arrived in the United States, having been sponsored by the Strecker family. The earlier unwed pregnancy of my grandfather's girlfriend and his parents' refusal to give permission for him to marry must have been a source of great stress. These multiple stressors may have set the course for an out-of-control emotionally conflictual union that produced 15 children. All but the last child survived into adulthood. The fusion of my grandfather and his parents is further suggested by the joint living arrangement on the farm of the new family, Jacob and Katherine, with his parents. It was reported by my mother that my Great-Grandmother Strecker asserted very tight control over the joint household, usurping much of her daughter-in-law's authority, even choosing the names of the first six children. My mother was number seven and claimed to be the first child that her mother was able to name. The timing of the early death of my grandfather in 1945 at age 57, within three years of his mother's death in 1942, and within two years of his father's death in 1943, is additional evidence suggestive of a high degree of interdependency in that primary triangle. The cause of his death was said to be gout. The lack of differentiation or the inability for my grandfather to be his own person with his parents, I believe, resulted in an angry, abusive parenting style toward his sons, overuse of alcohol, and a suspicious and domineering relationship with his wife, my Grandmother Strecker. All these behaviors are understood to have been supported by the adaptive nature of my grandmother, as she was frequently in the position of giving up self. The children even in later adulthood did not have a systems view of the relationship. They considered the father to be a demon and the mother to be a saint. In fact, upon the death of her husband, the mother was said to have blossomed, traveling alone by airplane to visit children who lived out of state, adopting a more cheerful attitude, and becoming more self-reliant.

Clarifying One's Own Beliefs and Values

Participating in the family nodal event of my paternal grandmother's funeral and reconnecting as an adult with family members on both sides of my extended family reinforced my thinking about the validity of the family values with which I had grown up. This experience provided a firm conviction for my transformative I-position. I had wanted a second child for several years but "could not talk my husband into it." The experience of the visit and the reality of being one of 200 relatives who followed the coffin down the aisle of the church helped me formulate an I- position in October 1975 in the airplane on my way to a Georgetown Family Center conference. Other shifts in triangles with my mother and father undoubtedly contributed to the increased clarity of my position. Upon returning home from the conference, I told my husband of my plan to have a second child, suggesting it would be most convenient if he would agree to be the father. Ten months later a second son was born, eight years after the first son.

Pregnancy as a Symptom of Anxiety in the Emotional Shock Wave

It is of interest to examine the symptoms of pregnancy in the light of the shock wave and multigenerational transmission process alluded to earlier. Victoria Harrison (2015, p. 201) has written that "the regulation of human ovulation reflects the counterbalance of reactivity to relationships and the ability to function as a somewhat independent organism." She suggests that "reactivity to relationships becomes the predominant influence over ovulation and mediates the impact of the natural environment over reproduction." The pregnancies of my sister and myself, mentioned earlier, all occurred at a time of early adulthood when individuals were struggling with the ability to function somewhat independently in the context of the intensity of family relationships.

Years later I was examining a family photo of the Strecker family, which I determined had to have been taken at the time of my great-grandmother's death in 1942. I identified myself as the infant in the photo by identifying older cousins and placing myself in the hierarchy. Unable to find any children of my oldest aunt, Lydia, I looked up the birth dates of her four children, my cousins. After a 16-year gap between her first two children, my aunt conceived a son, who was born nine months after the death of her grandmother. It's impossible to know whether that pregnancy was planned or not. However, the connection to the death of her grandmother seems a likely possibility.

Conclusion

From this experience I've reached the following conclusions: 1) an emotional shock wave after a death in the family can be disruptive to family relationships and to individual functioning; 2) knowledge of the possibility of an emotional shock wave can help individuals anticipate and manage the intense emotional process that can accompany a death; 3) staying in calm, respectful connection with family members after a death can lower the anxiety in self and in the system; 4) the opportunity to be "present and accounted for" provides a platform for managing self; and 5) defining self is more than thinking oneself into a position. Defining self involves integrating the lived experience in one's family with the objective knowledge of the family, of who one is, and of who one wants to be.

REFERENCES

Bowen, M. (1978). *Family therapy in clinical practice.* New York, NY: Jason Aronson.

Framo, J. L. (Ed). (1972). *Family interaction: A dialogue between family researchers and family therapists.* New York, NY: Springer.

Harrison, V. (2015). Emotional systems and the regulation of reproduction with ovulation as an illustration. In R. Noone & D. Papero (Eds.), *The family emotional system* (pp. 201–218). Lanham, MD: Lexington Books.

Reed, S. (1989). *Family reaction to death.* Interview of Dr. Bowen by Sydney Reed. Chicago: CFC Review Number 2.

6

A FATHER'S EARLY DEATH

A Family's Response

Kent E. Webb

Introduction

Bowen family systems theory views the human family as an emotional unit or system that developed through nature's evolutionary processes. When a family member dies, the loss of that individual will affect the functioning of each member and the family unit as a whole. Bowen defined "emotional shock wave" as:

> a network of underground "after-shocks" or serious life events that can occur anywhere in the extended family system in the months or years following serious emotional events in a family . . . It is not directly related to the usual grief or mourning reactions of people close to the one who died.
>
> (1978, p. 325)

The phenomena of emotional shock wave and after-shock, according to Bowen, account for the degree of emotional reactivity experienced by a family and the length of time needed to restore its equilibrium after one of its members leaves or when someone enters the family system.

My father's unexpected death in 1973 was followed by six significant life events. Nine months after my father died, in 1974, my mother married a man who was an abusive alcoholic; a man who, in short, was very unlike my father. My first wife had an affair in 1975, a second affair in 1981, and committed suicide two weeks prior to the finalization of our divorce in 1982. My brother's wife abandoned him and their two children in 1978, not to be heard from again for five years. In 1999, 26 years later, I acknowledged my homosexual orientation that led to a divorce from my second wife and the major disruption of my nuclear family. To say the obvious, these life events were not typical grief responses.

Throughout the chapter, the lens of Bowen theory and the phenomenon of the emotional shock wave followed by aftershocks and the related variables are utilized to account for two significant developments that occurred after the death of my father. The first development was the severe degree of emotional disturbance that erupted in the life of my mother, brother, and myself, and the second development was the fact it took over 40 years for all of us to reestablish emotional equilibrium.

The Earthquake: 8.0 on the Richter Scale

The phone was ringing at 6:00 a.m. on Monday, April 2, 1973, an ominous sign to the beginning of my day. Dr. Scarinzi, my hometown family doctor, was on the other end of the line. His message was brief and to the point, "I'm very sorry to tell you that your father died early this morning of a heart attack and you need to come home." After a few moments of silence, as I tried to absorb what he was telling me, I replied, "OK," and hung up the phone. I did not ask any questions and he did not provide any details. The entire conversation lasted less than a minute. I had just spoken to my father the night before about my parents' visit and plans for my upcoming college graduation the next month. I was 21 years old and my entire world, in the course of a minute, had changed forever. My father's death was a significant nodal occurrence in my life.

A major life goal and a dream of my father's was to have both his sons graduate from college. He viewed a college education as a sign of success, a way to have a better, easier, and more prosperous life. Fortunately, one of his goals was achieved: He was able to attend my brother's college graduation seven years earlier. Unfortunately, he wouldn't be attending mine. I was devastated he would not be present to see that dream fulfilled. My first wife's parents, my mother, and my brother were all present at our graduation. All of us tried to celebrate and enjoy the occasion, which signaled not only major accomplishments for my first wife and for me, but a dream of my father's being fulfilled. Even though we all wore a strong face, it was a sad celebration. The dreamer was absent.

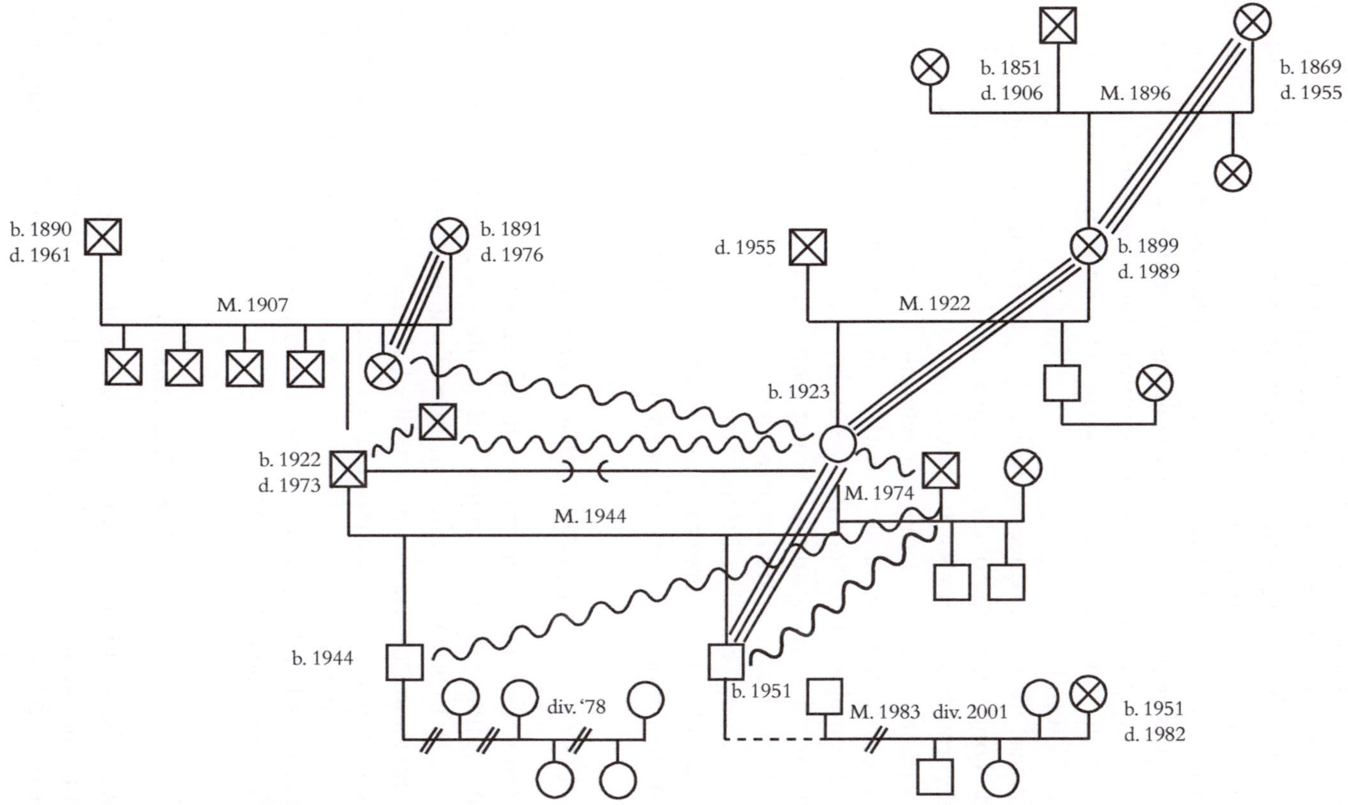

Figure 6.1 The Webb family diagram

In this chapter, Bowen theory and the phenomenon of anxiety are used to account for the degree of distress and disruption that occurred in my family of origin after the death of my father. To fully understand how such dysfunction could have occurred, I assessed my family of origin and extended family's multigenerational emotional process from the perspective of four variables associated with the emotional shock wave phenomena. I then examined this assessment through the lens of the interrelationship between differentiation of self and six other Bowen theory concepts.

Bowen identified three variables that are significant components underlying the notion of the emotional shock wave and its network of underground aftershocks. Bowen theory also identifies anxiety as an important variable affecting the response of a family to a significant life event such as my father's death. I therefore included anxiety as a fourth variable that affected my family's response to his death. The four variables are as follows: 1) the family level of differentiation of self, 2) the degree of anxiety experienced within the family system, 3) the functional emotional importance of the person who died to the family, and 4) the degree of denial in the family regarding its level of fusion/dependence between its members (1978, p. 325).

Variable 1: Differentiation of Self

Bowen believed that the manner in which a family and its members would function over the course of their life was determined, to a large degree, by their level of differentiation of self. In its most simple form, differentiation of self can be described as the degree to which one's functioning reflects their emotional maturity and self-sufficiency. In my assessment and in that of other Bowen coaches with whom I have worked, my family's level of differentiation was within the range of 35 to 40 on a scale of 0 to 100.

Variable 2: Anxiety

Bowen theory identifies two types of anxiety (acute and chronic) as significant variables that will influence a family's level of functioning over time. My father's death created acute anxiety for the family. The long-term, severe disruption in functioning experienced in the family following his death was generated by high degrees of chronic anxiety embedded within the multigenerational family relationship system.

Variable 3: Functional Importance of the Absent Family Member

The concepts of nuclear family emotional system and sibling position provide a perspective regarding my father having a higher degree of emotional importance within the nuclear family in which I grew up. As the nuclear family forms through marriage, the fusion created may be managed by one spouse becoming more emotionally dominant and the other more emotionally adaptive or submissive (Bowen, 1978, p. 473). In the marital fusion of my parents, my father was more emotionally dominant, whereas my mother was the more adaptive, functionally weaker spouse.

Bowen theory's sibling position concept, adapted from Toman (1969), states that the sibling position in which one grows up in the family of origin influences the development of particular personality characteristics and behaviors. My father was the fifth boy of seven children. A span of five years existed between him and the fourth son. My father was the oldest of the last group of three children and developed the personality traits of a functional older brother to a younger sister. This functional oldest position may have contributed to his characteristics of seriousness and caretaking, explaining why he was not competitive with my mother.

As the oldest sibling of a younger brother, my mother did not develop stereotypical dominant traits. According to Toman (1969), she may have realized her primary value to her parents was in taking care of, and protecting, her younger brother. My mother replicated the ways in which she engaged with her little brother with my father, my brother, me, and her second husband.

Variable 4: The Degree of Denial in the Family Regarding Its Level of Fusion/Dependence Between Its Members

My mother and father and their extended families were proud in their belief that they were emotionally strong and independent and had mottos such as, "Stand on your own two feet," "Pull yourself up,"

"Have a stiff upper lip," and "Be tough." To acknowledge a need for another was considered a weakness.

For two generations, nine nuclear families lived within 30 miles of one another. My family's functioning appears to be influenced by the emotional system to such a high degree that the family was blind to the amount of interdependency that it required in order for it to function reasonably. As a result of this emotional blind spot, the family automatically proceeded with its historical patterns of operation.

The Multigenerational Family Fault Line

The potent emotional forces within the extended family that created my multigenerational family fault line took many more generations to develop than the three generations I am describing. The forces that eventually created the fault line were generated by the interplay of the interrelated concepts of Bowen theory: differentiation of self, multigenerational transmission process, family projection process, triangles, nuclear family emotional system, sibling position, and emotional cutoff.

My parents owned and operated a small grocery store in Hugo, a small, rural town in Eastern Colorado with a population of 900. Overnight, at the age of 50, with her husband dead and her two sons married, the management of the store and their home became my mother's entire responsibility. In short order, she became emotionally and physically overwhelmed.

My mother grew up within a three-generation household that consisted of my great-grandmother, grandmother, grandfather, and my mother's younger brother. My great-grandmother became the family's matriarch and breadwinner after her husband, her first cousin, died. As a young widow, she moved her two young daughters by horse and buggy from Nebraska to Hugo in order to be close to her older brother and sister. As a schoolteacher, she taught in a one-room schoolhouse "out in the country" for many years.

My maternal grandfather, with only an eighth-grade education, had insufficient employment to support a wife and two children. As a result, my grandmother, not being too self-sufficient, turned to my great-grandmother for both emotional and financial support, and so they lived more of their lives together than apart.

My father's parents moved from Missouri to Eastern Colorado in 1910, to a homestead property just east of Karval, a very small country town near Hugo. In 1911, my paternal great-grandfather established a homestead one mile from my paternal grandfather. My great-grandfather's adult children moved to the Karval area, too. My paternal grandmother's younger sisters moved with her to Karval from Missouri. My father's parent's families were migrating together to this rural Colorado area.

My mother's and father's family systems had similar life principles and values. Both placed significant value on marriage, children, family, and hard work. Individuals in each family tended to marry at young ages, have two or three children, and did not divorce. Members of each family proudly identified as being part of a larger family clan.

The lower level of differentiation of self and the presence of higher degrees of chronic anxiety in my family system was characterized by the following: Life decisions and relationship interactions were driven more by feeling states than by intellectual principles; the need for togetherness, harmony, approval, and acceptance within relationships was high; individuality and action for one's self were less important than it was to act for the group; the degree of emotional interdependence was necessarily high in order for an individual to function with some degree of self; and each family member's pseudo self was significantly greater than their solid self.

The higher level of chronic anxiety was easy to observe on the maternal side of the family. For example, my grandmother expressed her worry externally and was considered by everyone who knew her to be a "worrier," and she often referred to herself as a "high strung." My father and his extended family appear to have managed their chronic anxiety through internal psychological and physiological processes, relationships, working, and smoking tobacco.

The lower basic level of differentiation of self of my parents was difficult to observe due to the seemingly adequate functional level of differentiation of self they demonstrated. By observation, the family functioned reasonably well, as determined by the fact my parents had been married for 27 years, owned and worked in a business together, and raised two children who completed college and married; there were no significant health, financial, or social problems; and reasonable emotional connection with their extended families existed.

The good functional level of differentiation of the family virtually melted away when my father, the more emotionally important one, was no longer present. The degree to which my mother, brother, and I borrowed self from my father was immediately apparent after his death and from the perspective of Bowen theory could be explained in the following way:

> The lower the level of differentiation or "basic self" in the spouses the more difficult it is to maintain reasonable emotional equilibrium and the more chronic the disability when adaptive mechanisms fail.
>
> (1978, p. 473)

The number of serious aftershocks, and the four decades it took for the family to sustain equilibrium after his death, illustrate my family's low level of differentiation of self.

The generational transfer of lower levels of differentiation on the maternal side of my family is easily observed beginning with the transfer occurring from my great-grandmother to my grandmother, then from her to my mother, and from my mother to me. The process just described is an example of the concepts of multigenerational transmission and the family projection process. The multigenerational transmission concept refers to how the undifferentiation of the family is passed along from one generation to the next via anxiety, emotional process, and the family projection process that occurs in the nuclear family (1978, p. 384).

The family projection process describes patterns in which the emotional immaturity of the parents is projected on to their children, usually one child more so than other children in the family. In my nuclear family, the projection process was of sufficient intensity that it appears to have involved both my brother and myself. It may be, however, that I received more of the projection process than he did. My father's emotional immaturity was projected to my brother, and my mother projected her emotional immaturity to me (Bowen, 1978, p. 477).

My maternal great-grandmother, who never remarried, shifted more of her attention to her oldest and more vulnerable daughter, my grandmother, and less attention to my grandmother's only younger sister. My grandmother became the more emotionally involved child in the nuclear family in which she grew up. My mother became the child more intensely involved in the parent–child triangle in her nuclear family and, subsequently, I was the more involved child in my family's child–parent triangle.

Triangles, according to Bowen (1978), exist in all families and form when the degree of tension or anxiety within a two-person system becomes too great and the more uncomfortable one will seek emotional comfort and support from a third person, or from a life situation, for example, work or an affair (Bowen, 1978, p. 373). The concept of nuclear family emotional system states that one way a nuclear family may manage too much fusion between the two spouses is to form a triangle that involves the children and parents.

The intense parent–child triangle pattern that developed in my mother's family of origin, and then replicated in mine, was a response to each husband emotionally pulling away, distancing from his wife who shifted attention that she would have directed at her husband to her child. From the concept of nuclear family emotional system, each husband's distancing behavior occurred because he was too uncomfortable with the degree of anxiety that developed from the intense marital fusion. According to Bowen theory, this degree of marital fusion and its associated elevated degrees of anxiety develop from the emotional lending and borrowing process, which occurs between each spouse for the purpose of forming a complete self. Similarly, my father's family of origin had a lower level of differentiation of self than that of my mother's family. However, in his family of origin, his only sister out of six boys became the focus of the parent–child triangle.

A Crack in the Family Fault Line

To me, there always seemed to be a noticeable degree of emotional distance and tension between my mother and my father's siblings and parents. The way my mother told the story, with its associated emotions, is that prior to their marriage my father left college during World War II to assist his father on the family farm. In exchange, his parents promised him that he would stand to inherit it when they retired or passed away.

After they married, my mother and father moved into a small house on his parents' homestead. They invested everything into this endeavor. At the time my brother was born, my father unexpectedly learned that his younger sister would be inheriting the farm instead of them. According to my mother, it was the only time she saw my father cry. It was a decision with which he went along. My mother believed that this blatant display of favoritism by his parents was unfair, even bordering on cruel. Of course, a triangle had been formed between my father, his sister, and their parents. My father found himself on the outside leg of the triangle by having lost his home and future farm to his sister. My father was resigned and my mother was angry.

In a very short time, my parents decided to buy a grocery store in Karval. Neither of them knew anything about the grocery business but they believed they could learn. Almost overnight, they found their way from farming to owning and operating a store.

Throughout my childhood and adolescence, my mother often seemed compelled to share confidential views and feelings with me that now seem wholly inappropriate. I heard her view about everyone in both her and my father's family, and in almost every instance she felt that she was the injured party. My father, on the other hand, simply did not talk about his emotions, and he certainly appeared to be less reactive to his family than my mother was. He was, however, reactive to the degree of closeness and influence my maternal grandmother had on my mother, on their marriage, and on me, but he did not do much to interfere with those relationships.

My mother's and my father's families began to emotionally disengage or cut off from each other after his death. It became clear that my father's family was not a resource for her. She did not ask for their assistance and they did not offer.

When my father died, my mother immediately began to worry that her mother would become more dependent and reliant upon her. It became clear that my mother's marriage to my father served as a way of establishing an emotional boundary to facilitate more separation between her and her mother. She was certain conflict would arise if she voiced these fears to my grandmother. Instead of confronting the situation directly, she passively modified behaviors to create the relational distance she desired.

The Bowen theory concept of emotional cutoff describes a way that people handle high degrees of emotional fusion within the generations. Families with lower levels of differentiation will be more likely to use the mechanism of cutting off from each other to reduce either internal or relational distress, or both (Kerr & Bowen, 1988, p. 171). My mother was cutting herself off emotionally from everyone—even me. I have realized that she would use the same emotional cutoff mechanism at age 50 that she used at age 20 to separate from my grandmother.

First Emotional After-Shock: 6.0 on the Richter Scale—January 3, 1974

On January 3, 1974, I received another unexpected call, this time from my mother. Out of nowhere, she announced that she had married the man she had met a few months earlier. This was truly a shock. There was no engagement, nothing to indicate that her relationship with him was anything other than a passing fling. According to my father's sister, her new husband was an abusive, controlling alcoholic. My father had died only nine months ago, and she was now married to a man I did not know and had never met. I did not know what to think, how to feel, or how to respond. I did not say anything to her. I just went along to get along.

The following months contained one rapid change after another. Her second husband decided that he did not want his wife to work so much and that he wanted my mother to sell her business and her home. To our shock and dismay, she quickly acquiesced and defended his every demand—because he was her husband. She was replicating, without rational thought, the automatic patterns of her emotional immaturity.

Clearly, she was demonstrating undifferentiation by creating a significant amount of fusion with a man for emotional stability that demonstrated her need for togetherness rather than trying to be a self-sufficient person. It appeared she was emotionally cutting off from her mother, my brother, and me to maintain the fusion with her new husband. Of course, I was not aware that these emotional processes were occurring; it just seemed like she was rejecting her life with my father and abandoning my brother and his family and me.

Second Emotional After-Shock: 5.0 on the Richter Scale—Fall of 1975

In the fall of 1975, after four years of marriage, my first wife told me that she was having an affair. I was scared, angry, and embarrassed. Feeling like a failure, I kept her affair a secret from everyone. Above everything, I knew that I did not want a divorce. With all of the chaos in my own nuclear family, it felt as though she and her parents were all I had left, and so I was desperate to keep that aspect of my life intact. I successfully talked her into continuing our marriage, which reflected my lower level of differentiation cloaked in insecurity and dependency.

Looking back, I believe part of my desperation to stay married was due to the absence of my mother and father from my life. Staying married helped me maintain the emotional fusion and togetherness I was trying to replicate from the emotional fusion and togetherness I had had with my parents.

From 1974 to 1978, I repeatedly asked my mother to visit us, but she always cited her second husband as the reason she would not be able to come. Even when my first wife and I received our master's degrees in the spring of 1978, she did not attend—because he needed her at home that week. Looking back, it's easy to infer that my mother had created a new triangle with her second husband. He had become the most important person in her life, and I had been replaced. All I knew was that my father would have attended my graduation. I was the first person in my extended family to obtain a master's degree. I was furious, hurt, and felt abandoned.

Third Emotional After-Shock: 4.0 Richter Scale—1978

In the spring of 1978, I received a phone call from my brother's wife. She informed me that she was running away and leaving Colorado with a man with whom she had been having an affair. She asked me to tell my brother because she was too afraid. She did not leave a note or a letter; she was just gone.

Out of concern for him and my nieces, I did call, and the conversation was surreal. Overnight, he became a single parent with two young girls. He desperately needed my mother's support and so did her granddaughters. My father would have driven to Denver in a second. My mother, on the other hand, did not offer help of any kind, emotional or physical, because her new life was entirely focused on the needs of her new husband. My mother's behavior again demonstrated her low level of differentiation through her emotional immaturity and her inability to be independent.

Fourth and Fifth Emotional After-Shocks: 6.5 and 7.5 on the Richter Scale—1981 and 1982

In the spring of 1981, my first wife announced that she had had another affair and wanted a divorce. Yet a month before the divorce was finalized, she requested to meet with me to ask that we reconsider and try to mend our marriage. I had anticipated the request, and in an effort to be more self-sufficient I was able to say no. A month passed, and one morning I received another ominous phone call—this time from my wife's parents. She had disappeared. She had stopped going to work and she was not answering her phone or responding to messages; therefore, I filed a missing person's report with the Denver police. A week later her body was discovered in the Rocky Mountains, an hour from Denver, at a spot well known to us both. Her legal cause of death was hypothermia. The coroner, however, hypothesized that hypothermia followed the use of alcohol and tranquilizers with the likely intent to die. In other words, suicide. Notes and letters found later indicated she was depressed and had had suicidal thoughts.

Her suicide, the fifth shock wave, was one that I never dreamed of, or even thought a possibility. I did not know how to make sense of it all. My identity was shattered. I had failed in my quest to be a typical heterosexual man and to become a parent. Her parents, with whom I had been very close, were devastated.

Efforts to Establish Family System Equilibrium

During these years, my brother, my mother, and I all utilized the forming of intense emotional relationships as a strategy to stabilize our lives. Marriage was automatically employed to regain footing in our lives. Our lower levels of differentiation continued as each of us made an effort to regroup and stabilize. Unfortunately, our functioning only deteriorated.

My Mother's Effort—A Marriage

My mother's marriage to her second husband was her effort to stabilize herself and her life. The two of them immediately formed a very intense fusion. Based on her previous actions of selling her business and her home, I believe she thought he would take care of her. She quickly learned that was not the case, and over time, she learned that he intended for her to take care of him. He was fired from his ranch foreman job just two years after their marriage and was never employed again. My mother, upon realizing he was dependent on her, chose, ironically, to open another store in Hugo, only selling clothes this time around. She both owned and operated the store for 20-odd years until she retired.

In her relationship with her second husband, the fusion manifested itself in him borrowing self from her. It was just the opposite pattern from her borrowing self from my father. Although she was the resourceful one, he maintained emotional dominance. In total, they were married for 40 years. I believe their high degree of fusion and the intense cycles of emotional closeness and distance they experienced allowed her to tolerate his alcoholism, his physical and emotional abuse of her, and his inability to help support them financially. He was very demanding of her attention and jealous of any amount of time spent with her children and grandchildren. Over the years, she continued to distance herself from her family to prevent disruption in the marital fusion. Her main concern was his happiness, and she was allergic to his disapproval of her.

In 2012, at the age of 85, she was medically hospitalized twice; the first time was due to extremely high blood pressure, and the second hospitalization occurred because of internal bleeding related to diverticulitis. When discharged, her physician, family, and friends pressured her to separate from him in order to be physically healthy. Reluctantly, she agreed, and with help and support from me, she obtained a permanent restraining order from the court to prevent him from living with her. Eventually, he was admitted to a specialized facility for residents with severe emotional and behavioral problems. He died in 2014 at age 84.

My mother at the age of 93 no longer takes medicines for hypertension, depression, or anxiety. She lived on her own for several years and now lives in an assisted living facility in Hugo. She acknowledges that her marriage to her second husband was a mistake and she should have divorced many years ago. She appears to have adjusted well to living without him.

My Brother's Effort—Marriages

My brother was divorced in 1978 and was remarried and divorced twice between 1979 and 1989. He did not marry again but had several unsustainable "live-in relationships." Eventually, he was "downsized" from a government managerial position after developing a significant alcohol and anger problem. His daughters married in late adolescence and did not complete high school. He eventually lost his home and spent his retirement savings. He survived an aortic aneurism in 2010. At 72 years of age, he works as a security guard, lives alone, and has limited contact with his children and grandchildren.

My Effort—Marriages, a Family, a Career, and a Little Individuality

I repeated my parents' pattern of utilizing a relationship to stabilize self. I intensely focused on the marriage to my first wife after my father died. I did take two independent steps and became more of a self when I decided to stay in Kansas rather than return to Colorado, and later when I made the decision to enter graduate school at the University of Kansas in 1976. After my wife's death in 1982, I had some emotional space to *think* as my mother focused on her marriage and my brother on his. I was not certain what to do next.

On the personal and emotional side of my life, however, I repeated a familiar pattern; I started a relationship with my second wife. We married in 1984, just 20 months after my first wife died. I needed to be married, to be a father, and to have a family. To me, this was equivalent to "The Holy Grail," a definite quest. My son was born in the fall of 1985. My daughter was born in 1988.

However, under the surface of all that activity and forward movement, I was avoiding, minimizing, and denying another aspect of self:

my homosexuality. I was aware of thoughts, feelings, and an attraction to men that I had rationalized, suppressed, and dismissed for decades. During this time, I found myself being increasingly anxious and angry. In August 1999, I met with a psychologist who specialized in working with gay men to discuss, for the first time, my belief that I might be gay.

I believe that as I studied Bowen theory, beginning in 1982, and applied it to my life, my homosexuality slowly came into better awareness due to the following: 1) my gaining more solid self, 2) having better awareness of my intellectual and emotional system, 3) working toward increased individuality, and 4) the fact that societal views were beginning to shift and become more accepting of homosexuality.

Sixth Emotional After-Shock: 8.5 on the Richter Scale—1999

Twenty-six years after my father passed away, in November 1999, I announced to the world that I was gay. I came out in my personal, professional, and public life, all at the same time. I consider this period of time to be the final emotional after-shock. To say the least, the entire process has taken an unfortunate and significant toll on my children and second wife. In many respects, I brought my nuclear and extended family out of the closet with me, and they had to deal with my homosexuality and its impact on them.

My low level of differentiation was more evident during this time than at any other time in my life. In my personal life, I was dealing with challenges associated with the loss of my marriage and my nuclear family as I had known it to be, a divorce, parenting as a divorced parent, financial and legal concerns, loss of identity as a heterosexual male, redefining myself, and living as a gay man. For several years, I was depressed, anxious, started smoking again, and misused alcohol. Not surprising, it was not long before I established a relationship, this time with a gay man. He and I have been life partners for 16 years.

It took approximately five years after coming out for me to reestablish a degree of equilibrium in my life. It has been humbling to learn the following: 1) that I have a relatively low basic level of differentiation of self, 2) that I have higher degrees of pseudo self than solid self,

3) that my functional level of differentiation of self is greater than I realized, and 4) that I, too, use relationships to establish my emotional stability.

Of course, time will tell, but I wonder about the future and how, with my lower level of differentiation of self, my decision to reveal my sexual orientation will affect the long-term functioning of my former wife and my two children. In my nuclear family, I was the person who created the earthquake and left.

Reflections

The emotional perturbation that developed within my family following my father's death was an illustration of how the emotional shock wave/after-shock phenomenon can play out in a family whose basic level of differentiation of self is low. The interrelated concepts of Bowen theory provided a comprehensive perspective that accounted for the dysfunction that occurred in my family for over 40 years.

Unbeknownst to the family was that each member had a high degree of need to achieve emotional security and stability, which would only come through a fused emotional relationship with another person. None of us realized that our emotional equilibrium could be restored, and our functioning resumed or improved, by working toward becoming a more defined, emotionally mature, independent self.

REFERENCES

Bowen, M. (1978). *Family therapy in clinical practice.* New York, NY: Jason Aronson.

Kerr, M., & Bowen, M. (1988). *Family evaluation: An approach based on Bowen theory.* New York, NY: W. W. Norton.

Toman, W. (1969). *Family constellation.* New York, NY: Springer.

7

MOM'S COMMITTED SUICIDE

Now What?

Anthony J. Wilgus

In speaking about death, Dr. Murray Bowen wrote: "Death is a biological event that terminates a life. No life event can stir more emotionally directed thinking in the individual and more emotional reactiveness in those about him" (Bowen, 1978, pp. 321–322). The suicide of a family member poses its own unique challenges both in the short run and in the long run. Generally sudden in timing, a host of issues ensue, including decisions on how to disclose the circumstances and whom to inform, how to manage oneself in the midst of the potentially intense reactivity of family and friends, whether or not to have a funeral, and how to negotiate the funeral home industry and the religious institution. Then, there is the anticipatory aftermath, as the novelist Hanya Yanagihara details in the words of an adoptive father of a son who eventually took his life:

> [I]f he killed himself, if he took himself away from me, I knew I would survive, but I knew as well that survival would be a chore; I knew that forever after I would be hunting for explanations, sifting through the past to examine my mistakes. And of course I knew how badly I would miss him, because although there had been trial runs for his departure, I had never been able to get any better at dealing with them, and I was never able to get used to them.
>
> (Yanagihara, 2015, p. 708)

How, then, can a person find a way through the obstacles presented by the untimely suicide of a family member?

Bowen theory can provide an opportunity for a little less emotionally directed thinking in this cauldron of anxiety. This chapter will describe the efforts of the son-in-law and his wife to incorporate a knowledge of the theory in the wake of the suicide of his mother-in-law and his wife's mother. Endeavoring to be a little more thoughtful and observant in the midst of this maelstrom, he hoped to contribute to a little more clarity and planning in the numerous pragmatic decisions that demanded attention. Drawing from Dr. Bowen's chapter, "Family Reaction to Death," the author will initially discuss the communication systems within the family member who took her life, within the larger family and friendship network, and within the religious institution and the funeral home industry (Bowen, 1978). The body of the presentation will highlight the implementation of theory as concepts take on the forms of key attitudinal shifts that translate into slightly more thoughtful behaviors in a predictably anxious relationship system. In conclusion, the author will mention some caveats relative to theory comprehension and application while underscoring the value of a framework for monitoring self in the immediate and the longer-term chaos of the sequelae of suicide.

Cast of Characters

Mrs. A, a 68-year-old woman attempting to rebalance her life after the demise of her 45-year-long marriage and the immediate remarriage of her former spouse, Mr. A, to a former high school friend, overdosed on a bottle of sleeping pills not quite two years after the announcement of the marital separation (see Figure 7.1). She had a daughter, Mrs. B, married to a man, Mr. B, familiar with Bowen theory, and a son, Mr. C, who lived with his family in the East. Her 95-year-old mother, Mrs. D, was still alive at the time of Mrs. A's death, living in the southern part of the United States. The eldest sister of three brothers, Mrs. A maintained contact with them until the time of her death. Additionally, she had four grandchildren, ages 9 through 21, and a step-grandson. Active in her community and her church, Mrs. A had a large network of friends and associates in the immediate geographic locale. Subsequent to Mrs. A's suicide in the fall of 2007, the bulk of the decision making fell to her daughter, son-in-law, and her son, with the daughter determining a good bit of the direction of the funeral

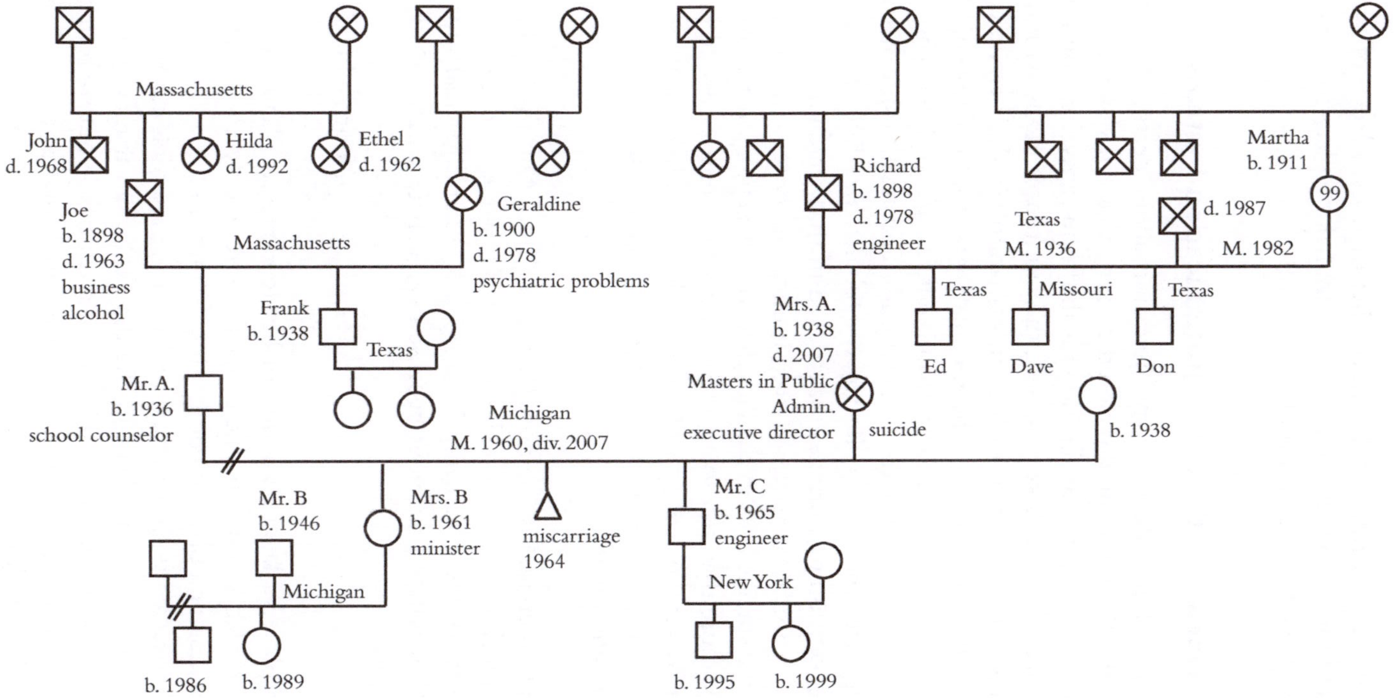

Figure 7.1 Mrs. A's family diagram

process. In that period, Mrs. B utilized her own knowledge of Bowen theory and the knowledge of her spouse in making plans for what was to occur in the wake of her mother's suicide.

Open and Closed Communication Systems

Noting the taboo nature of any discussion about death, Dr. Bowen outlined the three potentially closed communication systems operating around the terminally ill individual: the intrapsychic communications that the patient kept to self, the communications within the family and their tendency to hear information via their anxiety, and the communications within the medical system itself (Bowen, 1978, pp. 322–323). Secrecy can be a prominent feature in those who contemplate suicide and for the larger family and relationship network following that event (Cerel, Jordan, & Duberstein, 2008). This family was no exception to a process that moved in that direction.

Evidence for a more closed communication system in the family prior to the suicide rests in the fact that Mrs. A kept a journal over the course of more than ten years, with many of the entries occurring in the last two years of her life. Her own reflections offer a glimpse into how she managed her own thinking in isolation during the marital separation and divorce:

> People keep asking me how I am. I say 'fine.' And that makes them feel better, and it makes me sound stronger, and it makes me sound like something I am not . . . I can't get real support for where I am now, because I can't share where I really am now.
>
> (Journal 2007)

She displayed a keen awareness of her tendency to "shut down" in important relationships, unable to speak more openly about her sense of desperation and plans to end her life. In fact, on the morning of her suicide, she talked with her daughter by phone, not yielding an inkling of what would transpire later in the day (although it may have been more impulsive on her part). Her inability to talk about such matters may also reflect the reactivity of family and friends, as Dr. Bowen noted in his own discussions about death with suicidal patients: "They were eager to talk to an unbiased listener who did not have to correct their way of thinking" (Bowen, 1978, p. 323). This pattern of isolating self at the end of life was reflective of the closed communication systems within her own relationships with her husband, parents, siblings, and children over many years.

The daughter's initial discovery of her mother's death and the police report that the death was a suicide launched the family in a direction vulnerable to the more closed communication process that Dr. Bowen described. A myriad of difficult questions emerged for the daughter because she was the family member in the nearest vicinity to her mother's home community. She found herself pondering a variety of specific and time-sensitive matters. Who was going to be the person to identify Mrs. A's body, now in the morgue? Of the multiple family members, whom would she tell about the coroner's report, including her father and his new wife, her daughter and her son, her mother's mother and three brothers and their families, her brother and his family and the larger family and friendship network?

Then, there was the matter of whether or not to have any type of funeral service, complicated by the mother's requests long before her death that she did not want a funeral. If the daughter chose to have a service, then what form would that take? For instance, would there be a visitation at a funeral home? If so, would the casket be open or closed, or would the casket even be present? Should cremation occur even prior to a service? If there was a service, should it be simply at the funeral home or at a church or some other venue? If a religious ritual were to occur, there were questions about who would participate in the service, who would officiate at the service, the potential venue, and the degree of openness or closedness of this type of memorial.

Bowen Theory and Moving Toward an Open Communication System

Having a way of thinking that transcends cause-and-effect thinking, that goes beyond diagnosis and blame, and that focuses upon observation and management of self translates into a way of being that is clear and even precise. Upon hearing of her mother's death and the surrounding details that included a suicide note to her and her brother, the daughter simply KNEW that she would be the person to identify her mother's body in the morgue. Despite his professional responsibilities, the husband KNEW that he would accompany his wife, not knowing what they might encounter because the body was found almost 15 hours after the actual time of death. As distressing as it was for the daughter to witness this part of the death experience, she took comfort in coming face to face with the reality of what had occurred. No other family member requested to do likewise.

In the two-hour drive to her mother's hometown, the daughter and her husband not only learned from the medical examiner the cause of Mrs. A's death, but also discussed just how they wanted to handle this fact with the rest of the family. Historically, Mrs. A's family had managed some sensitive issues through secrecy, as manifested in her journals mentioned earlier in the chapter and the failure to disclose an adoption of a family member until that individual was in her mid-life years. The theme of this conversation was open disclosure, taking into account the sensitivity of time and place. For instance, the daughter did not disclose this information by phone with her brother, who was on route to the family home, wanting to wait until he and his family arrived. Shortly after this hospital visit to the morgue, the daughter's father and his new wife arrived at Mrs. A's home, where the daughter and her husband would remain for the week, unaware of the cause of death. The husband calmly conveyed the fact that Mrs. A, his former spouse, had taken her own life through an overdose of sleeping pills. When Mr. A questioned the accuracy of this information, the son-in-law told him about the report from the medical examiner and the finding of a suicide note near her body.

Waiting until her brother's family arrived, Mrs. A's daughter spoke to him in a private conversation, away from his wife and children, and sharing the information that she had garnered, including the contents of the suicide note, which had been addressed to both of them. The daughter found no need to disclose the specifics of the message, although she did indicate to others that a note had been found. Inasmuch as the brother's two children were ages 12 and 8 at the time, he made the decision to withhold the fact that their grandmother had committed suicide. Respecting her brother's wishes, she took a different route with her son and daughter, ages 21 and 18. As challenging as it was to discuss this emotionally laden situation, the daughter took each of her children aside, talking with them in a person-to-person manner. Both children had been quite close to their grandmother and their reactivity was high, but their mother was undeterred in the delivery of the facts of the death. Her daughter wept; her son stated that he was somewhat afraid that his grandmother's death was indeed a suicide, given her recent struggles.

Having had time to begin to absorb the nature of Mrs. A's death, her daughter and spouse discussed the merits of having a funeral service and the particulars associated with that. The husband drew upon his own experience with death and the writings of Bowen on this nodal event in a family. Although some funerals can actually deny death and contribute to a shutting down of the communication system within the family, Bowen offered a road to greater openness:

> I encourage involvement of the largest possible group of extended family members, an open casket, and the most personal contact that is possible between the dead and the living, prompt obituary notices, and the notification of relatives and friends, a public funeral with the body present, and the most personal funeral service that is possible.
>
> (Bowen, 1978, p. 332)

Despite the fact of Mrs. A's suicide and her wishes to have no funeral, along with the history of closed caskets in her family, the daughter's spouse stated his thinking on the importance of the funeral ritual, even going so far as to have the body displayed during calling hours. They agreed on having a religious service in addition to a visitation, out of respect for Mrs. A's faith tradition. The daughter, a cleric herself, knew of a thoughtful minister who could handle openly and sensitively a religious service that would honor the legacy of the dead woman while acknowledging the abrupt termination of her life. While the husband tried to simply state his position on these matters, his wife would later recall that he was somewhat "pushy" about the importance of the open casket. After some reflection, she assented, conveying her thinking to her brother upon his arrival from out of town the next day, and plans unfolded. Meanwhile, the daughter contacted each of Mrs. A's brothers, speaking openly about the suicide of their sister, whereupon they made plans to attend the funeral.

The Funeral Home and Communication Systems

Funeral directors are people, too, complete with their own set of emotional baggage and particular sensitivities. Again, having a way of thinking about death and funerals from a Bowen theory framework affords a path through the obstacles that will inevitably arise, sometimes from the most unexpected places. Although funeral homes are essentially service industries, the directors will vary in their own degrees of openness when it comes to the suicide of a community member. The daughter and her husband, together with the brother, arranged a meeting with the local funeral home in order to make plans for the calling hours and the funeral service. Again, they articulated their desires for visitation, an open casket, the obituary, and the religious ritual.

In short order, the young funeral director expressed his opposition to having an open casket in this situation, raising concerns about the state of the body and the unusual nature of the request under these circumstances. His reactivity was obvious. The daughter's husband remained firm in the desire for an open casket whereupon the director grudgingly agreed to do so but not without asking the daughter to purchase a dark-colored lipstick for her mother's corpse. The manner of the opposition, more than the actual logistics of the preparation of the body, was noteworthy here. Had the daughter and her husband been diffident or unclear about their stances, a different outcome would have occurred.

Next, the three family members received instructions on the preparation of the obituary. Much of the information focused appropriately on the history of Mrs. A's life, accomplishments, survivors, and affiliations. Again, the husband noted that there was no mention of Mrs. A's 45-year marriage and her former spouse. He brought this up in the meeting with the daughter and the son. They agreed to have some kind of mention of their father in the obituary. The funeral director proclaimed that it was not appropriate to include the name of former spouses in an obituary whereupon the family adamantly maintained their position. Later, Mrs. A's former spouse would note that he appreciated the fact that their marriage had been acknowledged in the obituary despite the recent divorce and his remarriage.

While the obituary stated that Mrs. A had "died unexpectedly," her daughter made every effort in her conversations with the myriad of family and friends who paid their respects at the funeral home to inform them of Mrs. A's suicide. Not surprisingly, a significant percentage of that network, although stunned by the timing, expressed the fact that they had indeed suspected as much. This openness of information permitted that network to extend condolences in a more nuanced manner, aware of the different circumstances of this death. In these communiqués, people were thoughtful and sensitive with the daughter and her family.

Upon the arrival of Mrs. A's three brothers from various parts of the country, there was an extended discussion of how and what to disclose to Mrs. A's mother relative to her daughter's death. The eldest son voiced concerns about what this information might do to their 95-year-old mother. Believing in thoughtful, direct, and compassionate communication, the daughter's husband gently staked his position in the midst of the three brothers and some members of their family. He then queried of the oldest brother: "If something similar had happened to one of your own children, how would you want the family to handle that with you?" This gave the brother some pause, although he never directly addressed the fact of his sister's suicide with their mother. Interestingly, several years later Mrs. A's mother asked her daughter about the nature of the death. The daughter gave her the facts. While she had a hunch that this was what had happened, she conveyed her anger and upset that her children did not come clean with her.

Perhaps due to the candor of the daughter and her husband, there was an outpouring of extended family presence and support, both leading up to the funeral and the gathering of the clan after the religious service. Prior to these events, Mrs. A's daughter-in-law's siblings arrived from all over the country, assisting in the extensive preparations for feeding people and providing activities for two grandchildren, ages 12 and 8. Their quiet efficiency and generosity alleviated the burden of these logistics dramatically. Additionally, the son-in-law's siblings and two of his daughters played instrumental roles in preparing the house for the overflow of guests and in ensuring that the chapel was appropriately decorated for the service that was to occur. People rearranged their busy schedules, flying in from various parts of the country, providing sustenance and comfort for each other in ways beyond measure.

Religious Service

In concert with her husband, Mrs. A's daughter saw the value of having a religious ritual. Mrs. A was the member of a small congregation for a good portion of her adult life; yet the place where church members gathered was far too small. The family secured a chapel in the community that would accommodate the relationship network, arranging for a minister who would structure the service. A friend of Mrs. A's daughter, this minister was familiar with the family and the circumstances of Mrs. A's death. What was noteworthy about her approach to planning the service was her desire to meet with the principal family members on a one-to-one basis. This permitted each family member to be as candid as they chose, filling in some of their own perceptions of the life and death of Mrs. A. These varying contributions from people who knew Mrs. A intimately resulted in a carefully crafted eulogy that highlighted the strengths and challenges of Mrs. A's life and the lessons that could be gleaned from that journey. There was little in the way of pathologizing Mrs. A and the manner in which her life ended.

In keeping with the personal nature of this service, the minister allowed for a brief period when the family and friends who so desired could come forward, saying some words of remembrance about the importance of that relationship. Two grandchildren, ages 12 and 8, stepped up to the front of the church, taking the opportunity to eulogize their grandmother in a poignant yet not maudlin fashion. They did this without the knowledge of their own parents whose reactivity might have deterred them from saying what they needed to say. The daughter's husband was one of the last to offer a few remarks, noting that he was one of those fortunate and unusual individuals to have *two* mothers-in-law at the same time inasmuch as his dead wife's mother was still living. In the midst of the grieving, there was laughter as he spoke to how she welcomed him into the family, despite not quite understanding some of his theory-inspired behaviors, such as arranging a meeting with his new wife's former spouse. Again, there were tributes to the accomplishments of Mrs. A's life along with the immense sadness at her far-too-abrupt departure from this earth.

In another indication of the openness of this process, Mrs. A's former husband of 45 years attended the funeral service with his new wife. Although there was a good deal of emotionality among various family members toward him and his spouse, he was welcomed both at the service and in the subsequent family gathering at the home. The daughter would later exclaim about her own behavior, "Nobody screamed at anyone and no one went to jail." Under certain conditions, this can be quite a remarkable feat.

Guiding Principles Emanating From Bowen Theory: Theory Informs Action

Central to a "new way of being" in the midst of anxious times and anxious families is having a new way of thinking that diverges from some of the automatic responses present in our species. It would not be uncommon, for example, for cause-and-effect thinking to predominate under such circumstances manifest in some of the following views: The divorce *caused* Mrs. A to commit suicide; Mrs. A's former spouse is responsible for her death; Mrs. A had a mental illness worsened by the shift in her marriage. The outcome of these ways of thinking might easily contribute to secrecy, exclusion, and blame. Villains and victims would be identified, making a family vulnerable to fragmentation and alienation. A wider view of these human behaviors intrinsic to Bowen theory, however, would transcend notions of guilt, blame, and helplessness and offer a new way of being in the throes of a family grappling with the suicide of one of its members. Moving beyond the location of this problem in any one person or relationship to the view of multiple players over many generations doing the very best that they can with what resources they have at their disposal leads directly to a new way of being with this family.

Throughout this narrative, a series of principles follow from the core concept of differentiation of self. Attention to this cornerstone of the theory would frame the suicide of a family member as a unique opportunity to become a researcher of the human condition. The research perspective can temper the "fix-it" perspective in the social worker self of the husband. To listen without preaching and getting on the backs of others by telling them what they should or should not do while being certain about where oneself stands is no easy task. Even for the long-time student of Bowen theory, it is critical to check the urge to be the "expert" on death and family funerals and rituals.

Thus, differentiation of self not only entails a studied observation of the entire relationship network in the midst of high anxiety but also continually focusing upon oneself and one's own reactivity to what is happening in the family.

In the midst of the pandemonium accompanying a family member's suicide are the tendencies to remove oneself either physically or emotionally from the scene. Differentiation of self challenged the husband, who has knowledge of Bowen theory, and his wife to be as actively present and emotionally engaged with as many members of the extended family and friendship network as possible. When intense feelings abound, escape seems a plausible solution, yet differentiation of self entails the counterintuitive posture of being in the midst of the fray while not becoming part of the fray. Is it possible to put the entire family in a bag and still stay connected to it, Bowen once asked an audience? In the 2015 commencement speech at Oberlin College, Michelle Obama, commenting upon the polarization and strife that seems rampant in this culture, cautioned students to fight the urge to run away, finding comfort in the bosom of their like-minded compadres. Instead, she exhorted them to run TOWARD the proverbial noise:

> Today I want to suggest if you truly want to carry on the Oberlin legacy of service and social justice, then you need to run to, not away from, the noise. Today, I want to urge you to actively seek out the most contentious, gridlocked, and polarized places you can find. Because so often, throughout our history, those have been the places where progress really happens.
>
> (Obama, 2015)

For most humans, those places of contention AND progress are in the midst of our families, especially in times of transition and loss. Being present and accounted for without getting "done in" by the cacophony of the herd is a feature of differentiation of self.

Attendant with being in the midst of the anxious group is having a clearly defined set of beliefs and positions while acknowledging that others may think quite differently. In this family, there was a history of keeping silent about difficult issues and avoiding painful disclosures.

It was no surprise, then, that a variety of family members preferred to avoid the mention of Mrs. A's suicide and to have a more discreet funeral process, if any. Believing in the openness of communication about the death and moving toward an open gathering of the entire family and friendship circle was a core part of the husband's orientation toward death, informed by Bowen theory and his own personal experience. While some of his immaturity emerged as his wife described his "pushiness" over having an open casket, she was thoughtful enough to get beyond his emotionality and see the merit of this suggestion.

When humans get anxious in their relationships, the tendency to look for allies, to gossip behind the backs of others, and to demonize or canonize certain individuals is amplified. The concept of triangles describes some of these processes. For Mrs. A's daughter, the triangle would manifest itself between her and her parents as vacillating between "feeling sorry for" her mother and anger at her father for the divorce and remarriage. Another version of this relationship would be the vilification of the new wife, holding her responsible for the demise of the marital relationship leading to the eventual suicide. The husband was certainly vulnerable to sympathetically siding with his wife in her feeling responses to her position in the primary triangle with her parents. Again, the husband felt sorry for his wife and pulled to intervene on her behalf during difficult encounters with her father. Once such incident occurred immediately after the father learned that his former spouse had taken her own life. The daughter and the father engaged in a tense conversation as he demanded to enter the old family home. The daughter refused to allow her father to come into the house, stating that this was no longer his home because he had left the marriage to her mother. The husband was sorely tempted to intervene on behalf of his seemingly beleaguered spouse. Stepping back for a moment, he thought to himself, "This looks like a pretty fair fight," embracing the notion that his good wife was well equipped to handle herself with her father. Curbing his almost reflexive action resulted in the eventual resolution of the immediate issue between the father and daughter. After the funeral service, however, Mr. A and his new wife attended a gathering for family and friends at the home where he had resided with his now deceased former spouse.

The presence of humor in the most dire of times can reflect a sense of perspective and an objectivity about these events while also providing a healing balm to the group. Mrs. A's three brothers were graduates and ardent supporters of the Ohio State Buckeyes; the daughter's husband was a Michigan graduate. Prior to the dinner for the family after the funeral service, the husband purchased three Ohio State–themed bandanas for the bereaved brothers. After some imbibing of spirits (indeed, the eldest brother indicated that he had not stopped drinking since he got off the plane), there was some merriment and laughter with pictures being taken and stories shared. Several weeks later, the daughter received a phone call from the wife of her eldest uncle. "I'm really upset with your husband." The husband wondered what faux pas he had made at the funeral, only to discover that the uncle would not stop wearing that college bandana around the house, much to his wife's chagrin. Lightening the tone in an uptight environment can be beneficial to the entire group.

The Aftermath and Human Variation

In his revealing research on humans and the grief process, George Bonanno purported that *Homo sapiens* is exquisitely prepared to manage death and loss with an often-overlooked resilience befitting our evolutionary heritage (Bonanno, 2009). Might suicide, however, be unique terrain for the bereaved? In other words, does the suicide of a family member automatically result in a more protracted grieving process for family members and significant relationships, or even contribute to the phenomenon of an emotional shock wave as described by Dr. Bowen?

The research is not unanimous or unequivocal on these questions. De Groot et al. found higher self-reported incidences of health and psychiatric difficulties among families in which a suicide had happened compared to families in which a death had occurred naturally (de Groot, de Keijser, & Neeleman, 2006). While Jordan underlined certain grieving themes unique to families in which a suicide had taken place, even noting greater isolation and stigmatization along with disturbances in the balance of family relationships, he concluded: "Given this conflicting data, we cannot say definitively whether the longer term trajectory of suicide bereavement is the same or different from other types of losses" (Jordan, 2001, p. 98). This statement closely parallels Dr. Bowen's observations: "Suicides are commonly followed by prolonged grief and mourning reactions, but the shock wave is usually minor unless the suicide was an abdication of an essential functional role" (Bowen, 1978, 328). The death of a 35-year-old mother with young children is far more likely, then, to result in a longer-term disturbance of the functional equilibrium of the family than the death of a 68-year-old woman.

Although it might be tempting in the case described to claim that the multigenerational family of Mrs. A negotiated the grief process with minimal reactivity due to the small efforts of one or two people trying to implement the tenets of Bowen theory during the immediate fallout of her suicide, that claim would be inaccurate. Tension and distance marked the relationship between Mrs. A's daughter and her father until the time of his death, six years after his former wife's suicide. The daughter and the new wife also remained distant, testimony to the power of triangles and the family process. This estrangement certainly had some impact on the other relationships within the family. Yet the disruption of the relationship between the daughter and her father did not interfere, with each of them maintaining a relationship themselves with the rest of the family.

A peremptory survey of four generations of the family confirms absence of an emotional shock wave. Some nine years after the suicide, marriages have remained intact; grandchildren and great-grandchildren have progressed in ways commensurate with their developmental ages; and there has been a relative absence of physical, psychological, or social symptoms. In fact, Mrs. A's daughter and son have developed a more open relationship with each other and their families, despite their differences in their relationship with their father after their mother's death. Additionally, Mrs. A's son and daughter-in-law did disclose the fact of the grandmother's suicide to the two children who spoke at the funeral, unaware at the time of the nature of her death. Although this information came to the grandchildren several years after their grandmother's death, this eventual openness is testimony to the longer-term impact of opening up the communication system within the family over time.

Perhaps some of the factors confounding researchers in their attempts to assess the magnitude of grief responses to sudden death, be it suicide or accident, is the nuance of human variation. In her work on animal grief, Dr. Barbara King elucidates and cautions:

> We humans have our own species-specific ways of mourning . . . Yet what stands out for me isn't human uniqueness, but the knowledge that animals other than humans do love, and do grieve. As I have stressed throughout the book, this statement shouldn't become a litmus test of emotional complexity for other species. Some dogs will grieve, depending on their personalities and contexts in which they live. Some dogs won't. The same is true for chimpanzees and other species who have mourned in a way that we recognize. The expression of animal emotion doesn't lend itself well to bold generalization across individuals—any more than the expression of human emotion would.
>
> (King, 2013, pp. 165–166)

Human families vary, then, in their levels of emotional maturity and in their ability to adapt to loss and transition. Some families simply have more rebound capacity than others, as discerned by Dr. Papa et al.: "resilience after loss appears to be contingent on the degree of flexibility in individuals' behavioral repertoire allowing engagement with an altered social landscape and access to positive reinforcement from their changed environment in self-relevant domains" (Papa, Sewell, Garrison-Diehn, & Rummel, 2013, p. 640). Assessing the short- and long-term impact of the suicide of a family member, then, would need to account for this individual variation. Bowen theory provides a lens for viewing those family and individual differences through the lens of both differentiation and anxiety.

Concluding Commentary

This description of how one family managed its way through the suicide of a family member is not meant to be prescriptive for other families, nor a blueprint of how to get through this major life event. For *this* family, Bowen theory offered an alternative way to think about what was occurring in the moment, which then led to a different way of being in the intense feeling throes associated with a suicide.

Observing, listening, focusing upon self, respecting the magnitude of the emotional process at work, clarifying personal stances on important issues, paying attention to blaming, and diagnosis can pave the way for behaving in a little more self-directed manner. Articulating positions on an open casket and speaking openly and directly about the fact of the suicide of a family member are not strategies or techniques applicable in all scenarios. They are concrete behaviors and ways of being in the midst of an anxious family that emanated from the thinking of an individual familiar with Bowen theory. Without having another way to think about the human condition, of which suicide is only one part, the husband and his wife would have behaved differently and more reactively to the event and the feeling responses of those around them.

Another caveat seems in order at this juncture. Among novices and even veterans to Bowen theory, the illusion can arise that the individuals who study the theory and all of their connected family members will somehow be immune from the mundane occurrences of daily living, such as divorce, extramarital affairs, chronic illness, substance abuse, or depression and suicide. *Wrong*. Bad things do happen to people and their families who study Bowen theory. Symptoms can occur in all families at any time and any place. Bouncing back from these disturbances in the relationship balance also varies. Some individuals and families do a little better—or worse—with it than others. For those so inclined, however, Bowen theory contributes to a way through the morass, with a little less reactive thinking and a little more wiggle room for being present and accounted for in the midst of the turbulence that is simply a part of being a member of this species.

Mrs. A had a fondness for daffodils, diligently planting them in her yard every years. Drawing from that tradition, her daughter and other family members distributed daffodil bulbs to all those who attended the funeral. People from all over the country returned to their respective homes with this floral token of Mrs. A's life. Each year since Mrs. A's death, the daughter receives pictures of those long-ago planted daffodils that spring to life in Oregon, Florida, Texas, Ohio, and elsewhere. Life ends for all humans in ways unpredictable and unknown. Death then yields to new life that continues in the ebb and flow of seasons. Children and grandchildren continue and flourish, heirs to the lives of those who came before them. Such is the cycle of life.

REFERENCES

Bonanno, G. (2009). *The other side of sadness.* New York, NY: Basic Books.

Bowen, M. (1978). *Family therapy in clinical practice.* New York, NY: Jason Aronson.

Cerel, J., Jordan, J. R., & Duberstein, P. R. (2008). The impact of suicide on the family. *Crisis, 29*(1), 38–44.

de Groot, M. H., de Keijser, J., & Neeleman, J. (2006). Grief shortly after suicide and natural death: A comparative study among spouses and first-degree relatives. *Suicide and Life- Threatening Behavior, 36*(4), 418–431.

Jordan, J. R. (2001). Is suicide bereavement different? A reassessment of the literature. *Suicide and Life-Threatening Behavior, 31*(1), 91–102.

King, B. (2013). *How animals grieve.* Chicago: University of Chicago.

Obama, M. (2015, May 25). *Commencement speech.* Oberlin College: Oberlin, Ohio.

Papa, A., Sewell, M. T., Garrison-Diehn, C., & Rummel, C. (2013). A randomized open trial assessing the feasibility of behavioral activation for pathological grief responding. *Behavior Therapy, 44*(4), 639–650.

Yanagihara, H. (2015). *A little life.* New York, NY: Doubleday.

8

DEATH AS A CATALYST FOR RECONSTRUCTING THE FAMILY EMOTIONAL SYSTEM

Catherine M. Rakow

This reconstruction of understanding a multigenerational family emotional system began as an effort to understand how my son's death, in a car accident in 1995, happened as a part of our family system. In this chapter I drew on many years of researching my family, using as a guide the concepts from Bowen theory that pertain to tracing the shifts in family functioning across generations, particularly before and after deaths in the family.

For this chapter, I have focused on just four generations in my maternal side of the family. I began this investigation considering nine interacting variables that I hypothesized might be important in the process leading up to and following my son's death. Here I focus on just four: 1) reconciliation with a mate, 2) nodal family events, 3) vocational instability, and 4) the multigenerational family process emerging within days of his death.

At the most personal level, I wanted to discover if it would be possible to address my participation in this emotional process with acceptance and, in so doing, learn what it would take to free myself from continuing to transmit this process to those who would come after me.

The Questions Guiding My Research

If the family does not move beyond the child's death toward a clearer definition of themselves, it is likely that confusing and chronic dysfunction will emerge.

(Hollister, 1975–76, p. 206)

Death can serve the function of opening a family system, bringing the potential to identify and perhaps resolve long-unresolved emotional attachments in a family system. Having a theory connecting the family's past and present allows for exploration of often disparate and seemingly separated events. Bowen (1978) specifically noted "that not all deaths have the same importance to a family" (p. 327). What would determine importance to a family of any one particular person? I postulated that it would be a family member functioning in alignment with particular elements of the family's ongoing, cross-generational emotional process. This involved the participation of family members dependent on the stability of the continuing triangle from my grandparents and my uncle on down to my mother, myself, and my son. And in the case I will describe here, the cascade of additional deaths in the aftermath of that death that revealed specific family emotional processes and family members' participation. Bowen (1978) has termed this cascade of events the "emotional shock wave" (p. 324), a process that follows the loss of certain family members central to the family's emotional process and one that marks the importance of dynamics previously denied.

It is one thing to know, conceptually, that triangles can carry emotional process across generations via the family projection processes and multigenerational process. Still, it is astonishing to be confronted with the reality that one's self was part of a process going back at least 90 years ago that played a part in a particular outcome—the death of one's child. Moreover, Bowen theory suggests that my family would likely continue this transmission to succeeding generations. As Kerr and Bowen (1988) explain: "The emotional functioning of one generation so programs the emotional functioning of the succeeding generation that levels of differentiation of self usually do not change markedly from one generation to the next" (Kerr & Bowen, 1988, p. 135).

Could the larger process be known? What was the part I played? Would it be possible to alter the programming of the emotional functioning of the succeeding generations in that particular way? Bowen (1978) offered hope, writing that the very essence of systems theory says "that unresolved emotional attachments between people that remain viable for life, that attach to significant future relationships, and that continue to direct the course of a life" are resolvable as "few human events provide as much emotional impact as . . . death in resolving unresolved emotional attachments" (p. 331).

How does one know when a particular process operating over generations in a family has ended? Could a death and the related cascade of deaths in the emotional shock wave bring resolution to unfinished business in a family? In this narrative, that unfinished business clearly related to the process in husband/wife/mother/offspring relationships and the content of a long-held wish, desire, hope, expectation that things could be set to rights in the family if a mother and daughter reconciled.

The Theory and Methods Applied

The study of my family has been guided in the past by Bowen theory (Bowen, 1978; Kerr & Bowen, 1988; Papero, 1990, 2015; and McCullough, 1987) and numerous others whose presentations I heard and whose readings guided my efforts. My intent was to continue this approach in the study of this particular path of my emotional system. The method was to gather as much factual and narrative information about the family as possible, noting patterns that have emerged over generations. Because the family that one researches is one's own, the gathering of such information is rarely a neutral experience for the researcher. To give an example of the emotional information transmitted in the family, here is the kind of comment made, for over 50 years, when there was mention of a particular cousin central to this discussion:

> Oh, poor Maria, you know her mother abandoned her when she was just a baby. That woman put that little child on a train all by herself at two years old, and sent her off (a hundred and fifty miles away). She has had a hard life ever since. What kind of mother would do that?

Over time, I collected family stories such as this one, stories certainly common to most families. I kept a journal to track thoughts as well as conversations with other family members. I videotaped and audiotaped interviews with my mother and other relatives. In this chapter, I present an abbreviated narrative of our family's history to provide

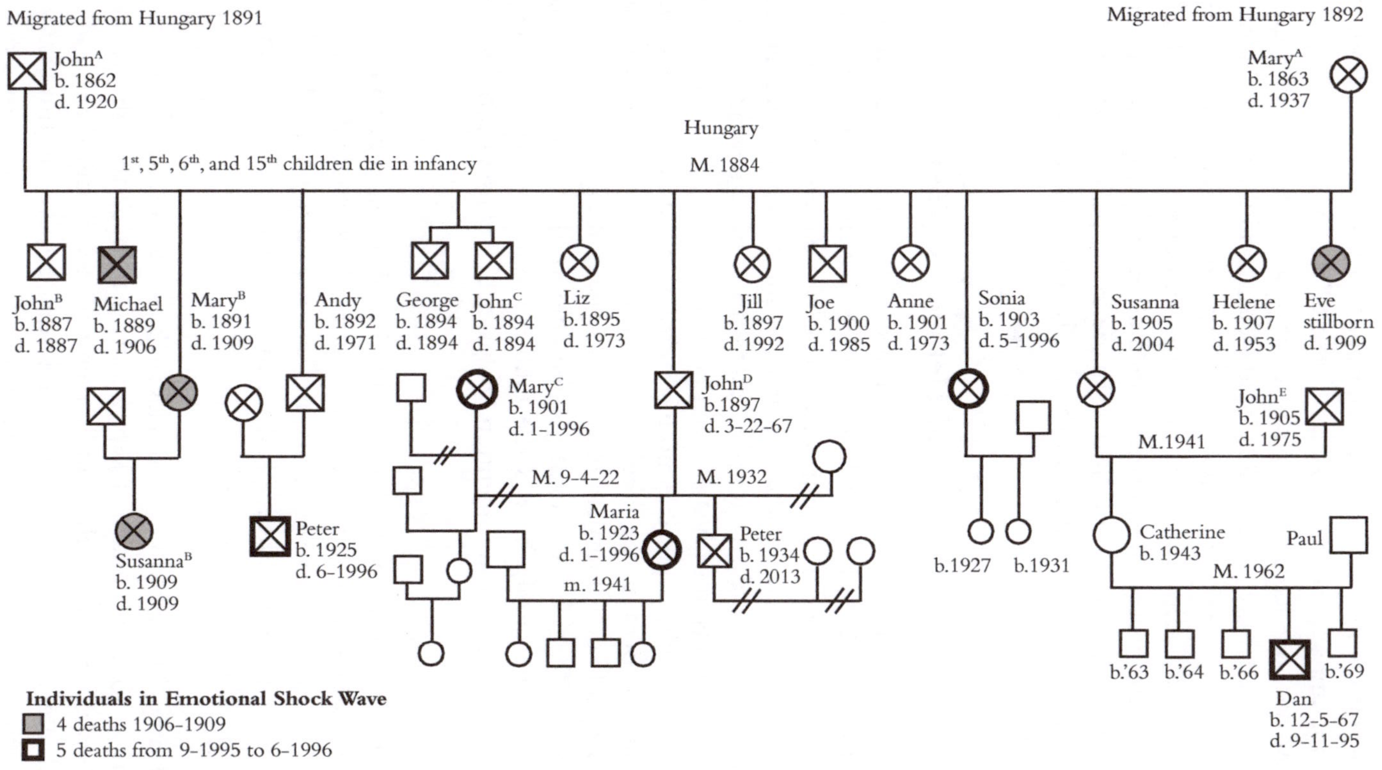

Figure 8.1 The Maternal Family

a context in which to examine certain patterns of interaction that seemed related to the multigenerational emotional process surrounding my son's death. I also made note of my own subjective experiences, including recorded recollections of odd, disturbing, and unwanted reactions that lacked a context for understanding them at the time they occurred.

By piecing together this information, birth and death dates, confidences and family secrets revealed in personal interviews, and my knowledge of the nature of past family relationships, a multigenerational process emerged. It had been there all along, like an underground river, only rising to the surface when family events and motivation were high enough to connect all of it. Unresolved issues among long-dead family members played out across generations via triangles. I found Hollister's (1975–76) article on "Families Who Experienced the Loss of a Child" to capture exactly what I was considering. She has written:

> [M]embers of families who in their mourning will be responsible for understanding their expectations of the child who died will serve future generations well, for they will make it less likely that the role this child played will remain active and always available to prevent examination and change.
>
> (p. 210)

There is repetition of names here. I have identified all those with the same name, either John or Mary, with a superscript to distinguish them.

The Maternal Side, Generations One and Two

While there is no "beginning" to any family history, this narrative will begin with my maternal grandparents whom I will refer to as the first generation. They married in Hungary and had three children before my grandfather left for a better life in America six years into the marriage. The first child, John[B], named after my grandfather, died in infancy. Two years later, my grandmother, Mary[A], and the two remaining children, Mike and Mary[B], arrived to join him. There were 15 children in all, 12 born in the rural Midwest town where they settled.

The first, John[B]; fifth, George; sixth, John[C]; and the 15th child, Eve, all died in infancy. The second child, Mike, born in Hungary, died in a coal mining accident at age 16. My mother, Suzanne, the 13th child, was born in 1905, a year before death hit the family hard. In response to her oldest brother's death in 1906, my grandmother went into a prolonged depression. My mother's oldest sister, Mary[B], then 14, became my mother's second mother during the next two years, a difficult family time and important developmental years for my mother. Sometime in these years, the family story says, Grandfather demanded his wife return to functioning. Death was not done yet with the family. After marrying at age 16, my mother's oldest sister, Mary[B], died in childbirth. Her baby, named after my mother, died within weeks of Mary[B]'s death. Grandmother was pregnant through this and several months later delivered her own stillborn child. Four deaths within three years.

Death and Birth Reconstitute the Relationship System

There were two distinct functioning phases in my grandparents' marriage. In the first phase, prior to 1906, the marriage was highly conflictual according to what the family reported generally about their parents' marriage. But while this contentiousness was remembered most vividly, careful exploration of the family's history over the years revealed that, following the deaths of the two adolescent children (the two remaining siblings born in the old country) in 1906 and 1909, the spousal relationship had changed. In the second phase of the marriage, there was instability in the parents. The stories of Grandmother's dysfunction after her oldest surviving son's death are numerous. Yet there are no stories—*none*—relating to her functioning after her firstborn daughter's and infant granddaughter's death. The birth of her stillborn child speaks poignantly to her distress in this year. What is known is this: The marriage settled to a form lasting the remaining 11 years of the marriage, that of dysfunction in Grandfather due to "black lung disease," overfunctioning in the form of caretaking of him by Grandmother, and intense reactivity and focus on the sixth son, John[D], then an adolescent, and the third son named after grandfather. Grandfather, John[A], was in the outside position with Grandmother and the sixth son, John^{D}, on the inside of the triangle. Bowen (1978) describes the function seen here:

> The child functions as a stabilizer for the parents, converting the unstable father-mother ego mass into a more stable triad. Parental stability depends on the child functioning as the "triadic one" . . . The triadic emotional process is adaptive and it can reestablish itself after most threats.
>
> (p. 127)

This holds true in my family.

With the marital relationship managing its anxiety by involving a child, other relationships in the family responded. With her oldest sister/second mother, Mary^{B}, dead, my mother, then age four, shifted to a close position with Grandmother, possibly filling the void left by her sister's death.

Death Further Realigns Relationships

When Grandfather died of chronic black lung disease in 1920, four children were still living at home: the older, troublesome brother, John^{D}, age 24; another brother, Joe, age 20; my mother, Suzanna, age 15; and her younger sister, Helen, age 13. Soon after Grandfather's death, my uncle, John^{D}, began a relationship with a woman who happened to have the same name, Mary^{C}, as my grandmother. This woman was married to a minister at the time. Grandmother predicted (to others, not to her son) that the marriage would be punished by God. Grandmother's response to this unacceptable marriage was to host the wedding in her home and have the newlyweds move in with her. Two months after that marriage, the oldest surviving brother, Andy, came and moved Grandmother and the remaining siblings, including my mother, from their rural Midwest home to live in an industrial city 125 miles away where he was living. In a departing act of caring for her son, Grandmother left the family home to her newly married son and his wife, John^{D} and Mary^{C}, even though she believed the marriage was cursed due to "taking a minister's wife." It is evidence that energy in the group was going into the relationships.

After the move to the city, my mother, then age 17, made a decision to care for her widowed mother as long as needed. She did not want Grandmother shuttled from one sibling to another. It was a life principle lived out by caring for her mother for 12 years until Grandmother's death. After that, consideration could go to beginning her own family. This is an example of a nonnegotiable life principle, as well as part of the family emotional process. It is also an example of a "don't go far from your mother" theme, and it shows up as a feeling in me toward my mother. This mother–daughter piece of the emotional fabric of the extended family exists in every other mother–daughter pair across the second and third generations of the family.

Generations Two and Three

Ten months after my uncle's marriage, a daughter, Maria, was born. My grandmother and my uncle's siblings had all moved away. The marriage heated up quickly after the birth of the first child. Kerr and Bowen (1988) note, "A nuclear family can be stabilized by outside relationships, particularly by those with the extended family" (p. 267). Kerr also described destabilizing factors: "An event, or more likely a series of events, can disturb the balance of a relationship system and trigger symptoms. The event may be the addition of something new that has to be dealt with or the loss of something old that was relied on" (Ibid). Both were present here: a new baby was added and Grandmother was not nearby. As my uncle, John[D], worked two jobs in another city 90 miles away, his wife began another affair. The new paramour wanted nothing to do with someone else's daughter. My uncle left the marriage, seeking solace in his mother. This is the description as told by my mother to me:

> My brother came to Pittsburgh. He came into the house where mother lived. He threw himself at her feet and buried his head in her lap saying he was sorry and that she was right, he never should have married her. He said he did not want to go back to his wife but he could not live without his daughter. [Grand]Mother said to bring her (here). Two days later, before he told his wife this, his wife called the family and told them to go to the train station as she had put the child on the train

> to Pittsburgh. She was two years old. This story of this child being put on the train alone at age two has always been a big emotional story in the family. The family vilified her mother for this.
>
> (December 6, 1994, conversation)

My uncle's wife, Mary[C], then married her lover and began a new family. This is a culmination of the emotional process changes in reestablishing an equilibrium as far back as 1906. I consider this a convulsion in the family system as its ramifications shadow far into the future. Kerr and Bowen (1988) note the impact of such disruption: "After system equilibrium has been distorted, it may not be possible to restore equilibrium without introduction of a chronic symptom" (p. 114). This chronic, unfinished emotional issue, the cutoff between mother and daughter, reactivated prior to the time of my son's death. The family view of my uncle, John[D], after this divorce was that "his life ended when his wife left him" (Personal conversation with family members). The psychological oneness of the family considered him incompetent to manage his own life without his wife. This illustrates Papero's (2015) point: "The members of the family . . . share a common mindset and . . . look at the world through the same lens" (p. 17). The rupture of my uncle's marriage and his wife's abandonment of their daughter generated a sense of deep sorrow across the family, paradoxically coupled with perpetual hope that reconciliation between mother and child would restore the heart strength of the family. Good evidence that this relationship was entangled in the family emotional process was evident in the involvement of all family members in placing their continued happiness on him. No one was neutral. All family members blamed both John[D] and Mary[C]. The difference was that their brother was pitied whereas his wife was despised.

Maria was sent to her father, John[D], who brought her to his mother and his sister, Suzanna, my mother. My mother assumed maternal care for Maria, leaving her job to stay home the seven years Maria lived there. This relationship mirrors what happened with my mother early in her life when an older sister stepped in to care for her when Grandmother was functionally absent. (A repeating pattern that probably increased chances of adapting to the new circumstances.)

When my uncle remarried, his daughter returned to live with him and his second wife. Two years later, a son was born to this second marriage. In a repeating pattern, the addition of a new baby brought disturbance to the marriage. Blame goes to Maria, now a preteen, who is again sent away. She went to my mother's next older sister, Sonia, living 400 miles away on the East Coast. Another of the patterns noted at the broader level in this family is that in mother–daughter pairs there is some symptom outbreak in a daughter prior to the mother's death. Sending my cousin Maria away occurs when my mother needed thyroid surgery and she was not available to resume the surrogate mother function. In the intense togetherness here, there was a symptom cluster between the two siblings most involved: marital disturbance between my uncle and his second wife, an inability of my uncle to keep his own child with him, and my mother developing thyroid problems, all coinciding with grandmother's decline. My mother went with my cousin Maria to the eastern seaboard city where her sister's family lived. She had her thyroid surgery there. Mother's older sister had two daughters of her own, younger than my cousin, and this older sister, Sonia, and my mother decided that this family environment, with close-in-age would-be siblings, would best serve my cousin. Distance from her father's troubles in his second marriage was considered a benefit. It is unknown if my uncle abdicated his paternal responsibility or asked his sisters to take over. The sisters always told the story as their decision.

The involvement of my mother's older sister Sonia in this reconstruction of the family emotional system is important; she was one of the deaths in the emotional shock wave. During the five years my cousin Maria lived with Sonia, Maria's biological mother, Mary[C], attempted contact with her daughter (more than a decade after putting Maria on the train alone). Sonia blocked this effort, keeping it secret for 50 years from all the family, revealing it to me when I visited in the early 1990s. She said she had never told anyone, including my cousin, out of fear of criticism and losing the relationship with Maria. Contrary to the positive regard between my mother and my cousin Maria, the relationship between Maria and my mother's older sister Sonia, who raised my cousin over five years, was twitchy. How much had to do with that secret is a guess. In contrast, my cousin cherished my mother as the closest person to a mother that she had. My mother spent considerable time nurturing, comforting, and counseling Maria throughout my cousin's life. I think now that this attention diverted a more enhanced focus toward me.

In the year following Grandmother's death, my uncle's second marriage ended. Another lifelong cutoff is in place between my uncle, his second wife, and his son from the second marriage. My uncle never again functioned at a level that could sustain a relationship. He had the minimum of contact with his daughter and no contact with his son. Neither the second wife nor son had any further contact with my family with one exception, my mother, who maintained a yearly holiday contact with this nephew until her death, though she had no further contact with her brother. That nephew married twice, did not reproduce, and this branch has dead-ended. From Grandmother's death forward, there was no direct contact between my mother and my uncle. Later I will speak to the energy remaining in that relationship that then transferred to my son at this uncle's death and the odd thoughts at his birth, prickliness between him and me in his adulthood, and the exchanges between my mother and myself about him. My mother never expressed to me any desire for contact with her brother, although my mother was in good contact with all other family members. Any information about either my uncle or my mother came through others' contacts with each of them or hearsay. Comments by other siblings about my uncle were that he was to be pitied. Life had done him wrong. There were no comments on his strengths or his capacity to solve his own problems.

Thirty Years of Unsettledness

From 1906 to 1937, there was a prolonged period of unsettledness in the family that swirled around my grandparents, John^{A} and Mary^{A}; my uncle, John^{D}; his two wives, Mary^{C} and his second wife; his daughter, Maria; my mother, Suzanna; and in the last few years of this time, my mother's older sister, Sonia. This duration of system disturbance, symptom eruption, and managing of relationships through extreme distance speaks to the intensity of the upset that then goes dormant. The next 30 years were a time of little disturbance. There are no family stories of memorable upset from these years beyond the ordinary births, deaths, and marriages common to any family.

Nuclear Family of Origin

As noted, emphasis is on my mother's side in elaborating details, as it is on this side of the family that the multigenerational process, from my maternal grandmother to my son, came to stand out from the general fabric of the family. My parents married in 1941. My mother married distinctly out of her ethnic group, the only sibling to do so. I was born in 1943. My father was incapacitated four months after my birth and unable to work for several months. Mother's story is that the doctor told her she should prepare to take over the function of securing the family's future. Their marriage was characterized as one of low conflict, chronic symptoms in my father of stomach ulcers and diabetes, and deep attachment of each to their only child. After my father's death, I became aware of my dependence on him and his moral compass. His death in 1975 was a growth point for me and led to my first major effort to define who I was long before I came to Bowen theory.

I married at age 18 and moved several hundred miles away until giving birth nine months later. I then returned to where my parents lived and purchased the family home from them. Within six years I gave birth to five sons. In one of the conversations after my marriage, my mother told me, "I lost your father when you were born. He came back to me after you married and moved away." I had no way of conceptualizing this as an emotional triangle process back then. I simply recorded it. My husband married a "package." He got a wife and mother-in-law as a unit, illustrating Bowen's (1978) point: "Spouses may maintain their most important relationships to the past generation, their parents" (p. 126). And illustrating Toman's (1976) point, "A man who takes an only child for his wife would be well advised to consider her mother . . . (who) often comes as a part of the package" (p. 186). In the early years of my marriage, with children arriving so quickly, I would ask myself, whose life am I living?

Death and Birth, a New Thirty-Year Cycle

In March 1967, my uncle, John[D], died in the state hospital with a diagnosis of organic brain disorder. His daughter, Maria, attended his funeral. Neither of his wives attended, nor did his son. The birth of my fourth son, Dan, followed nine months later, in December 1967.

A death followed closely by a birth sustains a systems equilibrium. There is a continuing representation in the triangle managing the original unresolved issues in the system. None of that was thought about back then. Kerr and Bowen (1988) speak to functioning positions within a family system that seem apropos here:

> People are born into and occupy functioning positions in a family, positions that have an important influence on many aspects of their biological, physiological, and social functioning. These functioning positions are molded over many generations and are anchored in emotional, feeling, and subjective processes.
>
> (p. 50)

This birth did not fit into the reproductive sequence of my nuclear family. Other births were 18 to 24 months apart. This one was 12 months between births and 9 months after my uncle's death. This birth prompts the first awareness in me of some connection to the larger family system though it was not understood as that at the time. On seeing the baby, my son, for the first time the thought came instantly that he looked like his maternal great-grandfather along with panic that this was not good. I had never seen the man beyond photos and, other than listening to family stories, I had never thought of him. He had died 47 years before my son's birth and 23 years before my own birth. This odd thought was powerful enough to remain in my memory until after my son's death. I now consider it evidence that I was a conduit for anxiety transmission and the thought was an intuitive[1] rapid cognition of the automatic emotional process not understood then. McCullough has asked, "What was the emotional significance of the person who died? The next person who's born gets some of that significance," noting that a family's unfinished emotional issues, the ingrained reactions, will come forward at time of death (McCullough, 1987). Both Bowen and Kerr touch on this automatic experiencing as part of the emotional transmission process. Kerr and Bowen (1988) write, "One of the major revelations of the study of the human family was that the functioning of individuals, including internal psychological and physical functioning as well as behavior, was far more regulated by relationships than previously thought" (p. 39). Bowen (1978) also notes, "The emotional system operates through all five senses, and most often through visual and auditory stimuli . . . I believe the automatic emotional process is far more important in establishing and maintaining relationships than verbal language" (p. 348). Epigenetics is moving toward explaining how real and PERCEIVED trauma in one generation can cross three generations without personal contact (Jones, 2014, pp. 105–127).

Realignment of Relationships After a Birth

When my mother's perception was that I needed her to assist in caring for the growing brood of grandsons, she retired "to help Cathy with the kids." This coincides with the birth of my son whose death is integral to this telling. This would fit with the description of an only child's dependence on parents if there were multiple children (Toman, 1977, p. 187). It was after this birth that I began to consider life goals other than mothering. It was also now that I moved to the outside position of the triangle that was now composed of my mother, myself, and my son, representing his grandfather, John^{A}, and his uncle, John^{D}. Mark Twain (1874) has sagely described this: "History never repeats itself, but the Kaleidoscopic combinations of the pictured present often seem to be constructed out of the broken fragments of antique legends" (p. 430). An unanswered question is how this transmission got into my family and not that of my cousin Maria who had four children of her own? The only answer I have is the anxiety was bound elsewhere in her family and they were not part of the triangle with my mother, my son, and me. Anxiety has left its mark in their lives but not from this specific triangle.

As to my son's growing-up years in our family, there was nothing out of the ordinary beyond what has been mentioned. He moved into adulthood with no difficulty or particular concerns and left home at age 24 to move into his own home. On reflection, it comes to me that my son was a "focused-on child" only in the grandmother–mother–son triangle, not in the nuclear family. He was the connective tissue of triangles from the past in the present. My son's birth filled a functioning vacancy in the triangle within a family field of chronic anxiety. There was some awareness in me of a sensation I now would identify as chronic anxiety. Back then it was experienced as fear that he resembled his maternal great-grandfather. That chronic anxiety expressed itself over the years as a prickliness when we were around each other. I described our relationship as that of a "prickly pair." This was a sensation within me without an understanding of its origin. My son was aware of it too, and each, mother and son, tried over the years to be able to tolerate this inner tension in the presence of the other, without any way of understanding it before his death. As an adult, my son also put it into words: "I don't know why but I feel tense around you. I really wish I didn't." How does chronic anxiety play out generations removed from the original upset in the triangle in the past? After my son's death, I knew these sensations and relationship patterns were a remnant of relationship process and unresolved emotional attachment transmitted down the generational line.

A repeating, predictable pattern in this triangle took the form of the inability of speaking with my mother about my son. I would bring up my son in conversation with my mother, who then shifted immediately to negative comments about her brother and her father. This recurred many times. I made note of this, recognizing it as a repeating pattern, after beginning the study of Bowen theory in 1982. I noted both confusion and fascination with this chain reaction. I did not note as important the change this produced in me, wariness in any further discussion with my mother regarding my son. I found myself speechless, and the conversation ended when this occurred. Bowen (1978) and Papero (2015, p. 18) both define such a pattern as an emotional reflex. "The closed communication system is an automatic emotional reflex to protect self from the anxiety in the other person" (p. 332). Not recognizing this pattern as such is another example of being blind to what was right in front of me. I only came to understand it after my son's death.

1994–1995 Activation of the 70-Year Cutoff

In December 1994, my long-gone aunt, Mary^{C}, from generation 2, recruits her granddaughter to find her firstborn daughter, my cousin Maria. This is her dying wish. Mary^{C} had told no one she was married to my uncle and had a daughter she gave away. Beyond her second husband, this was a secret in her second family. The granddaughter searches, finding a male cousin with the family name in the city where I lived. The male cousin, Peter, sends the granddaughter with her grandmother's dying wish directly to my mother now living in my home. They speak and information is exchanged to reach Maria directly. The granddaughter quotes her grandmother: "There isn't a night that I go to bed that I don't wonder where my daughter is." The first in this link of possible reconnection, the male cousin, Peter, was the nephew who was born at the time of the convulsion in the system in 1925. He is also the cousin who gave me the gravesite where my son is buried. This is just fact. I would have no way presently to attach greater meaning to the timing of his birth and his subsequent death in this narrative. Following this call, my mother spoke directly to my cousin Maria. It is during this phone call that Maria first hears the family story of her arrival on the train 70 years ago. I asked my mother how it was possible Maria never knew this when it was such a big story in the family. She said, "We just never told her." The emotional impact of these calls was later observable when my mother said her legs were numb, she felt done in, and she had to go lie down. Another example of the intensity is the relief my mother expresses later, "I have been waiting for this all my life."

For the first time in 70 years, two of three original participants in a convulsive episode in the family's history, Mary[C] and Maria, were in a position to address unresolved differences. The third original participant, my Uncle John[D], was dead but the system did have an unknowing representative in my son Dan. The intensity level of emotional arousal rose in those who had been present 70 years ago and were still living. Letters, phone calls, and many discussions between my mother, my cousin, and my mother's sister Sonia, the second surrogate mother, occurred reviewing the years of the family's grief and helplessness with the situation. Bowen (undated) confirms that bridging cutoffs releases bound-up intensity: "The intensity of the emotional reactiveness in making contact with the past is directly related to the intensity of the emotionality that was buried in the original emotional cut off" (Bowen, undated). At a system level, this potential connection opens up the possibility of bridging a long-awaited reconciliation. During these months, my son, working nearby, had lunch daily with my mother. How much was directly discussed between them of this matter is unknown to me. I do know my son would have been responsive to his grandmother's distress. In addition, I do know her criticalness of me toward my son increased during this time.

Confluence of Similar Life Events to the Original Convulsion Prior to My Son's Death

It is the who, what, when, and where that can make a difference in the ability to manage the reality of a death. My son's death on September 11, 1995, occurred in a perfect storm of colliding variables. The multigenerational transmission process activated by the effort to bridge a 70-year cutoff had the extended family holding its breath in apprehension and fear—fear it would occur and fear that it would not. Our nuclear family system and my son's life in the present moment were also in flux. Two brothers had moved away, one became engaged, and while his brothers' lives were moving forward, my son's was stalled. I was in a wait-and-see place with him. I had concern for where he was in life and was waiting for an indication he might accept some discussion with counsel from me.

Confluence of Life Events Similar to the Original Convulsion

Variables in my son's life replicating the original cutoff during these immediate weeks preceding his death were a reconciliation with a mate initiated two weeks before his death and then her subsequent departure to the West Coast on a planned visit four days before his death. His activity the day of his death would have been different had she been nearby. My son had serious difficulties at work the week before his death due to external complications out of his control and internal upsets about those. Bowen (undated) has referred to clinicians making promises to clients that cannot be kept as a "breach of unconscious promise." Substituting his employer for the clinician, his upset at work meets that definition. There was a personal betrayal in a close friendship. There was an upset between my son and me three days before his death. My perceptions were that this was a regression prior to a growth spurt in him. If I could just stay present but noninterfering to him, he would find his way. I invited him to stay in contact. He did, contacting me the day before his death to make amends. It was a solid conversation of two people who care about each other. There was none of the old "prickles" between us. Without consideration of the multigenerational factors, his death was an outcome far removed from my expectation. The day after our amends, my son died in a car accident. It is useless to speculate on wondering what the trajectory in the family would be if my uncle had died back in 1925. As others noted, his life ended then. Just as the odd thought of extended family connections came at his birth, when going to see my dead son for the first time at the funeral home, I had a distinct awareness that his death was connected to my ancestors' lives and something of import was ending—another intuitive rapid cognition.

Emotional Post-Mortem

Following my son's death, no action was taken on the cutoff between my aunt and my cousin. Within four months, the deaths of people actively involved in the sustained chronic anxiety began. In December 1995, my mother informed my cousin Maria of my son's death. What was the delay in telling my cousin of this? Speculating, I would say my mother's functioning was so affected by my son's death she did not write or call Maria and apparently, her older sister, Sonia, did not either. Sonia lived only 20 to 25 miles from my cousin. She was the aunt who took her in and raised her for five years, and she also knew of the attempt to reunite by her biological mother both early in life and in 1995. Reflecting on this now, it illustrates how isolated and overprotected my cousin was in the family. No one told her the facts of her mother giving her away, and no one told her of my son's death until the end of December when my mother wrote to her. On January 2, my cousin Maria died unexpectedly. Her biological mother, Mary^{C}, died on January 4, with no notification that her daughter had died. Five months later, May 1996, my mother's older sister Sonia died unexpectedly. A month after this, June 1996, my male cousin, Peter, died. He was mentioned earlier for giving me my son's grave and being the first family contact in the reconciliation effort. Peter's gift of the grave solved a thorny, chronic issue in his own branch of the family. It was an action that could be conveyed as be careful what you wish for, as it might have powerful consequences when you get it—a theme that fits with the family emotional process presented here. All these people were healthy when my son died with the exception of the long-gone aunt, Mary^{C}. Who knows how to weight such things? Considering an emotional shock wave as directly related to the chronic anxiety stream in the family is illustrated here.

The only other prominent participants remaining alive were my mother and myself. I wish I could explain that beyond the two of us being still tightly bound. The cross-generational "clumping" of not knowing where one person begins and one person ends was addressed between my mother and me after my son's death. The rest of the original "clump" were dead. The lens shifted directly to my understanding the relationship with my mother, who was 90 years old at the time of my son's death, living with my husband and me. I saw how each of us, in our togetherness, was a variable in his death. I was working on my relationship with my mother for many years but never put together all these pieces: the thought at my son's birth which, later at his death, I interpreted as my being a conduit for transmission of anxiety, the life course changes in my mom and myself at his birth, the prickliness between my son and me as he approached adulthood and launching his own life, and the predictable emotional reflex when I mentioned my son to my mother and she shifted immediately to her brother and her father. The course our relationship took after my son's death was further evidence. His death surfaced the depth of unresolved emotional attachment between mother and offspring over four generations and specifically between my mother and me. It defined the context to my efforts for further separating a self.

My mother wondered why I was not a comfort to her as I wondered the same about her. I wanted her acknowledgement that I had lost my son. This led to conversations such as Mom saying, "I feel empty inside. I feel like a ghost" or "I feel like a walking skeleton." In the months and year following my son's death, I asked, "Why can't you comfort me? Why can't you say 'I'm sorry your son died?'" Her response was "He was more my son than yours" or "I've experienced much more death in my life than you have." This reflected the emotional process around deaths from the earliest days in my mother's life from the time of her brother's death back to 1906 and to my son's birth following her brother's death in 1967 when she retired and I moved more on my own life path. For myself, I was clear now about the fusion between us. It was important to me to know if my mother had it in her to 1) recognize the boundaries of the generations and who was the mother and 2) offer me motherly solace. I kept this in my heart without negativity; I just wanted to know if it was possible. I thought my chances in life would be better if she could. On Mother's Day 1997 she accompanied me to the cemetery. Standing at my son's grave, my mother expressed her sorrow that my son died. So simple, so profound.

I consider this another nodal point in the resolution of the chronic anxiety of 70 years. My mother lived with us 17 years, 8 of those years before my son's death and 9 years after it. She died at age 99 in 2004, outliving all her siblings and many of her nieces and nephews. She died in her own bed, as was her wish. I understood my place in her dying as walking beside her on this last transition, being a resource and comfort to her. Her strength in her own dying and the openness of our relationship through that time left me with no awareness of grief after her death. Our living relationship was done. My admiration for what she made of herself in her life has continued to grow. Having a theory to offer enlightenment, she did the best she could.

Reflecting From a Systems Perspective

> The period immediately following the death of a child is often a time when family roles and expectations change. It is also a time when members of a family can more clearly perceive each other as individuals, can examine the role each person plays, and can interrupt the process by which disabling roles are passed on to future generations . . . After a child has died, a seat is empty and a role is vacant.
>
> (Hollister, 1975–1976, p. 205)

In the preceding pages, we have seen one distinct aspect of an otherwise far more complex family emotional process over a period of 90 years (since the first destabilizing death). Across those four generations, this family managed to sustain a number of unresolved emotional issues with the cooperation of multiple individuals. For so many years, the family lived in a state of concerned uncertainty about the reconciliation among a father, mother, and daughter that never arrived.

Within this family process, I focused particularly on the multigenerationally transmitted process as lived in the triangle of my mother, my son, and myself. While I did look as closely at other parts of the extended family system, at my own nuclear family emotional process, at my husband's extended family, and at the myriad of other variables that were part of my son's and others' deaths in the shock wave, I have not included that here. By shedding light on just this one pathway of family chronic anxiety—projected across four generations—I found it characterized by:

1. A history of unresolved mother/offspring separation carried forward across generations through interlocking triangles that persisted even after the original participants were dead and upon which the family's togetherness balance depended.
2. Chronic anxiety from the distant past felt at a primal level of intuitive rapid cognition and kinesthetic experience, which included a chronically anxious mind-set among family members involving persistent distortions of perception. Jones (2014) has noted "that a person's perceptions of the social environment can reach deep into the genome and alter cellular level processes even if the threat is only imagined" as it was here (p. 117).
3. An emotional shock wave response to death involving those persons connected to this particular thread of chronic family anxiety via the aforementioned triangles, which guided me to understanding my son's death in this larger context as well as my role in the process.
4. A cutoff binding the unresolved anxiety from the first generation that, when bridged, released that anxiety with such force that, in this case, it drove the shock wave.

In the sequence of deaths called a shock wave, a reverberation occurred throughout the family attachment network related to the functional position of individuals living the inherited triangles and the activation of the original disturbance. My son replaced my Uncle John[D] in a cross-generational triangle. My son's death released the energy bound in that triangle when the issues in the original cutoff became active in the present. The system then adjusted to a new reality about an old, long-held experience in the family, the long-held intense desire/

question as to whether my cousin Maria and her mother would reconcile. They would not. What remained was would another mother (mine) and a daughter (me) reach some resolution in our relationship, the remaining remnant of the fused relationships in this cross-generational anxiety stream, or would things continue predictably with some other family member filling in the triangle gap?

For me, as an active participant in this process, understanding the family as a system explained what previously had been unexplainable. It taught me how chronic anxiety operates across decades and how it is revealed in the triangles of a relationship system.

Since the death of my son and the subsequent shock wave, my family has stayed with its developmental tasks. The family has grown to include seven grandchildren. Each of them knows their Uncle Dan's name, has visited his gravesite, and has a sense of who he was. In studying my family, I have considered the idea that nature abhors a vacuum and without resolution, emotional issues will be projected into the future. In my own efforts to define a self I came to see my part as being a conduit for the chronic anxiety; a fused daughter; a participant in the unresolved emotional fusion operating in the triangle between mother, daughter, and son; and denying what the process revealed even as I was diligently studying theory. Before my son's death, my entrenchment in the emotional process and "observational blindness" allowed me to dismiss the clues of that participation. Has this small piece of the chronic anxiety process in my family ended due to resolution of a piece of the unresolved fusion between my mother and myself? How would one confirm that? A little change toward separation can have long-reaching impacts. Only time and additional attention to family process will reveal if this piece is no longer driving its way into the future. I have noted two 30-year cycles in this family. Only 20 years have passed so far.

> ...he who learns must suffer. And even in our sleep, pain that cannot forget falls drop by drop upon the heart, and in our own despite, against our will, comes wisdom to us by the awful grace of God.
>
> (Aeschylus, 525 BC–456 BC, translated by Edith Hamilton, 1930)

NOTE

1 Intuition is understood to be an information signal from the family emotional system. The response to the intuition would be reflective of the recipient individual's emotional maturity. In this case, were I more of a separate self and had I understood the intuition as an informational signal of present emotional process, there could have been a different internalization of it. The unanswered question regarding intuition is whether generating/receiving an intuition serves a function for the emotional system.

REFERENCES

Bowen, M. (1978). *Family therapy in clinical practice.* New York, NY: Jason Aronson.

Bowen, M. Undated correspondence. Acc. 2004–013, box 4, folder: U Tenn. (Awards), Papers of L. Murray Bowen, History of Medicine Division, National Library of Medicine, Bethesda, MD.

Bowen, M. Undated correspondence. Acc. 2005–055, box 3, folder "Murray Bowen, M.D. Position Statements." Papers of L. Murray Bowen, History of Medicine Division, National Library of Medicine, Bethesda, MD.

Hollister, M. (1975–1976). Families who experience the loss of a child. In R. Sagar (Ed.), *Georgetown family symposia, volume III (1975–1976), a collection of selected papers.* Washington, DC: Georgetown University.

Jones, A. (2014). Toward a science of human behavior: Epigenetics, social genomics, and Bowen theory. *Family Systems: A Journal of Natural Systems Thinking in Psychiatry and the Sciences, 10*(2), 105–127.

Kerr, M., & Bowen, M. (1988). *Family evaluation: An approach based on Bowen theory.* New York, NY: W. W. Norton.

McCullough, Paulina G. (1987). *Differentiation and the death of a parent.* Presentation at Western Pennsylvania Family Center.

Papero, Daniel V. (1990). *Bowen family systems theory.* Boston, MA: Allyn and Bacon.

Papero, Daniel V. (2015). The family emotional system. In R. Noone & D. Papero (Eds.), *The family emotional system: An integrative concept for theory, science, and practice.* Lanham, MD: Lexington Books.

Toman, W. (1976). *Family constellation.* New York, NY: Springer Publishing Co.

Twain, M. (Samuel L. Clemens) & Charles, D. W. (1874). *The gilded age: A tale of to-day.* Hartford, CT: American Publishing Company (Google Books Full View).

9

TERRITORIAL BEHAVIOR

Inheritance and Death in the Family

Anonymous

Introduction

Territorial behavior can be observed as the possession and disposition of property within and between generations. The property may be real estate, cash, personal property, or investments. Property distribution and family emotional process reciprocally influence one another. Few studies have addressed variable ways of understanding emotional process.

This chapter uses territorial behavior as one important clinical tool for the assessment of emotional process. It reports one person's efforts at differentiation of self over several years and demonstrates the value of observing territorial behavior among family members as a way of monitoring emotional process in the context of death.

Part I: Territorial Behavior

Six generations of the family appearing in Figure 9.1 have been studied over time by the author. In generation II through IV the surviving spouse allied self with the youngest child for the disposition of marital property. The manner in which the disposition was managed parallels the degree of emotional fusion of the youngest child to the surviving parent. Additionally, the parents in generation II used property to enhance the functioning of dysfunctional children. They gave land during their lifetime to their most dysfunctional children: siblings 7 and 13.

However, the territorial behavior of generations IV to VI is the focus of the chapter. The first section of the chapter highlights the

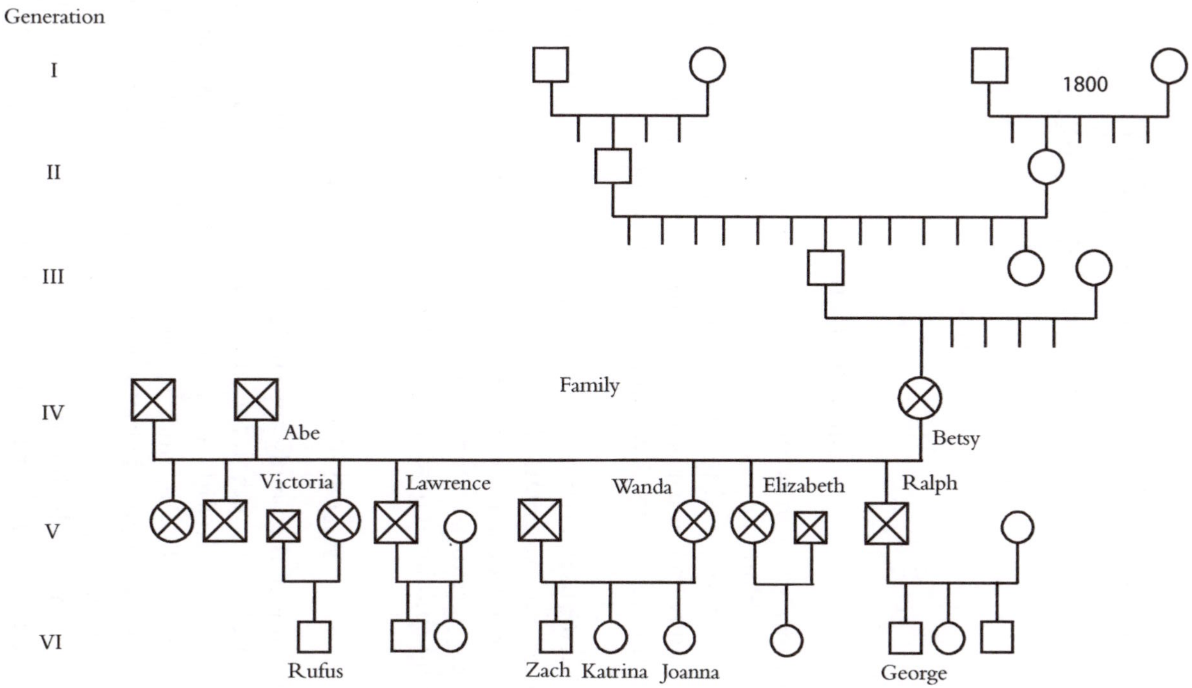

Figure 9.1 Six generations of the Smith family

territorial behavior of generation IV. This couple, Abe and Betsy Smith, established a homestead in 1906. When they died, the couple divided their land equally among their five children, excluded the two children from Betsy's prior marriage, and gave the house on their land to Abe and Betsy's youngest son, Ralph. The land Ralph received with the home was contiguous to the homestead, carved out with a small number of acres surrounding it. The youngest son, Ralph, stated that he was determined to rebuild the home as a memorial in his father's name and he refused assistance from all his siblings.

The "protection" of territory in the name of a memorial to his father created the following problem: The home could not be rented without the surrounding land to farm. The land could not easily be farmed without a home in which to live. The adult siblings believed they could not enter the home in which they grew up without permission of their younger sibling, Ralph, who now owned the homestead. Zach, Abe and Betsy's grandson and author of this narrative, understood that Abe and Betsy's children and grandchildren never discussed the origin of the division of property, except to say that Abe and Betsy wanted it that way. Zach hypothesized that the territorial complexity might have a comparable nuclear family and multigenerational emotional complexity.

Efforts at Differentiation of Self: Gather the Facts

Zach gathered facts about the family to determine the origin of this division of property, providing clues to each nuclear family emotional system and multigenerational projection process. Betsy had two children by a prior marriage. Her first husband died. Abe and Betsy, grandparents of Zach, had a conflictual marriage but together had five children: Victoria, Lawrence, Wanda, Elizabeth, and Ralph.

After the children left home, Abe was hospitalized for a period of time in the state mental hospital. The events and the process that led to the hospitalization served as an emotional earthquake that divided this family for decades. The family did not discuss the hospitalization or the impact on any member of the family.

Zach determined that the hospitalization and the distribution of the homestead, which were the culmination of a long-standing marital conflict, were indicators of the family emotional system. This emotional process was likely the basis of the territorial behavioral conflict described earlier. All family members distanced from discussing the origin of the territorial impasse. Zach set out to understand the origin of the impasse with the goal of testing his hypothesis that some change in the family emotional system might create a new resolution to the territorial impasse.

Efforts at Differentiation of Self: Establish a Plan of Action

Zach needed a plan to obtain the family's well-hidden history. He wrote the state mental hospital asking for the records of his grandfather, Abe, who had been hospitalized nearly 40 years previously.

Zach learned from the records at the time that all the adult children lived away from the home, Betsy filed assault charges against Abe, and the case went to court. Betsy asked the court to commit Abe to a hospital based on his alleged assaults. The court committed Abe to a state mental hospital, and Betsy required the oldest son, Lawrence, to drive Abe hundreds of miles to the state hospital for commitment. Abe stayed in the hospital for one to two years. The youngest son, Ralph, ultimately went to the hospital and requested that Abe be discharged, and Ralph drove him home. Ralph received the homestead as a reward for his loyalty to his father, Abe, and was thereafter perceived by the other siblings as their father's favorite child.

Efforts at Differentiation of Self: Develop a Hypothesis

Zach believed that if the family became less reactive to known facts about the family emotional process, the family was more likely to be able to resolve its territorial conflicts and the inheritance impasse. He wrote to each family member in generation V stating that he had the hospital records and that he was willing to meet individually with each of them to discuss the records and answer any questions they might have about them. This communication reversed the emotional polarity in the cutoff. Rather than Zach pursuing others, he hypothesized others would now want to talk with him.

Zach began to develop productive conversations with each of the surviving children of parents Abe and Betsy. Zach's uncle Lawrence said he "never got over" having to hospitalize his father, "the hardest thing he ever had to do."

Over time and with these individual interchanges, Zach could see and hear that each of the adult children had a more balanced view of the events, their parents' marriage, and their reaction to Abe and Betsy and the conflict between them. Family members also discussed with one another similar issues in their own lives and marriages. Zach was able to observe that the system became much more open and less reactive.

Efforts at Differentiation of Self: Territorial Assessments

Zach communicated personally and by letter that Generations IV and V should resolve the home and homestead problem and not "gift" the emotional or territorial problem to Generation VI. Zach repeatedly stated to all at different times that he did not care how the issue was resolved, only that the preceding generations reach agreement in how to manage their property (the homestead and land).

Although he discussed this opinion with everyone in the family, he discussed it most often with his mother, Wanda, one of Abe and Betsy's five children. Over time, Abe and Betsy's youngest son, Ralph, and oldest son, Lawrence, died, leaving the unresolved territorial problem with their children. The oldest daughter, Victoria, also died, leaving the issue to her son, Rufus.

Wanda and Elizabeth were the two surviving children in generation V. After Lawrence and Ralph died, Elizabeth replaced the oldest son, Lawrence, as the titular manager of the land. After Ralph died, the homestead lay in disrepair. Lawrence's daughter, Lucy, represented her branch of the family in discussions about the property. Lucy reported that the meetings were intense discussions between two strong-minded women, Wanda and Elizabeth. Ralph's children were only peripherally involved in the family discussions.

Wanda, Zach's mother, developed criteria for the property resolution. If possible:

1. Keep the land and homestead in the family;
2. Sell to someone in the family who could afford to restore it; and
3. Select someone seriously interested in taking care of the property.

Ralph's oldest son, George, was finally identified as the family member who best met these criteria. He now owned the home on the property and, by purchasing the land, both would be consolidated under one person. George restored the home built in 1910 to its original state and built an adjoining home for his own family.

After the homestead restoration, George invited the extended family for a weekend party and all branches of the family were represented. Evidence of more functional differentiation included the fact that family members "returned" items back to their grandparental restored home, including heirlooms and a framed copy of Abe and Betsy's wedding license.

Zach believes that the fact that Generation V was able to talk with Generation VI about the intense conflict between their parents (Generation IV) was a significant step toward everyone's being more open about the facts. The party represented the family's reuniting as an emotional group and discussing events that had separated them. The youngest son, Ralph, in Generation V had a wish to establish a memorial to his parents. His wish was accomplished not by him as an individual in conflict with his siblings, but rather by the family acting via principle and in relationship to one another.

Part II

After the resolution of the homestead impasse, Zach reports a ten-year effort anticipating and planning for the deaths and funerals of Abe and Betsy's two surviving daughters, Wanda and Elizabeth, both living beyond 100 years of age. These were the two independent-minded women who had agreed on the decision about what to do with the homestead property. This multigenerational process (between Betsy, Wanda, and Elizabeth—replicated between Wanda, Katrina, and Joanna) reflects emotional interdependency between generations and influences territorial behavior. The interdependency is evident in the territorial behavior. The reciprocity in this process may be most fluid during death and dying and in the behavior of survivors. In calm periods interdependency may appear functional. Yet the stress of death and dying can reveal the emotional fusion and conflict within emotional interdependency. The lack of emotional resolution in one generation enhances projection of the problem to the next generation.

Territorial Behavior: Predictions for Generation VI

During the ten-year period of his efforts, Zach hypothesized that if the multigenerational emotional process (between Betsy and Wanda and Elizabeth and later between Wanda and Joanna and Katrina) is accurate, conflicts over territorial behavior will occur in the next generation. Zach predicts to his mother, Wanda, that similar behavior will occur with her children in Generation VI as did with her siblings, Generation V. Wanda decided that leaving clear directives that she had consistently discussed with her children before she died might be helpful. Zach clearly told his mother that he did not wish to be the recipient of any property but only to have the best quality relationship with his mother.

Zach's Family History

Zach's family had a rather intense negative, competitive, and conflictual emotional fusion between their mother, Wanda, and her two daughters, a reflection of a similar triangle in Wanda's Generation V. Zach was an outsider in both triangles. The two sisters in Generation V, Wanda and Elizabeth, even competed as to who would live the longest and have the healthiest life. Zach was able to observe from the outside position in both triangles that he had a less intense but positive relationship with all the women in both Generations V and VI (Figure 9.2).

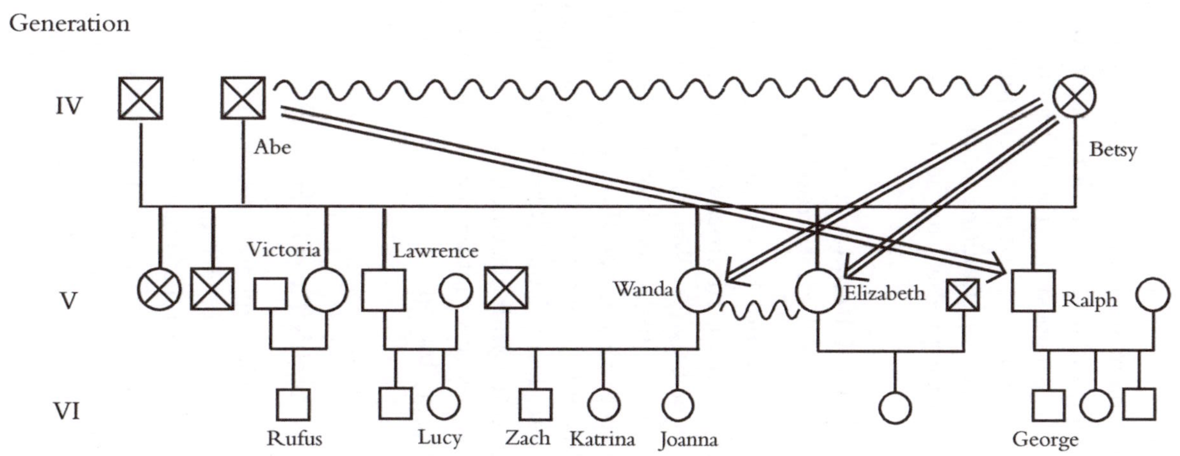

Figure 9.2 Emotional fusion, conflict, and projection in Generations IV and V

Zach's Efforts at Differentiation of Self: Prediction Based on Facts

During the last ten years of her life, Zach spoke almost daily with his mother, made biannual visits to see her, and for the last three years of Wanda's life visited every three weeks for a weekend. There were numerous discussions about long-term care planning, funeral plans, and the disposition of her personal and real property. Zach's mother established a revocable living trust into which she placed all her property, both real and personal. Upon her death, the assets were to be sold and the proceeds divided equally among her children. These wishes seemed clear.

Zach predicted conflict between his siblings after their mother's death. The prediction was based on the chronic conflictual and competitive relationship patterns established among his siblings and between each of them and their mother, Wanda. Moreover, their mother's death would present the siblings many immediate issues about which to disagree.

Zach's mother wrote a letter to Zach agreeing with his predictions of post-death conflict, and asked him to be in charge of all matters pertaining to her funeral. Zach circulated copies of Wanda's letter to his siblings. For the last ten years of her life, Zach's mother made him her medical power of attorney/health care agent.

Zach's younger sister Joanna regularly communicated and visited with her mother, Wanda. After Zach's circulation of their mother's letter, Joanna and Wanda visited Wanda's lawyer, removed all the property except the mother's house from her revocable trust, and made Joanna the person nominated to be the executor/personal representative of their mother's estate. In a lengthy letter to her older brother and sister, the younger sister opined that these changes simplified their mother's property disposition. Subsequently, after Wanda told the older daughter, Katrina, about the changed documents, Katrina informed Zach that Wanda had stated to her that she did not understand what she had been asked to do by younger daughter, Joanna.

Zach gave the benefit of the doubt to both Joanna's intentions and Katrina's comments. He concluded, probably erroneously, that the document changes and comments were just another manifestation of the sisters' historic sibling rivalry that he had observed on other

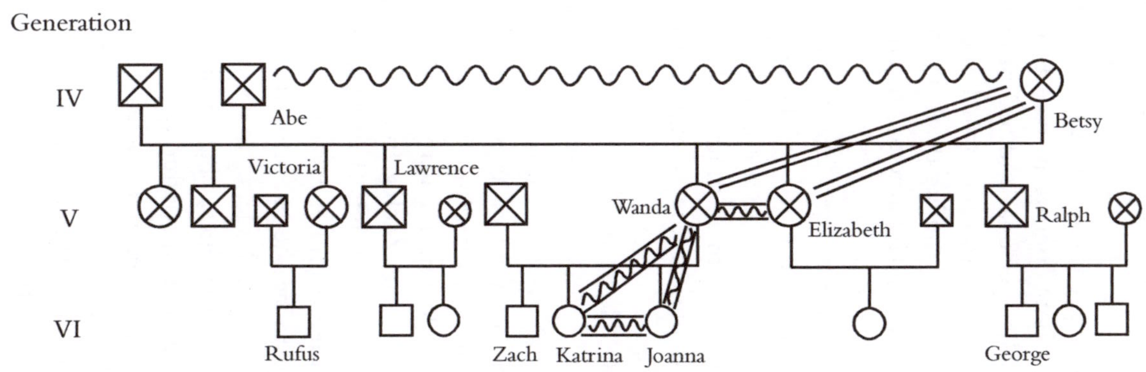

Figure 9.3 Emotional conflict, fusion, and projection in the next generation

occasions. With more time and thought, and a view from the family history perspective, Zach realized the terms of Wanda's trust had been changed after he circulated Wanda's letter putting him in charge. Zach finally recognized the intensity and purpose of Joanna's making a planned territorial move—a move that would allow her to exercise future control over all her mother's property and avoid any "supervision" by her older siblings.

Zach's Efforts at Differentiation of Self: Post-Death Behavior

At age 102, Wanda fell, broke her hip, and died within a four-day period. Joanna, the younger sister, with agreement from her siblings, arranged for cremation. They also agreed that Zach would make burial and funeral arrangements as previously expressed by their mother in the letter Zach circulated to his siblings.

Within a few days of Wanda's death, the younger sister, Joanna, announced that because she had been nominated to be the executor/personal representative of Wanda's estate, she had a plan for the disposition of all the property, and the siblings needed to sign a document agreeing to its disposition. Joanna picked a date that everyone would meet in the mother's home for implementation of Joanna's plan, and everyone agreed to meet. Zach and the other sister Katrina told Joanna that they were not willing to sign the document, citing the need for further discussion. Within the next few months Joanna:

1. Refused to attend the mother's scheduled burial service or provide her mother's ashes for burial;
2. Implemented a plan to divide the tangible personal property without making a list of the property that existed prior to the division;
3. As the trustee of the revocable trust, she sold the family home and kept the proceeds, stating that she needed to pay for a potential legal defense; and
4. Announced that she was legally entitled to keep all the mother's cash assets as she was the surviving owner of the joint checking account.

Zach observed that his younger sister moved forward with plans very quickly. He complimented her efforts and stated that it need not all be done immediately. She retorted, "Do not tell me how to grieve."

Territorial Behavior: Possession of the Ashes

Joanna announced to Zach and her sister that she would meet at the mother's house to divide the property, but could not stay for the burial. Zach stated that he expected their mother's ashes to be present for burial. Joanna said she would not provide them and would not attend the scheduled burial.

Zach clearly stated to Joanna that if she could not make the meeting date she selected, he expected that she would provide their mother's ashes. In her grief it seemed conceivable that Joanna might not be able to allow her mother to be buried.

Zach wrote to his sister, Joanna, and the funeral home saying state law provided that each of the children owned an equal share of their mother's ashes and that if the younger sister would not provide all the ashes, then the funeral home should send the other two-thirds to the burial. After a lengthy deliberation, Joanna agreed to attend her mother's burial and to bring the ashes, provided she could pick the date for the memorial service. She said that their mother's handwritten letter requesting Zach be in charge of funeral arrangements was not "a controlling legal document." She further asserted she had not promised her mother she would be cooperative with her siblings.

Territorial Behavior: Division of Property, Cash, and Real Estate

Zach and his two sisters met for five days to pack up their mother's home and divide her personal property. There was no properly prepared list of items. Jewelry, china, and silverware had disappeared.

Following the burial, Joanna, despite their mother's written wishes as to Zach's involvement, announced a date and detailed plans for their mother's memorial service. Zach decided it was emotionally more important for his sister rather than for himself to plan the memorial service. Zach knew his sister would do a good job and he chose to "cede" territory to the younger sister who had anointed herself as Mom's favorite after Mom's death.

As the substituted trustee of the revocable trust, Joanna sold the home, did not divide the proceeds in thirds as directed in Wanda's trust, and retained the cash against possible legal suits from her siblings. Two weeks after the memorial service, Joanna sent out a proposal stating that she was entitled to keep all her mother's cash. She had "given considerable thought to how her mother would designate the balance of her checking account." Her mother was deeply appreciative of her visits and care she provided to her. She planned to pay herself $20 per visit or $20,000 for the burdens that fell on her to care for her mother. She was willing to give the remainder to Zach and exclude the other sister whom she thought did not visit sufficiently. Zach, who was neutral on the distribution of property, was now placed in the middle of the sibling conflict. Zach determined that receiving the money was legal but not morally correct. Doing nothing was taking a side.

Efforts at Differentiation of Self: Establish a Hypothesis

Zach was witnessing an emotional quagmire as exemplified by Joanna's territorial behavior, among other things. He believed he had been neutral about the division of property but now he had been thrust into the middle of the sibling conflict. He surmised that Joanna saw herself as the underappreciated youngest. She perceived herself as having assumed most of the burden in caring for Wanda. This position emotionally resonated with the one that occurred when her siblings went off to college and Wanda returned to finish two years of college and was away during the week. Joanna perceived that Wanda left *her* with a directive to care for her father.

Her father was in good health, owed his own business, was the trustee of a local bank, and served on the city council among other civic organizations. He died ten years later after a short illness. Underappreciated and feeling abandoned, Joanna perceived herself to be in the center of the family emotional system. Joanna appeared to have the least sense of resolution about the relationship with Wanda, her mother, who had predicted to Zach that Joanna would have the most difficulty with her death.

Joanna had managed to assign herself as the person in charge of her mother's personal affairs, get the majority of the personal property, propose keeping most of the cash assets, and refuse to disburse the trust assets to her siblings.

Zach's Efforts at Differentiation: Develop a Plan

Zach soon determined that his efforts to work with his sisters were futile. Zach's repeatedly saying yes to Joanna's proposals brought further conflict over a newly manufactured set of details.

Zach understood this process as the reversal of the projection process. Joanna was now engaging in territorial behavior to rewrite her emotional place in the family. She was placing herself in the center of family conflict, and was in a position to dictate the results of the territorial behavior. All of this behavior was justified under the guise of carrying out her perception of her mother's wishes. This behavior is similar to Ralph's in memorializing her place in the family in relationship to a parent, as Ralph had done.

Zach was determined to step outside the process. He had no interest in the personal property, but that may have served only as a red flag to make the sisters work harder to involve him as they managed to do. After becoming bogged down in his family impasse, Zach proposed three options, any of which were acceptable to him. He acknowledged that Joanna had been nominated but not been legally designated by their mother's will to be the personal representative of the estate.

Zach believed the sister who had claimed the estate distribution territory had not behaved in a responsible fiduciary manner. Zach told her that 1) she could start over and make a proper inventory and arrange for distribution in a fair and equitable manner, 2) the family could hire a neutral person to do it, or 3) she could file probate and have the court appoint someone. The decision was hers. None of these alternatives were acceptable to Joanna. To Zach it appeared that Joanna's goal was continuing the disagreements, prolonging her place in the center of the conflict and therefore exercising domain over the most important sibling territory. None of this behavior appeared to be resolving grief.

Zach and his older sister, Katrina, had no interest in further conflict over property. They drafted an agreement giving half the cash to

Joanna, dividing the proceeds of the house equally, and allowing her to keep all the property she had taken but returning copies of important family documents and photographs to share with Zach and Katrina. The agreement signed by Zach and Katrina indemnified all three from any legal suits against each other. Zach and Katrina signed the agreement and sent it to Joanna. They further stated they were not willing to engage in any more discussions or negotiations about the matter.

Joanna refused to sign the agreement. In essence Joanna refused to accept yes as an answer. Over the next six months Joanna sent four different ultimatums with timelines. If Zach and Katrina did not sign her revised document by a certain time, she was taking further specified action. One demand followed another. Zach and Katrina never responded.

After several months Joanna implemented most items in the Zach and Katrina proposal, while still refusing to agree to it or sign it. Joanna retained a sum of money stating the need to ensure against a potential lawsuit from either of her siblings. This sum was approximately equal to the amount she thought she should be paid for the alleged "extra" caretaking of Wanda, their mother.

Zach and Katrina were not willing to engage in any more discussions or negotiations about the matter. After another 18-month period of limited superficial communications and no negotiations, Joanna proposed an equal distribution of the retained money with a mutual hold-harmless agreement. Both Joanna and Zach signed the agreement; however, Katrina, despite knowing the terms of the proposed agreement, was either unable or unwilling to open the letter containing the agreement.

At this point there were two virtually identical agreements: the one proposed by Joanna which she and Zach had signed and the one Katrina and Zach had proposed and signed. Neither sister was willing or able to sign the agreement proposed by the other sister despite their being virtually identical agreements. Zach had signed both of them.

Zach wrote to both sisters saying:

> Under our circumstances I think the proposal is a way to deal with the remaining money. I have signed the proposal and forwarded it to the lawyer. I thank both of you for your efforts in working on this issue. I look forward to getting beyond

> dividing up the money and hope we can resolve in the future other issues important to each of us.
>
> I know this process has been very difficult for all of us. I am certain that you have found me, or my behavior, to be a problem for each of you at various times. If I have offended you, I ask for your forgiveness so that our relationships can move forward.

Zach anticipated one of two reactions from his sisters. Either they would be angry and say, "No way, you SOB. I am not going to agree" or "Yes, it is sensible to acknowledge our agreement and move on to other issues." Instead, neither sister responded to him or to one another. There was once again in the family total verbal silence, which probably reflected emotional impasse or paralysis!

This polarization was precisely what Zach and Wanda, his mother, had feared and predicted 15 years earlier based on family emotional process. The lack of resolution in the property agreement parallels the lack of emotional resolution in the original parental triangle between Wanda and her daughters, Katrina and Joanna. Three years following Wanda's death, her children had reached the earlier described rigid emotional triangle. All three agreed on the territorial disposition, but the two sisters were unable emotionally to implement the agreement. Zach had signed documents produced by each sister, but the sisters remained unable to accept each other's document.

Observations: Ongoing Nodal Events in the Extended Family System

Well-differentiated directives regarding one's death and funeral can plan only so far into the future. Wanda, in Generation V, made significant efforts in her relationships and estate planning. She wanted to avoid in her own estate for Generation VI the problems passed down to her and her siblings from Generation IV with the homestead property. The family projection process, the lack of emotional resolution of a relationship, and post-death emotional interdependency can interfere with the best of plans.

In the three years following the deaths of two women, Wanda and Elizabeth, the larger extended family worked on two family celebrations. The first was a celebration of the lives of the five siblings (Victoria, Lawrence, Wanda, Elizabeth, and Ralph) in Generation V. The second was a civic celebration in Katrina, Zach, and Joanna's hometown for Wanda and her husband.

Generation VI survivors planned a large extended family reunion at the homestead now owned and refurbished by Ralph's oldest son. The extended family met at the homestead for a weekend and planted five different trees commemorating the lives of each of the five siblings, their parents, in Generation V. More than one member of each branch of the family was present. Zach brought his children and grandchildren. Despite six months' advance notice of the celebration, Zach's sisters Katrina and Joanna did not attend. Joanna sent a speech to a cousin to be read at the tree planting ceremony but the trees were planted in silence as the cousins and Zach agreed that words would not improve the ceremony. The larger extended family gathered with a remarkable absence of anxiety and friction despite the degree of emotional turmoil apparently confined to the Wanda family triangle.

One year later there was a public ceremony in Wanda's hometown honoring civic contributions by Wanda and her husband, among others, over the prior 60 years. Zach made certain his siblings and all his extended family were notified months in advance. He invited his children and grandchildren, and some were able to attend. Extended family made efforts to attend, and all sent greetings. Neither Katrina nor Joanna attended or communicated about the event.

While attending the ceremony honoring his parents, Zach visited the family home sold three years earlier to a young schoolteacher. Pleased with the changes made, he asked permission to photograph them. The new owner also gave him notes that his mother had left around the house to remind herself of tasks. Zach sent photos to his sisters with a description of the celebration honoring their parents. One sister wrote, "I am so grateful mother is not alive to see what this man did to her house." The other sister said she could not bear to open and look at the photos.

The Future

Although the siblings in Generation V sold the homestead land, they all individually maintained the mineral rights. Over 100 years after acquisition of the homestead now owed by Ralph's son, he made a well-informed decision to drill for oil. The prospect of discovering oil had the potential to ignite regressive territorial behavior. He performed all the necessary seismographic and geological testing and shared the information with everyone. He made it clear that everyone would share both information and profits.

One of Zach's cousins said, "Let us hope our generation learns from those before us, on what NOT to do when it comes to oil." Another said, "The anger and disappointment our parents felt is long in the past. I just wanted to share the information that I have and do not begrudge any family anything that might come their way."

Results

The management of territory and possessions reflects level of differentiation pre- and post-death and is often solid evidence of the emotional level of resolution in a relationship. The good news: When the larger system is together in a family celebration or decision making, there is less emotional reactivity. Attendees at celebrations may be self-selected for a lower level of reactivity. Nonattendees may stay away as a function of higher levels of emotional reactivity or more emotionally unresolved family relationships. The regressive polarized territorial behavior in the Wanda nuclear family appears to occur in other branches of the family. When it surfaces, however, it remains confined around issues emotionally important to that specific nuclear family. Emotional contagion between branches is reduced. Every individual family member could learn from observing the functioning of the larger extended family.

The not-so-good news: As is clear from the latest conflict in Zach's family, in which the younger sister refused to sign and Zach and Katrina haven't yielded, there is no conclusion to this story. This impasse is a characteristic of family emotional process. The family continues, and although most of the property is distributed, the remainder sits . . . for now. We will see what the next generation brings.

The elements of Bowen theory abound: Money, property, and family objects play a large part in the emotional process after a death in the family. Variation in differentiation of self manifests itself in multigenerational family and nuclear family emotional process, projection process to children, emotional distance and cutoff, and sibling triangles. These mechanisms are significant factors in the manifestation of emotional fallout after death in families. Territorial behavior is one important clinical tool for the assessment of this emotional process.

Conclusion

At the death or disappearance of a nuclear family member, the management of territory and possessions reflect level of differentiation pre- and post-death. It is also evidence of the level of emotional resolution in a relationship. Unresolved grief and unresolved emotional relationships can lead to complicated interactions. Families and individuals do not uniformly resolve these relationships.

III

CHRONIC ILLNESS IN THE THERAPIST'S OWN FAMILY

10

A SYSTEMS VIEW OF CHRONIC ILLNESS IN A SPOUSE AND FAMILY

Eileen B. Gottlieb

Introduction

The purpose of this chapter is to explore a systems view of chronic illness. It will focus on three ideas derived from Bowen family systems theory in the effort to understand the origin, expression, and impact of chronic illness on the family. First, systems theory provides a broader view of chronic illness than a cause-and-effect, individual, symptom-focus perspective, which includes the relationship system and the family emotional process. Second, systems theory views chronic illness as a multigenerational process with origins observable in preceding generations long before the actual expression of the disease. Finally, systems theory suggests that chronic illness may be unpreventable and the management of the relationships around it is significant to the next generation.

Bowen theory views chronic illness as derived from the family emotional process and also considers how relationships influence individual behavior. Togetherness forces bind family members together as well as drive them apart. The intensity of the togetherness process interacts with chronic anxiety to create patterns of emotional functioning that automatically regulate the behavior of individual family members. Over time these patterns become repetitive and fixed, resulting in a reciprocity whereby one person overfunctions and the other underfunctions. This reciprocity is more pronounced in an anxious emotional field in the face of challenges, which exceed the capacity of the family to adapt. Each family member plays a part in the emotional process that results in the impairment of one family member. Through a series of interlocking triangles, anxiety and emotional reactivity can be passed from one family member to the other, with consequences for all. The two-against-one nature of the triangle calms the insiders and does in the outsider in an effort to manage the chronic anxiety that drives the system. This process, while observable, operates outside the awareness of the family until such time as someone begins to recognize and address it. In the case of chronic illness, this is usually long after the symptoms have been expressed.

From the perspective of Bowen theory, the solution to this dilemma is the development of self-awareness and self-regulation within each individual that directs him to be responsible for his own functioning as well as a resource to the others. It is a delicate balance between individuality and togetherness. The ability of the family to strike this balance and improve its functioning, especially in times of extraordinary challenge, plays a part in the viability of the system.

Living for ten years with a chronically ill family member has given this author the opportunity to observe the family emotional process, to see her part in it, and to find ways to manage herself effectively in the key triangles that contribute to this problem. It has been a difficult but enlightening journey.

While she has become clearer as to her part in this process, she still works to manage herself in a manner consistent with the principles of differentiation of self with the belief that this is a way through the dilemma of chronic illness and premature death.

This chapter is an attempt to present what the author has learned to date about chronic illness as a family emotional process and the questions that still persist in her effort to stand with the family and lead through unchartered terrain with Bowen theory as her guide. She will present her observations of the family relationships as they have evolved since the onset of symptoms in the impaired member, as well as the multigenerational context in which they developed. Nodal events, facts of functioning, patterns of relationship management, and triangles will be emphasized. Finally, attention will be given to the value of differentiation of self in the management of chronic illness and the observable difference it may make to the functioning of succeeding generations.

Systems Thinking Versus Individual Thinking About Chronic Illness

Chronic illness is viewed very differently from a system thinking point of view than from an individual perspective. Systems thinking views chronic illness as a derivative of the family emotional process. The family is observed to be an emotional unit, characterized by functional interdependence, and influenced by competing forces for togetherness and individuality. Emotional reactivity and triangles play a part in symptom development. Systems thinking considers the interaction of chronic anxiety, level of differentiation, and patterns of relationship management in the expression of chronic illness. The functional position of the most projected-upon family member in the key triangles is considered to be a factor in vulnerability to disease and chronic illness. This family emotional process is believed to be multigenerational. Evidence of similar relationship patterns can be seen in previous generations. One such pattern observable in chronic illness is an overfunctioning/underfunctioning reciprocity that contributes to a learned helplessness in the impaired one. Chronic illness is one outcome of emotional distance and a closed emotional system that contributes to fewer viable relationships as resources for effective engagement of life challenges and problems.

Systems thinking takes a broad view of man and his evolutionary heritage, a product of nature, governed by its laws and principles. In individual thinking, man is viewed as unique, separate from the natural world, and unrelated to his evolutionary heritage and the broader emotional process that governs living systems.

Individual thinking views chronic illness as a derivative of the individual. The problem is seen as existing in one of genetic, organic, or hereditary factors. It is believed to be the outcome of the interaction between the individual and a set of stressors emerging at a point in time. Chronic illness from this perspective focuses on the symptoms in the individual and the appropriate remedies, including medication and surgery. No consideration is given to the role of the relationship system in the development and expression of the problem over multiple generations.

Family Emotional Process

The interaction among level of differentiation, chronic anxiety, and the multigenerational process plays a part in the expression of chronic illness. Chronic anxiety, the basic and functional capacity to manage self, and the generational patterns of relationship management, all play a part in this process. Families with more chronic anxiety, a lower level of differentiation, and a high degree of emotional fusion are more likely to experience chronic illness in a family member.

Emotional fusion is a process in nature. It functions to bond organisms together for purposes of reproduction and survival. The intensity of fusion affects its role in symptom development. Intensity characterized by significant emotional reactivity contributes to an anxious emotional field. Variation exists in the degree to which unresolved emotional attachment, or fusion, plays out in the expression of chronic symptoms in a family member.

The greater the degree of emotional fusion, the lower the level of differentiation and the more chronic illness can emerge. Fusion drives the relationship process when an anxious focus on one family member relieves the anxiety of the rest at the expense of the other. An emotionally reactive family projects anxiety to its most vulnerable member. This is usually one who gives up most self to the family and absorbs the family problem at cost to him or her. The symptomatic family member protects the family from chronic anxiety.

With chronic anxiety coming to rest in one, others are freer of the problem and are thus able to function more for self. Those family members are able to pursue their own life goals with less involvement in the family dilemma. They appear to be higher functioning than the impaired one. However, observations of this process point to the degree of interdependence that underlies this pattern.

The family is an emotional unit. Reciprocity protects some family members and disables others. Both overfunctioner and underfunctioner contribute to the family problem, including the development and expression of acute and chronic disease. The greater the degree of emotional interdependence, or emotional fusion, the more likely individual behavior is less differentiated and more relationship driven. Ultimately, one party in the relationship takes on the more dominant functioning position reciprocated by the other being more subordinate. Both functioning positions are expressions of the reciprocal nature of the relationship.

Triangles both calm and undermine the relationship system. Involvement of a third party in the relationship between two temporarily calms the system at the expense of the other in the triangle. The more fixed the positions in the triangle, the less flexibility in the system, which results in patterns of functioning driven by the anxiety and emotional fusion in the relationships.

Variation in vulnerability to chronic illness is observable at a point in time as well as across time. A more anxious family member interacts with stress to increase vulnerability in the moment. Repeated patterns of managing the anxiety associated with a person's position in the triangle are observable across the generations. The family member who relinquishes more self to the family than is available to manage himself is the most likely candidate for a chronic illness.

A more anxious family produces more symptoms such as chronic illness with limited recovery. The level of chronic anxiety adds to the susceptibility to stress and impairment over time. Chronic anxiety is the outcome of too much emotional fusion that inclines family members to function less independently. The less responsibility each takes for himself or herself, the more anxiety for all. The family as an emotional unit can both increase and decrease anxiety in each member.

Chronic illness reflects a multigenerational process that is rooted in triangles in previous generations. Examination of family emotional process across generations reveals the function triangles play in the impairment of a family member. An anxious system in contact with a neutral third party lowers anxiety and affects functional level of differentiation. A calm, neutral, and objective person who relates to each side of the triangle without taking sides becomes a resource to the family struggling to manage itself.

Definitions

To summarize, chronic illness can be defined as a long-term physical, emotional, or behavioral disability that severely undermines functioning. It can be irreversible, degenerative, and progressive, and in some cases may lead to permanent incapacitation and/or premature death.

Bowen (1978) defined differentiation of self as follows:

> The concept of differentiation of self is important. At the more differentiated end of the scale is the person who can "know" with his intellect, and who can also "know" or "be aware of," or "feel" the situation with his emotional system. He has reasonable ability to keep an operational differentiation

> between intellect and emotions and to take action on the fact of intellectual reasoning, which opposes his feelings and the truth of subjectivity.
>
> (p. 441)

Chronic anxiety can be defined as *that which one imagines may be* as opposed to *that* which *is actual in real time.* It is acquired from previous generations and from anxiety present in one's own family. According to Gilbert (2004) in *The Eight Concepts of Bowen Theory*, chronic anxiety summons the outer cells of the adrenal gland, or cortex, secreting cortical stress hormones and setting into motion "cascades" of other hormonal secretions and effects, including anti-allergic and anti-inflammatory processes (p. 8).

The Process of Chronic Illness: What? How? Where? When?

Bowen wrote (1978):

> Systems theory attempts to focus on the functional *facts* of relationships. It focuses on what happened, how it happened, and when and where it happened, insofar as these observations are based on fact. It carefully avoids man's automatic preoccupation with why it happened.
>
> (p. 261)

What is the emotional field in which chronic illness develops? The emotional field that breeds chronic illness includes the following: 1) high degree of chronic anxiety, 2) low level of differentiation, 3) high degree of emotional fusion, 4) multigenerational pattern of overfunctioning/underfunctioning reciprocity, and 5) projection of anxiety onto a particular family member.

Bowen (1978) defines a family system as:

> The family *is* a system in that a change in the functioning of one family member is automatically followed by the compensatory change in another family member.
>
> (pp. 154–155)

Bowen (1978) provides an example of overfunctioning/underfunctioning:

> For instance, the underfunctioning of a family member who is temporarily ill will be automatically compensated [for] by the other family members who overfunction until the sick one recovers. If the sick one becomes chronically or permanently disabled, the overfunctioning of the others becomes a long-term imbalance in the family.
>
> (p. 260)

According to Bowen theory this is how chronic illness comes to be: 1) anxious focus is projected upon a vulnerable family member, 2) the most projected-upon functional position in key triangles plays a part in vulnerability, 3) fixed interlocking triangles permit other family members to operate as if they are outside the problem, 4) emotional distance exacerbates the process, and 5) the projected-upon member becomes isolated from the rest of the system.

Kerr (Kerr & Bowen, 1988) wrote:

> Chronic symptoms are more likely to be a feature of poorly differentiated relationships, because the lower the level of differentiation, the more prone *both* spouses are to accommodate to the presence of chronic dysfunction rather than to address the underlying process that creates dysfunction. A harmonious "togetherness" can exist between an overfunctioning spouse and a dysfunctional spouse, but there actually tends to be more emotional distance in a marriage with chronic symptoms than in one without chronic symptoms. Greater distance exists in relationships with chronic dysfunction because for relationships to get to that point, the emotional sensitivities of people must be fairly great and the list of issues to be avoided must be fairly long.
>
> (p. 175)

According to Bowen theory the context in which chronic illness is more likely to occur involves the following: 1) a chronically anxious family, 2) an emotionally reactive family, 3) an emotionally cutoff family, 4) a multigenerational pattern of dysfunction in a spouse, and 5) projection on to a child.

Kerr (Kerr & Bowen, 1988) wrote in *Family Evaluation* about the role of the family emotional process in symptom development:

> Chronic symptoms are associated with long-term disturbances. Symptoms are rooted in the undifferentiated togetherness aspects of human functioning. In other words, the more members of a relationship system function *in reaction* to one another, the more likely someone in the system will get into a position emotionally that impairs his functioning.
>
> (p. 256)

According to Bowen theory the process that contributes to the expression of chronic illness in a family member involves 1) fixed and persistent triangles, 2) unawareness of the part family members play in the process, 3) a family perceptual framework of the impaired member that governs the manner in which they interact with him, each other and in which he reacts to them, and 4) a family inability to adapt to existing challenges without projection onto another family member. Kerr (Kerr & Bowen, 1988) wrote:

> A disturbance in the relationship balance of an emotional system, both within an individual and within his relationship system, can trigger the development of symptoms.
>
> (p. 256)

Undifferentiation is the fundamental emotional process that interacts with chronic anxiety in the face of environmental challenges to undercut functioning. The greater the degree of emotional fusion and the higher the level of chronic anxiety, the more reciprocity governs the relationship system. This process results in functioning that is regulated more by the individual's position in relationship to the other than his capacity to think for self and act on the courage of his convictions. Lack of differentiation in the face of environmental challenge contributes to the togetherness process. Decisions are driven by the anxiety and uncertainty of the group at the expense of the individual. He or she is unable to stand up to the demands of the system and succumbs to the pressure to be for the others. The combination of a failure to define self and extraordinary stressors over time can evolve into chronic illness.

What is the role of "functional helplessness" in the expression of chronic illness? Bowen (1978), in his paper on family psychotherapy, discusses the issue of "functional helplessness" and the importance of finding a family leader:

> In my opinion these families are not really helpless. They are functionally helpless. The parents are adequate, resourceful people in their outside relationships. It is in relationship to each other that they become functionally helpless. When the family is able to be a contained unit, and there is a family leader with motivation to define the problem and to back his own convictions in taking appropriate action, the family can change from a directionless, anxiety-ridden, floundering unit, to a more resourceful organism with a problem to be solved. (p. 56)

Family History

Mr. and Mrs. G met when he was 21 and she was 16 years old (Figure 10.1). They were introduced by her younger brother, who was working as a lifeguard at a swimming pool that Mr. G was managing during summer break from college. They remained friends through both of their first marriages, each of which ended in divorce after ten years, his in 1972 and hers in 1980. They began their courtship during her separation and married the day after her divorce was finalized. Their attachment was intense and interdependent, as were their relationships with their former spouses, parents, and siblings.

He had a son born in 1969 and she a daughter in 1973 and a son born in 1978. They spent the first year of their relationship living together with her children in his home, with joint custody of his child who moved between his parents' homes. A year later they married and moved with her children to the state she had been living in before her divorce, closer to her children's father, but farther from Mr. G's son. Mr. G left his entire extended family and lived close to her family until his death. His son did relocate for college to the state where his father

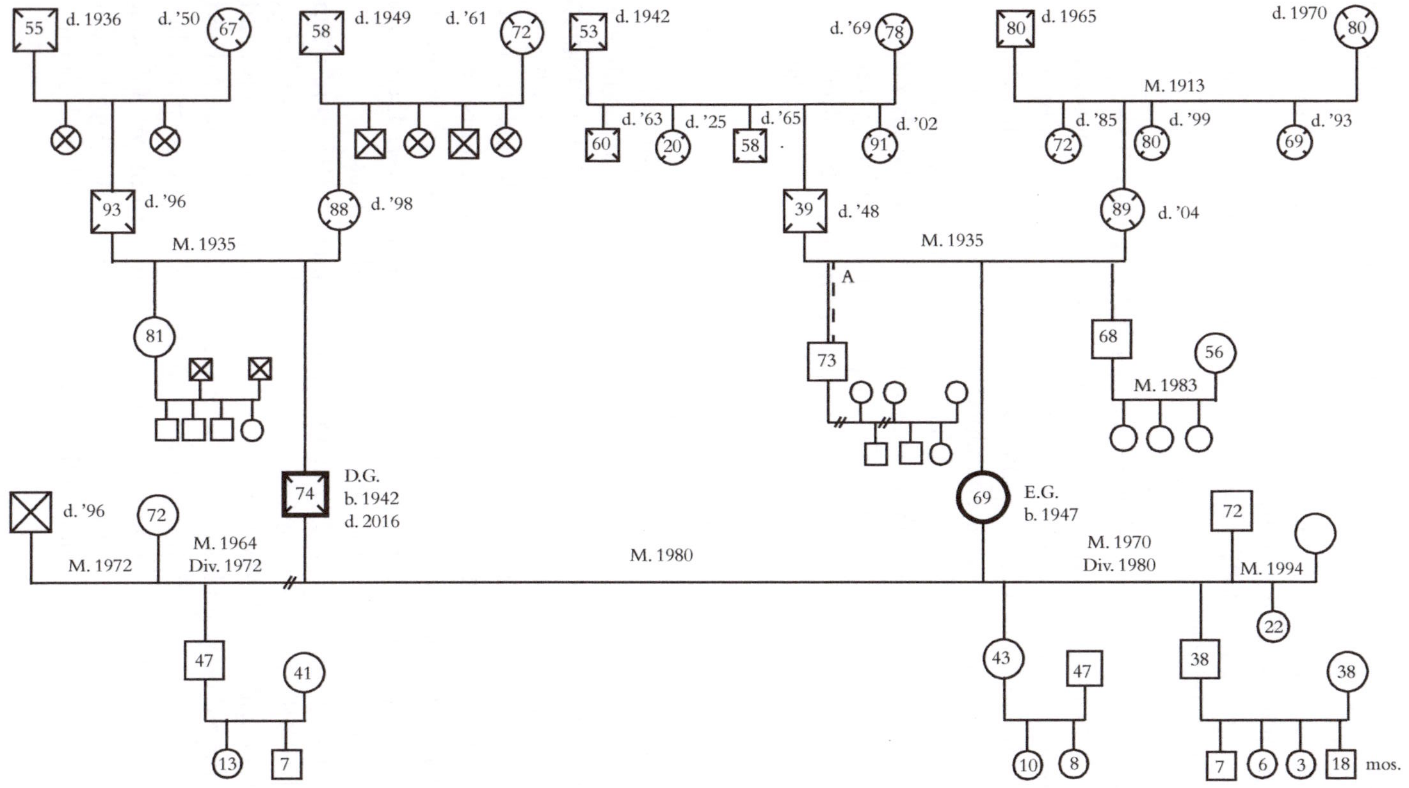

Figure 10.1 G family diagram

resided, closer to his stepmother, stepsister, and brother and remained there after his marriage and the birth of his children.

Mr. G was the youngest of two children with a sister, seven years older. His parents were married for 62 years. His father was the middle child and only son of Eastern European immigrants who resided in Brooklyn. The marriage was distant with periods of conflict, characterized by an overadequate/underadequate reciprocity in which the husband displayed physical, emotional, and behavioral symptoms, ultimately predeceasing his wife by 14 years.

Mr. G's father joined the Coast Guard at age 14 and sent money home to help support his mother and two sisters. He eventually married, retired from the Coast Guard, and took a position in the government close to where his wife's family resided, raised their children, and retired there. Mr. G's mother was the oldest daughter of five children whose parents immigrated from Eastern Europe and resided in Washington, DC. The marriage was distant but harmonious with focus on the children, especially the oldest and youngest daughters. Mr. G, his sister, and mother lived together with his maternal grandparents during his father's time at sea and throughout WWII.

Mr. G became very close to his maternal grandfather until he died prematurely in 1949, 12 years prior to his wife. Both of Mr. G's parents were emotionally important to their mothers as he was to his mother before her death in 1998 from dementia. A case can be made for how a distant marriage, managed through a focused-upon child, existed and intensified from one generation to the next. This pattern may have played a part in his loss of self and in his susceptibility to chronic illness.

Mrs. G is the middle child and only daughter with an older and younger brother. Her older brother was adopted at birth after her parents were unable to conceive in the early years of their marriage. Four years after the adoption, two births occurred, 18 months apart.

Mrs. G's father was the fourth of five children, two older brothers and an older and younger sister. His parents emigrated from Eastern Europe and settled in Baltimore. His father emigrated before World War I, leaving his family to manage for themselves for nine years. The separation intensified the relationship between his wife and children, particularly the older sons, who helped protect and provide for the younger son and daughter. The older daughter died in childbirth prior to her father's departure for the United States. Mrs. G's father predeceased his mother by 23 years. She remained deeply attached to her children, who always looked after her throughout their lives. Mrs. G's father had a history of heart disease and high blood pressure from his young adult years. He smoked, was overweight, and worked very long hours, seven days a week as a pharmacist in several drug stores that he owned. Mrs. G's father died of a cerebral hemorrhage at the age of 39, leaving his wife, age 32, with three children under the age of 4. At the time of his death, he and his wife had relocated to Washington, DC, bringing her entire family from Baltimore over a ten-year period while his family remained in Baltimore. Over time he saw them less frequently while becoming very involved with his wife's family until his death.

Mrs. G's mother was the second of four daughters whose parents both emigrated from Eastern Europe when they were children. They met as young adults in Baltimore where they married and lived. They relocated to Washington, DC, after the marriages of their two eldest daughters to pharmacists who had been fraternity brothers in college.

Mrs. G's mother was deeply attached to her parents who had always struggled financially during her childhood, with her father frequently unemployed and having to move when they were unable to pay their rent. Her mother left high school in 11th grade to take a job in an effort to help provide for her parents and younger sisters. At 19 she met her husband, age 26, and shortly after his graduation from pharmacy school, they eloped before leaving Baltimore for Washington, DC. Over the course of her life Mrs. G's mother remained devoted to her parents and siblings, always contributing her time and resources to ensure their well-being, as her husband had done for her family before his untimely death. As a single parent she struggled and succeeded financially, supporting three children, one with significant emotional issues who left the family at age 21 never to return.

Mrs. G and her younger brother remained very connected to each other and their mother until her death in 2004, 55 years after her husband's death. Mrs. G, like her mother, relocated after her second marriage to live in proximity to her mother. From childhood throughout her life, the relationship between mother and daughter was harmonious and intense, perhaps the most influential of both their lives. As with Mr. G, a case can be made for the role of a distant marriage and child-focus as primary forces in the intense emotional process over several generations that played out in her family of origin and both marriages.

The marriage between Mr. and Mrs. G could be characterized as distant, with alternating periods of harmony and conflict and the development over time of an overfunctioning/underfunctioning reciprocity resulting in physical symptoms in Mr. G, culminating in his ten-year chronic illness and premature death at age 74. Mrs. G, at 70, lives independently; still works at her profession; is self-supporting; and is closely connected to their children, eight grandchildren, and extended family. She has assumed the leadership of her family in the aftermath of his death, and the family appears cohesive, strong, and resilient. Time will tell.

Facts of Functioning

2005 Mr. G has accident on spinning bike.
Peripheral neuropathy diagnosed.
Chronic pain.
Medication.

2009 Mr. G loses ability to walk without poles.
Dismissed from teaching position.
Begins substitute teaching.
Nine months later removed from list.

2010 Pain management.
Medication.
Implants.
Surgery.
Physical therapy.
Alternative medicine.
Multiple specialists.

2012 Access long-term care.
Aide four hours per day.

2013 Walker.
Wheelchair.
Bedridden.
Diminished eyesight.
Falls.

2014 Eldercare attorney.

Qualified for government assistance for additional care at home or eventual placement in care facility.

Awaiting evaluation and assignment to waiting list based on necessity.

Cost to be shared by government and long-term insurance.

Protection of family assets to secure support of spouse.

Mr. G referred to hospice for evaluation.

Declared nonterminal and sent to full skill nursing at end of October.

Difficulty adjusting for first six weeks. Depression, suicidal thoughts, problems with caregivers and roommate. Change of room and decision to seek help with eyesight and pursue a change of facility improves disposition and functioning.

2015 Mr. G takes himself on Palm Tran (public transportation for disabled) to Baskin Palmer Eye Institute for evaluation and treatment of loss of sight. Correction is achieved which permits him to read with improved prescription glasses and a patch.

Mr. G takes himself on the Palm Tran again to tour Morse Geriatric Center and decides this is where he will be most comfortable.

Family and eldercare attorney assist with application for government assistance and admission to the new facility.

Acceptance held up by psychiatric evaluation done in early November when Mr. G was diagnosed with bipolar personality disorder with no follow-up since.

Family requests follow-up psychiatric evaluation as well as interviews with current nurses and caregivers regarding his functioning three months post admission.

Psychiatrist deems him a “miracle” entirely appropriate and fit to manage well in new facility and agrees it is a better fit for him.

Admitted to Morse Geriatric Center on March 9, 2015.

Reads, attends religious services, interacts with fellow residents and staff, takes pleasure in eating, physical therapy, rest, and sleep.

Speaks daily to family and friends. Welcomes visitors.

Arranges own transportation on Palm Tran to Liam Joseph Rubin's bris, doctors' appointments outside facility, and other family events.

Teaching Hebrew to 25 residents, some of whom wish to prepare for bar and bat mitzvah in their 80s and 90s.

Learns to use iPad for communicating to family and friends as well as writing projects.

2016 Mr. G teaches Judaic studies weekly at the Morse Geriatric Center.

Despite his increasing chronic pain and progressive physical deterioration he manages, with help, to get from bed to wheelchair to teach whoever shows up for class. Some students sleep through his lessons and discussions but he persists. "I just keep talking, even if no one is awake!"

On January 23, 2016, Mr. G travels in wheelchair and van 75 miles each way to be present at the bat mitzvah of his eldest grandchild. As his condition worsens he continues to accept visitors, read, converse, think, write, and openly discuss his condition and the fact of his death. He discusses with his wife plans for his funeral, including who will speak, what music will be played, and what to do about burial or cremation. At the end of one such conversation he remarks, "It sounds so exciting I hate to miss it!"

Mr. G dies on May 8, 2016, following 16 hours in an unconscious state surrounded by family. The family, individually and collectively, organizes his funeral and cremation in accordance with his conversations with each family member. They support one another emotionally, financially, and physically. Everyone does his part. There are no disagreements, tense moments, or unpleasant encounters. It is exactly as Mr. G wanted it to be and consistent with the example he set during the ten years of his impairment and decline. The communication between family members is person-to-person, thoughtful, and open. The family appears to be a more cohesive, efficient, mature emotional system with no indication of significant symptoms in any member.

Nodal Events

It is important to note that during the 15-year period leading up to Mr. G's chronic illness and death there were many significant nodal events, including the death of both of Mr. G's parents, the death of Mrs. G's mother, the marriages of both of her children, the birth of eight grandchildren, and Mrs. G's diagnosis of acinic cellular carcinoma of the parotid gland.

Managing Self in Key Triangles

The triangles involving their siblings, children, extended family, and friends became opportunities to manage self through principles of differentiation of self.

Bowen emphasized the observation of one's part in the triangle, ability to maintain person-to-person relationships, and capacity to be neutral in the relationships between the others. Over the course of Mr. G's chronic illness, the usefulness of these ideas became more apparent as the level of anxiety diminished and the communication between family members became more open despite Mr. G's declining condition and ultimate premature death.

In an effort to manage the key triangles in her family, both during the ten years of Mr. G's chronic illness and in the aftermath of his death, Mrs. G developed a list of principles based on Bowen theory. Judging from the manner in which the family handled his illness and his death, they appear to have made a difference in the overall functioning of the family.

Bowen (1978) described three principles for defining a self: *person-to-person relationships; becoming a better observer and controlling one's own emotional reactiveness; and detriangling self from emotional situations* (pp. 541–543).

Mrs. G found the following 20 principles helpful for her and the family in dealing with the lengthy chronic illness and eventual death of Mr. G:

1. Observe self;
2. Seek clarity of thought and position;
3. Distinguish fact from emotional reactivity;

4. Work toward emotional neutrality;
5. Person-to-person communication;
6. Be present;
7. Stand beside but not in the way of the other;
8. Determine real from imagined needs of self and other;
9. Assist when asked, if necessary and possible;
10. Ask for assistance when necessary and possible;
11. Stay in contact;
12. Communicate facts;
13. Contain feelings;
14. Focus on functioning;
15. Set goals;
16. Determine a direction;
17. Evaluate progress;
18. Make adjustments as needed;
19. Address the immediate;
20. Maintain a broad perspective.

Conclusion

A systems view of chronic illness extends the lens beyond the focus on the individual symptoms and cause-and-effect thinking. It considers the broad emotional field in which the illness develops with particular emphasis on the family emotional process. The functional position of the individual in relationship to the family is observed to play a part in the vulnerability of certain people to chronic illness. It is not the nature of the relationships that causes impairment, but it is in a relationship context that impairment occurs. A more emotionally fused family generates a higher degree of chronic anxiety that must ultimately be managed within the relationships in patterns that are observable over the generations. Intense relationship patterns interacting with the challenges of life may contribute to the expression of chronic illness in a more vulnerable family member.

Chronic illness and in some cases, premature death, may be predictable and unpreventable. An understanding of the multigenerational emotional process that operates across time, outside of awareness, but is observable upon examination, may provide the facts necessary to inform the family of its part in this problem. An ability to take responsibility for one's part in this process opens avenues of cooperation and solution not otherwise available in an anxious, uninformed, closed system.

Finally, a broader understanding of the role of the family in the development and expression of chronic illness is a way to ensure the viability of the next generation as it prepares to face its share of stressors and life challenges. The ability to take on the responsibility for one's own life as well as be present to the family increases the potential for effective problem solving in the generation to come. Ultimately the family unit is only as strong as its weakest member. The stronger each member, the more viable the unit, and thus more of a resource in times of extraordinary challenge.

REFERENCES

Bowen, M. (1978). *Family therapy in clinical practice.* New York, NY: Jason Aronson.

Gilbert, R. M. (2004). *The eight concepts of Bowen theory.* Falls Church, VA: Leading Systems Press.

Kerr, M. E., & Bowen, M. (1988). *Family evaluation: An approach based on Bowen theory.* New York, NY: W. W. Norton.

11

UNRESOLVED EMOTIONAL ATTACHMENTS IN A FAMILY WITH CHRONIC ILLNESS AND DEATH

Selden Dunbar Illick

> *Few human events provide as much emotional impact as serious illness and death in resolving unresolved emotional attachments.*
> (Bowen, 1978, p. 331)

Bowen observed that all people have some degree of unresolved emotional attachments to their parents. The unresolved attachments present challenges to growing up and better managing one's own anxiety and emotional reactivity. The essence of my work with Bowen theory emanates from Bowen's following statement:

> The life pattern of cutoffs is determined by the way people handle their unresolved emotional attachments to their parents. All people have some degree of unresolved emotional attachment to their parents. The lower the level of differentiation, the more intense the unresolved attachment. The concept deals with the way people separate themselves from the past in order to start their lives in the present generation.
> (1978, p. 382)

People avoid and cut off from each other when they cannot manage the unresolved emotional attachments and themselves in relationship to one another.

The focus of this chapter is on how chronic illness and death provide a continuing opportunity for further resolving degrees of unresolved emotional attachment in the family system. The first section includes unresolved emotional attachment, anxiety, and differentiation of self. The second section includes efforts to resolve degrees of the unresolved emotional attachment within the primary triangle between mother, father, and self. The third section includes the patterns of unresolved emotional attachment between myself and my mother and my father that were repeated in my marriage. The fourth section includes resolving some degree of the unresolved at the time of my husband's death following a serious illness. In the last section, I conclude with my awareness that the efforts to resolve the unresolved patterns of emotional attachments do indeed continue after the deaths of important others. This continuing process brings hope for better functioning in the present and for future generations.

Unresolved Emotional Attachment

Resolving the degrees of unresolved emotional attachment is a lifetime of work requiring awareness of the "simple bones" of the theory. As Bowen states, "The simple bones of the theory are: Number one: reduce the anxiety and number two: Work on differentiation of self" (Videotape: Bowen & Kerr, 1979).

Bowen's description of emotional development in the human beginning at birth is as follows:

> Every human infant starts life fully dependent on others, specifically on the family of origin. Growing up involves progressive development of individual characteristics, and aspects of increasing independence. The development of self occurs, in the case of each person, in and through networks of relationships with other members of the family system.
>
> (Bowen, 1991, p. 89)

The emotional attachments formed at birth are initially necessary for physical as well as emotional survival. At some point these attachments are no longer necessary for survival. As the development of self occurs within the network of relationships with the family system, the fundamental challenge is to manage a self, both as an individual and as part of a group. This challenge has its origins in the parental triangle.

Bowen posited that this triangle "is the most important primary triangle in life, and the one in which a person develops the triangle relationship patterns that remain relatively fixed in all relationships" (1978, p. 531).

The primary triangle between mother, father, and infant lays the groundwork for relationship patterns that remain, as Bowen stated, relatively fixed throughout life.

Some of these developmental patterns, particularly the patterns developed in the primary triangle, can serve an individual and the family well over time. Other patterns that do not function so well can be better managed by resolving degrees of unresolved emotional attachments.

Bowen talks about the anxiety that "goes along with" the unresolved emotional attachments. What is the definition of anxiety? What are unresolved emotional attachments?

Anxiety has been described by Bowen as the automatic emotional reactiveness to a real or imagined threat. He states that the reactivity is the manifestation of anxiety (Videotape: Bowen & Kerr, 1979). Often, what were *real* threats to the human infant become *imagined* threats when the infant becomes an adult.

Bowen theory posits two kinds of anxiety, two kinds of automatic emotional response to threat: acute and chronic. "Acute anxiety is fed by fear of what is. Chronic anxiety is fed by fear of what might be" (Kerr & Bowen, 1988, p. 113).

An infant begins life dependent on others with basic needs that must be fulfilled for survival. The infant's crying signals these needs: "I am hungry." "I am cold." "I am wet." "I am bored." As the infant develops and becomes more conscience of these basic needs and the concern that they need to be filled by another, acute fear can develop into chronic anxiety. Emotional dependence continues as physical independence develops. Awareness of the importance of relationships brings more concerns: "Do my parents like me?" "Am I doing what they expect?" The child's experience of dependence in the parental triangle can promote chronic anxiety, the fear of what might be, that can be carried over into adulthood. "I do not agree with my parents on this or that." "I have a different life course than the one expected of me." "If I do certain things, I will be rejected and alone."

What are unresolved emotional attachments? As I understand it, elements of unresolved emotional attachments include:

- The degree to which people look to others to regulate themselves;
- The degree of sensitivity to others that comes from adapting to the parental family in childhood; and
- The degree to which people are unsure about self.

These elements fuel the anxiety that goes along with the unresolved emotional attachment. Bowen posited: "All things being equal, the life course of people is determined by the amount of unresolved emotional attachment and the amount of anxiety that comes from it, and the way they deal with this anxiety" (1978, p. 537). Bowen used the term "unresolved dependency" interchangeably with "unresolved emotional attachment" in his writings (1978, p. 113). In my view this is an important message suggesting in large part how much anxiety comes from the unresolved emotional *dependency* on others. In other words, the unresolved emotional attachments are, in essence, the emotional unresolved dependencies that generate chronic anxiety over time. The challenge is to be less constrained by the relationships and therefore freer to be a self.

Bowen was known to ask the following question: "Do you have the ability to see your parents more as people than as 'emotionally endowed images?'" (1978, p. 531).

When people begin to resolve degrees of unresolved emotional attachments, they can begin to see their parents more as real people than the emotionally endowed images developed from infancy, childhood, and young adulthood. These "emotionally endowed images" contribute to and perpetuate chronic anxiety. Representing more of a self to one's parents reduces the perception of parents being "emotionally endowed images." This not only helps to better see one's parents as real people, it also contributes to lessening the degree of chronic anxiety in the system.

Degrees of anxiety and levels of differentiation vary from person to person and family system to family system. The process of growing up involves the ability to move toward increasing emotional independence and maturity. An important step in the process is becoming aware of one's sensitivity to important family relationships. It is the development of this sensitivity that can generate the unsureness—the unsureness that comes from focus on the other for validation rather than on self. In other words, developing awareness of this sensitivity enables a person to work toward being less regulated by the unresolved emotional attachments developed in childhood and more regulated by self. Another variable in this sensitivity is the degree of intensity which waxes and wanes over one's life. This idea is consistent with Bowen's statement, "One of the most important functional patterns in a family has to do with the intensity of the unresolved emotional attachment to the family" (1978, p. 433).

What degree of intensity challenges your efforts to manage yourself in your parental triangle? How much does self adapt and accommodate? How much self gets lost in the process?

Further questions:

- Under what emotional conditions are you more apt to seek approval?
- Under what emotional conditions are you more prone to distancing?
- Under what emotional conditions are you more likely to become conflictual?

Something to think about:

- What would it take to be willing to engage in the opportunity to resolve unresolved emotional attachments?
- What would it take to move toward increasing independence?
- What would it take to respect the other and know the other is up against it too?

There are many ways to apply theory to self and family. For me, it is important to think about how the degree of unresolved emotional attachment is linked to chronic anxiety. The challenge to manage myself and deal with anxiety is at the heart of my efforts in my family system. Back to the "simple bones"—reducing the anxiety enables a person to think more clearly. When one can think more clearly, one can act more from self and less from constraints from others. My premise is that the more dependent one is in seeking approval from important others, the greater the challenge of becoming more mature.

For the purposes of this chapter, I am focusing on the imagined threats that drive the anxiety that comes from the unresolved emotional attachment. In other words, this has to do with the degree of unresolved emotional dependency in the parental triangle. In my case, much of the fear and anxiety that challenged my ability to be more of a self was lodged in fear of disapproval. Embarrassing to say? Yes. Nevertheless, it is true.

It is uncomfortable to face and admit these kinds of things. However, there is a kind of emotional freedom that comes from seeing *what is*. Bowen stated, "All people have an emotional attachment to their parents that is more intense than most permit themselves to believe" (1978, p. 433). Denying the emotional attachment keeps one from seeing *what is*. Bowen also said,

> However the issue is handled, *the denied emotional attachment to the past replicates itself with one's spouse and one's children.* This can be said another way: *The more one denies the attachment to the past, the less choice one has in determining the pattern with his own wife and children* (as if he has much to begin with).
>
> (1978, p. 433)

Efforts to Resolve Degrees of the Unresolved Attachment in the Parental Triangle

I have listed a brief history here of my efforts to resolve the degrees of unresolved emotional attachment in the parental triangle, which involves working on differentiation of self. This work involves using one's ability to think and observe the more automatic reactive response to real or imagined threat.

- Noticed that I avoided taking a position with my mother and my father.
- Noticed that it was hard to think, particularly if my mother held a strong position and the intensity between us mounted.

- Learned that when I had difficulty thinking, it was related to the need for approval and the degree of anxiety in me and in the family system.
- Learned that I needed to manage the anxiety.

While being respectful of differences with my parents, I needed to find ways to lower the anxiety in order to think through my position. This involved finding ways to shift from avoidance and silence toward contact and finding ways to have conversations about difficult subjects.

An example of bewilderment and emotional reactivity was evident the day I graduated with a master's degree in social work. A friend invited my family and friends for lunch following the graduation. My mother and father had not seen each other for the 11 years following their divorce. My mother initiated the divorce and married another.

The following is a parental triangle dynamic: My mother walked over to my father with her arms outstretched and a smile on her face. My father put out his hand. He did not smile. My mother's face fell. The next thing I knew my mother was commanding me to stand still so she could take my picture. I reacted to the command and instead of stating my position—I do not want you to take my picture at this time—I said, "It is muddy here," she said, "Then go over there!" Deflated. I went. She took my picture.

I lost self again. What was going on?

I later realized that saying "it is muddy here" was my inability to merely state my position. Such a simple thing to say, "No thanks, not now." It is so hard to think and talk when old patterns not resolved get activated! There remained lots of emotional awareness and learning still to come.

As the years went on, my mother was still trying to get my father's approval. I was working on resolving degrees of emotional attachment and managing my fear of disapproval. My mother noticed a shift in my behavior as I was learning Bowen theory and working with a coach. She came to me. She said, "Every time I see your father at these family events, when I approach him, he avoids me. Can you help me?"

Is this a trap or is this for real? Trapped because often as a child, as I saw it, I would get pulled in to the emotional struggle between my parents, feel great because I was "important" and could "help." Then things would get better between my mother and my father, and if I had something still to say, I would be told that this was none of my business. Stunned and confused, I would back off, only to eagerly engage the next time my mom needed me. The pattern was an automatic dance.

I decided I was grown-up enough to venture into these emotional waters and try to hold my own. My mom and I talked. I asked what she was trying to accomplish by going toward my father. She said she just wanted things to be friendly between them at these family events. I suggested that she was seeking my father's approval. After all, she left him. This was not his choice. Their divorce had not been resolved within and between my parents. I further suggested that she not go near him at the next family event. Be your charming self and engage with others. My mother did just that at my niece's engagement party. Afterward on the phone, my father said, "I did not talk with your mother yesterday. How is she?" I said that she was fine. I reported this to my mother and congratulated her on backing off.

My parents actually flirted with one another at my niece's wedding. For me, it was a relief to see them getting along. That was a brief moment in time. After the wedding until right before their illnesses that led to their deaths, what was unresolved between my parents and between my parents and myself in the parental triangle was somewhat quiescent, listing along without much progress. Although I had no idea that my mother's diagnosis of pancreatic cancer was a few months away, fortunately for me, I decided it was time for me to stop avoiding listening to my mother's side of the divorce. After hearing my mother's side, I was better able to understand the challenges they were both up against with each other. I was then able to tell my father that I listened to my mother and am no longer taking his side in the divorce. His response, "That is good. I thought daughters were supposed to support their mothers." Although that was an important step toward resolving degrees of the unresolved, it was only a step. What follows illustrates how the emotional process continues throughout life, especially in times of heightened tension such that chronic illness and death can bring to a family system.

Picture this: My brother, sister, and I were all with my mother in Virginia following her recent diagnosis of pancreatic cancer. My mother chose not to have the Whipple surgery. She chose instead to be on morphine in order to stay out of the excruciating pain she had been experiencing prior to her diagnosis. While we were sitting on her bed talking with her, a phone call came from a mutual friend of my parents in Pennsylvania. The friend said that she thought we would want to know that our father had been admitted to the hospital. Sitting on our mother's big bed, we called our father. After we all talked with him, he asked me how my mother was. I told him she was doing remarkably well and that we were all in awe of her brave choices in facing her death. I acknowledged that she was right here and did he want to speak with her. Much to my amazement, he said, "Yes!"

Their conversation was animated in tones of kindness. He was on Percocet and she on morphine. From then on during the three months before her death, my mother seemed quite smitten with my father. She even said the hell with the second husband, she and the first one were on a "race to the pearly gates." We gently reminded our mother that our father was happily married and that perhaps he was not as sick as she.

My mother's request in Virginia several weeks before her death: "When you see your father, will you please give him my phone number and ask him to call me." Simple enough request for some, but not for me! I was on my way to see my father in a rehab facility for his stroke in Pennsylvania.

When my mother asked me to intervene on her behalf with my father, the intensity of my anxiety in this triangle increased. I felt pressured. In my opinion, my mother wanted my father to understand why she left him. My mother wanted my father's approval. I was the conduit. I *did not* like this. And although I made steps to get out of the middle with my parents, I continued to get triggered.

Before the divorce, I took my mother's side. After the divorce, I took my father's side. As mentioned earlier, even though just a few months before my mother's diagnosis, I was finally able to listen to my mother's side and was able to talk with both parents about no longer taking sides, degrees of sensitivity to their approval remained unresolved.

Back to my mother's request to give my father her phone number. I said to myself, "Uh-oh. My father is *not* going to want to hear this." And, besides, I consoled myself, my mother is really too sick for me to ask her to call him herself.

Back in Pennsylvania I said to my father, "Mom wants me to give you her phone number. She wants you to call her." In a surprisingly gentle way (not always the case when referring to my mother), my father said to me, "I do not need your mother's phone number. I won't be calling her. I have nothing to say to her." Despite the gentle delivery, this was *not* a message I was looking forward to taking back to my mother.

I watched my father do his routine rehab exercises. Before the routine was finished, he collapsed. The nurses put him back into bed. I sat with him. Before I left to go back to Virginia, my father handed me a new pair of hospital socks. He asked me to, "Please give these socks to your mother."

At this point, I was somewhat relieved. I had something to give to my mother from my father. But this is an easy way out for me. Unresolved chronic anxiety about getting their approval was driving me. I did *not* have the courage to tell my father that my mother will *not* like to hear that you will *not* be calling her. I did *not* have the courage to tell my mother that my father would *not* be calling her.

In other words, these degrees of chronic anxiety and unresolved emotional attachments, unresolved emotional dependencies, were going every which way in this triangle. My parents were challenged in their inability to talk with each other, and I was challenged by my inability to better represent myself to either my father or my mother. In this process of resolving degrees of unresolved emotional attachments to my parents, to what degree did I still see my parents as "emotionally endowed images" as opposed to real people?

Thinking about my mother's question: "When you see your father, ask him to call me." What was the threat? At face value, my mother was asking me to do her a favor. So what was the big deal? Was this a real or imagined threat? At the time, I was 50-some years old. Was my survival really at stake? Although this was an imagined threat, I reacted as though it was a real threat.

What is unresolved in this situation?

- Degree of anxiety and fear of disapproval.
- Feeling pressure to do it my mother's way.
- Feeling unsure—should I be taking this request from my mother to my father? Whose job is this anyway?

And so the emotional process went from Virginia to Pennsylvania, from Pennsylvania to Virginia. Back in Virginia, I gave my mom the socks. The next thing I knew, they were on her feet. I never brought up the phone call request. She never asked. However, opportunity to grow up kept knocking.

During our parents' illnesses, my brother, sister, and I took turns making sure that at least one of us was with each parent. The morning of the day my mother died, she began an incessant groaning. It was my turn to be with her. All attempts to figure out what was wrong failed. The hospice nurse could determine no pain. Nothing the minister could say stopped the groaning. The disturbing groaning persisted. Then I had an idea. It occurred to me that she needed a message from my father. "Oh dear," I thought. There were various people in her room and some in the kitchen with a monitor. I asked the people to please leave her room and to turn off the monitor.

Those things done, I knelt down beside my mother and stroked her forehead. I knew what I was going to say. After telling her that my brother, sister, and I all benefited greatly from her love and her challenges as our mother and that we loved and appreciated her, I concluded by saying, "My father wishes you deep peace." With those words, my mother pulled her hand up to her chin. She closed her mouth and did not groan again. She died eight hours later. I was with her. She was wearing the socks from my father.

But . . . it was not over yet. The parental triangle was, and is, alive and well. I now have to tell my father what I told my mother in his name! Up from Virginia to Pennsylvania, I told my dad the story. When I got to the part about "my idea" that involved him, he leaned forward from his propped-up pillows and with a look of intense inquisition, asked, "And . . . *what* did you tell your mother I would say?" I took a deep breath and said, "My father wishes you deep peace." My father put his head back on the pillow and said, "Thank you. That is exactly right." My father died 23 days after my mother.

What happened during the dying process? The parental triangle that had been somewhat quiescent in our geographical distances was activated in the proximity of our togetherness. In the togetherness, when difficult subjects and tension arose, our inability to deal with each other in a person-to-person way became evident. The intensification of the anxiety in the parental triangle revealed how caught

I was. Curiously, this level of being caught in the parental triangle also brought with it a degree of objectivity to see more clearly the inability of each of us to make person-to-person contact with one another.

What changed in me? Increased awareness of the anxiety triggered by the emotional unresolved dependencies manifested in the fear of not getting approval. And alas, an increased awareness that I am not nearly as resolved as I thought I was!

What changed in the parental triangle? An awareness of the intensity of the attachment slowly increased over time. Although the emotional elements of the divorce between my parents were not resolved, the fact that their messages regarding one another softened somehow enabled me to fill in some of the gap between them. The intensity in the triangle had decreased, which seemed to help my mother and father die with some modicum of increased connection to one another.

Bowen stated, "The basic relationship patterns developed for adapting to the parental family in childhood are used in all other relationships throughout life" (1978, p. 462). People resolve as much as they can with their parents. After the deaths of one's parents, the family systems beat goes on. And there are always those in all the other relationships that can trigger the unresolved emotional attachments in self and in the family system throughout life. For better or worse, illness and death can bring emotional intensity to the surface, and with that comes the opportunity to resolve degrees of emotional dependencies in ways that can lower the level of anxiety in self and in the parental triangle.

Unresolved Emotional Attachments: Understanding the Relationship of the Parental Triangle and Marriage

The anxiety I felt within the parental triangle often left me in a state of confusion (Figure 11.1). At times I would feel loved by my parents; at other times I would feel dismissed. To manage the anxiety and to feel calmer, I would work hard to seek approval. If this failed, I would cave and end up feeling furious. Although much of the unresolved dependency was with my mother, it was also challenging for me to engage with my father. As an adult in the parental triangle, I worked to be in better emotional contact with both my mother and my father.

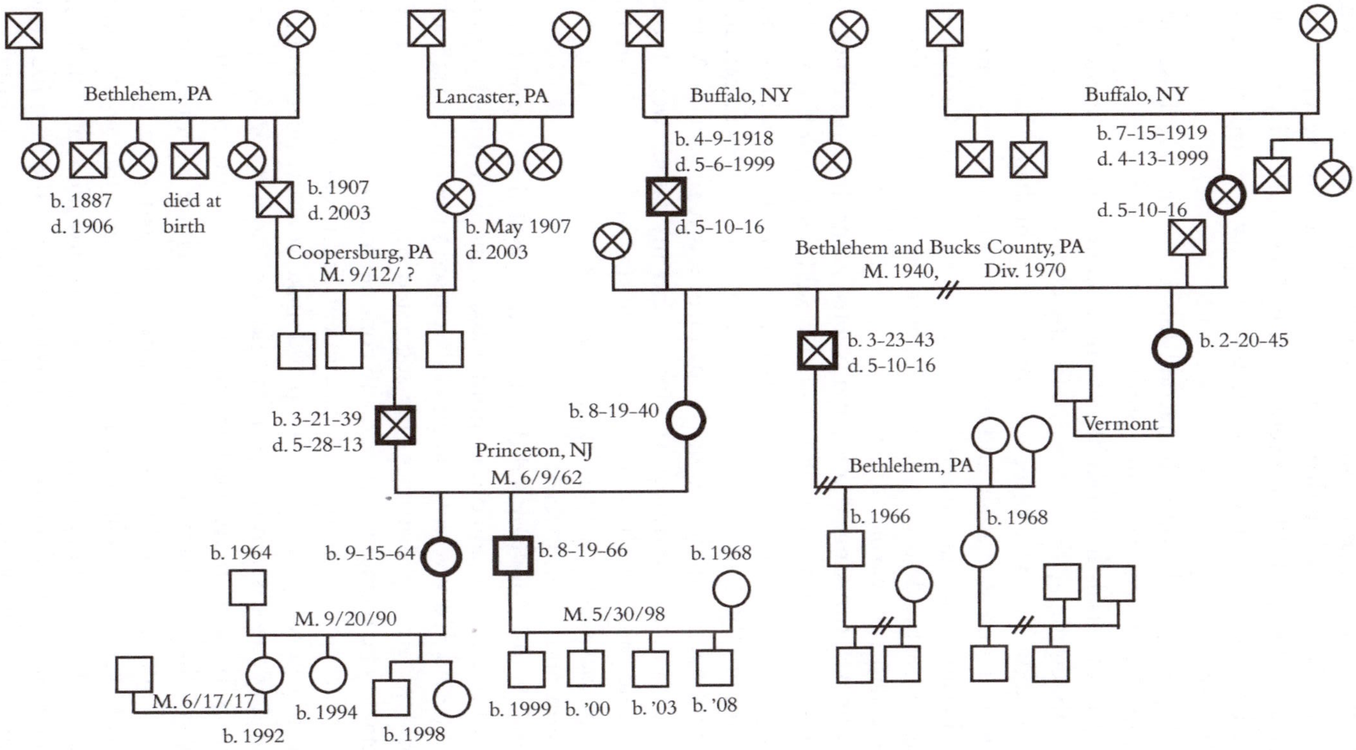

Figure 11.1 The Dunbar Illick family diagram

My husband and I started our married life several states away from my parents. While my husband finished his last two years in law school, I taught school. After several years in New York City and two children later, we moved to New Jersey where we settled about 50 miles away from our parents in Pennsylvania.

We bought an old house. It needed lots of work. My husband's father founded a construction company. He offered to help. I did not like the materials he brought. I wanted something different. My mother offered to pay the difference for my choices.

Very quickly the unresolved attachment my husband had to his father in his parental triangle and mine to my mother in my parental triangle became a battleground between my husband and myself—each still too dependent on our parents, both emotionally and financially. We had not learned to make our own plan and find ways to convey our best thinking to our parents. His father threatened not to help unless we did it his way. My mother would not pay unless we did it her way. In the activation of these triangles: my husband, his father and me; my mother, my husband and me; my mother, his father, and me; my mother, his father, and my husband, intensity mounted. As the intensity mounted, my husband's mother and my father were more or less comfortable on the outside of all the uncomfortable triangles whirling at that time. We were in the swamp of unresolved emotional attachments and dependencies.

Meanwhile our four-year-old daughter was enrolled in a wonderful nursery school that we could not afford. I asked my mother if she could help us. She did. However, our daughter developed a resistance to school. We talked with the pediatrician. He suggested my husband and I go into therapy. The therapist observed and commented on my attachment to my mother and my husband's attachment to his father. She asked, "When are you two going to grow up and make your own decisions?"

While that made sense to me, I had no idea how to grow up. In fact, things became more challenging and chaotic before calming down somewhat. I remained in therapy. Our daughter went to school. The house construction finally got finished. I began to see my emotional dependence and reliance on my mother. I not only wanted her approval, I still wanted her help. I could see that my mother's thinking took preference over my husband's thinking. I began the long journey of making efforts to be a self. It was not easy and it was not pretty.

As a young child, I saw my mother in a very positive light. In fact so positive that if there were disagreements, I became unsure of myself and assumed I was wrong. As I began to think more for myself, I could see how much I wanted her approval. The focus on my mother and trying to get her approval actually *raised* my anxiety. This emotional reactiveness would manifest itself in confusion, anger, and blame. I would become defiant or give in to her point of view. It is so fascinating to me to see how much focus on the other intensifies anxiety. And how when the focus shifts to self, anxiety lowers over time.

I distanced from my mother. I cut off. I was "polite." I did not represent myself. I did not engage. A strikingly similar version of this pattern—the emotional dependency, the fear of not getting approval, the anxiety generated from the unresolved emotional dependency—was being repeated in my marriage. And, like my parents, my husband and I were often challenged in having person-to-person discussions on difficult subjects.

Enter Bowen family systems theory. It provided a way to think more for myself and not to blame others. In addition, it provided a way to get a grip on my immaturity and take responsibility for myself and grow up! It took a lot of effort to apply Bowen theory in order to make changes in my relationships with my parents.

Bowen found that rather than transferring emotional attachments to the therapist, a great deal of progress could be made if people would go back to the original triangle and make efforts to be more of a self with one's mother and father. In cases where the mother and father are deceased, people can observe and make efforts to manage their reactivity and anxiety patterns to others in their social and work relationships.

At a training session, I asked Dr. Bowen what one could do with anger. My recollection is that he said, "Work on self. The more you are a self, the less angry you will be." I found that to be true. Instead of blaming my mother for my misery and cutting off from her, I made efforts to be more accountable, more of a self, in her presence. It was and is amazing to see the parallels in relationship patterns adapted in the parental triangle repeating in marriage.

In spite of an abundance of love and good will in a family system, when people are more emotionally driven than thoughtfully directed, emotional turbulence can take the lead. Over the years, even though I made efforts to think more and react less, in times of rising anxiety, the automatic unresolved emotional reactiveness embedded in original hard wiring would inevitably come to the forefront.

Efforts to Resolve Degrees of the Unresolved Attachment in the Marriage

Eight years after my parents' deaths, my husband underwent a failed heart ablation, ending up in open-heart surgery. The trauma of these events, which included lack of oxygen and two lengthy stays in the intensive care unit (ICU), is thought to have triggered the onset of Alzheimer's disease, which is progressive disease with no cure to date. Following the diagnosis our two children came to visit. Family discussions were introduced around financial planning and ways to proceed as the disease progressed. Before this family was aware of Atul Gawande's remarkable book, *Being Mortal*, our children also asked what seemed to me to be brave and somewhat awkward questions about their father's end-of-life wishes. Was there a point in the progression of the disease where he would think he no longer had quality of life? My husband was also asked what was important to him and what plans would he like to make in the present that would be pleasurable and meaningful to him. With my husband, we made plans that would be modified as the disease progressed. It was also important to him to contribute his brain for continuing research into this horrific disease. As was discovered, not only did he have Alzheimer's but he also had Lewy body, another form of dementia.

My husband's decision was to stop eating. How he pulled it off when he was in the advanced stages of dementia remains a question. Hopefully, the answer will lie in the research of his brain at Massachusetts General Hospital, available to researchers around the world.

My husband was in Hospice House for the ten days leading up to his death.

Two nights before my husband died—after all the children and grandchildren had been with him—a hospice nurse pulled me aside and remarked, "Your husband seems to be stuck. Is there anything you have not said? Is there anything you can think of to say?"

Like my mother separating from my father, I had separated from my husband. Unlike my parents, my husband and I did not divorce. Nevertheless, degrees of unresolved emotional attachment were alive and well in our marriage. Too much of my focus over the years had been on getting my husband to see his part in the marital problems rather than focusing more on my part. Whenever my focus was on him in an effort to get his approval and understanding of *my version*, I had lost sight of taking responsibility for myself. The nurse's question nagged at me. I needed to get clear, very clear. This was a poignant moment.

Deep down, I knew there were unresolved issues between my husband and me. And I knew I needed to deal openly and honestly. I realized that I had been hoping that all the "good stuff" I had done would override my having to go back to this challenge of needing approval and not taking *full* responsibility for myself in the marriage, which had been persistent components of my unresolved emotional attachment. I needed to deal with my truth. My truth—that is, that I was more invested in getting his approval than taking responsibility for my actions and accepting the consequences. It was important to me to become as objective and thoughtful as possible. A consultation with my Bowen coach helped me think more clearly, focus on facts.

The next day knowing what I needed to say came out of a realization that I was, in fact, not taking *full* responsibility for my part in the marriage. When the subject of our separation would come up, I was not able to be enough of a self, to take *full* responsibility for myself in these discussions. There seemed to be a persistent part in me that wanted my husband to get the focus off of me and talk about himself. If he could see his part in the relationship challenges, maybe he would better understand me. As all this was coming more clearly into focus for me, it was obvious that it was my job to take more responsibility for my part and to make efforts to be more understanding of him! If I could be more of a self in the marriage—take 100% responsibility for me—not operate out of a need for approval, he might be freer of the pressure of the burden, spoken or not spoken, in or out of awareness. Through it all, I gained clarity in knowing that it is easy to become blind to the degree of unresolved emotional attachment that can live on out of awareness in a person's life. In other words, the-out-of-awareness unresolved emotional process that led to my need for approval with my parents lived on in my marriage with my husband. Although I had made strides of resolving degrees of this with my parents, I nevertheless unwittingly brought that unresolved emotional attachment pattern into our marriage.

As I thought about the relationship between my husband and me, I could see that when we were challenged, we were up against the degree of unresolved emotional attachment that we both brought to our marriage. But, and this is the important essential part, I can only take responsibility for *my* unresolved emotional attachments. It was useful to see this. What a relief! I could now describe what I was seeing to my husband. Perhaps this awareness could help to release my husband and me from this stuck place.

The next morning, I sat beside my husband and said,

> I am here to say that I am seeing the subtle, and not-so-subtle ways that I have never stopped putting pressure on you to approve of me and understand why I separated from you. I have not been clear enough about *my* responsibility in the problems that emerged between us. Until now, I did not see how my focus on your part in the problem got me off the hook. What I am seeing is that my focus on needing your approval and not taking *full* responsibility for myself—my unresolved stuff from my family—was the part I played in our inability to better communicate with each other.

That said, that finally understood, the leap over this somewhat formidable emotional hurdle was followed by a stream of expressed gratitude for and love of our life together. My husband died the next morning with our daughter, our dog, and me at his side.

It is so interesting to me how this emotional process operates within a family. I think that the work that went into trying to better understand the parts that each person played in the parental triangle, my mother, my father, and myself, helped me to better see the parts my husband and I were playing in our marriage. Better managing one's self does in fact lower the anxiety in the relationship system. Lower anxiety does in fact make more room for thoughtful direction. Although I could see both sides, I am only responsible for one side, my side. It is also fascinating to me that when I can see both sides, I can better understand and be more respectful of what the other is up against, not only with me, but also in the other's own life.

As I look back, I believe that something significant shifted as I made efforts to become more aware and more accepting of my part in the emotional process in my marriage. Becoming more accepting of my part also enabled me to see and accept the similarities in my parents' marriage and in my marriage. I think that this ability to see and accept has the potential to make room for all relationships in the family to be more open and flexible. I think that this has to do with developing a more accurate perception of self as separate from the other, which is a significant part of the process of resolving degrees of the early emotional attachments. If I can continue to be this way with others in the family—especially my children—then I believe everyone can potentially benefit.

Efforts to Resolve Degrees of Emotional Attachment With My Adult Children

As Bowen posited,

> The degree of unresolved emotional attachment to the parents is equivalent to the degree of undifferentiation that must somehow be handled in the person's own life and in future generations.
>
> (1978, p. 382)

How might the resolving degrees of unresolved emotional attachment described in this chapter affect the family system going forward? I believe that making an effort to do a little better—even though it may only be a little bit better—does make a difference for self and future generations. With that in mind, I will describe what I have observed in the relationship with my children as I continue in my efforts to resolve the emotional attachments developed for adapting to the parental family in childhood.

Following my husband's death, I have lived independently. As with many people who are in their 70s, I live on a fixed income. As anxiety increased around my financial future, my children became more involved—sometimes in a low-keyed way, sometimes not so low-keyed. As these conversations began to take place, I began to *feel* that something was not right. I stepped back to think about *my* emotional reactivity and noticed old patterns emerging.

Fortunately, my efforts over the years to become more aware of family emotional patterns helped me to more quickly see my emotionally reactive response to discussions about my financial future. My shifting from being less driven by emotional reactivity to being more thoughtfully directed has enabled me to represent myself more clearly in challenging conversations. I continue to be reminded that while others can present emotional challenges, it is *my* work and nobody else's to manage myself in the emotional field.

Will my lifelong efforts in this area make a difference for future generations?

I am hoping that it does. At this point in time, it would appear that unlike my parents' marriage and my marriage, my children's marriages are more open. My children and their spouses appear to be better able to represent themselves, are less focused on approval seeking, and are better able not to blame the other for their problems.

Does increasing awareness and the effort to resolve degrees of unresolved emotional attachment challenging those in one generation make a difference in the next? The answer, in part, may lie in how well the present generation continues to make efforts to become more aware of anxiety and emotional reactivity in self and in the family system. These efforts can help people better manage the unresolved emotional attachment to families of origin and the anxiety that "goes along with it."

I would like to thank Peg Donley for her essential content editing, Dan Papero for all the years of incredibly respectful coaching, and Elizabeth Utschig for her excellent copyediting.

REFERENCES

Bowen, M. (1978). *Family therapy in clinical practice.* New York, NY: Jason Aronson.

Bowen, M. (1991). Diversity from unity. In E. Joseph (Ed.), *Individuality and cooperative action.* Washington, DC: Georgetown University Press.

Bowen, M., & Kerr, M. E. (1989). *Anxiety and emotional reactivity in therapy*, [videotape]. Washington, DC: Georgetown University School of Medicine.

Bowen, M., & Kerr, M. E. (1979). [videotape] Bowen Center for the Study of the Family. Washington, DC.

Kerr, M. E., & Bowen, M. (1988). *Family evaluation.* New York, NY: W. W. Norton.

12

ALZHEIMER'S DISEASE IN THE FAMILY

Peter Titelman

This chapter describes my effort to define myself in my relationship with my father during the time of his life when he had Alzheimer's disease (Figure 12.1). The chapter also describes my sister's Alzheimer's and the reaction in her nuclear family; the Alzheimer's of one of my first cousins, who is no longer living; and my own chronic anxiety that I may end up with Alzheimer's disease.

In the first section I describe the history of my father's Alzheimer's disease from the time I first recognized it in 1979, until his death in January 1993. Section two describes my cousin's Alzheimer's disease. The third section describes chronic anxiety, Alzheimer's, and me. The fourth section describes my sister's Alzheimer's and the reactions in her nuclear family. The final section provides reflections on Alzheimer's disease and ways that family members can relate to the one who has Alzheimer's.

The History of My Father's Alzheimer's Disease

Looking back at my father's functioning prior to the onset of his Alzheimer's disease, it should be noted that he had experienced bouts of mild to moderate depression during his adulthood, although for the most part he was a handsome, vibrant, energetic, intelligent, generous, loving man. He functioned well in his work, but in 1967 at age 56 he retired, having become unhappy as the sales manager of the paternal family business in New York City. He and my mother moved to the south of France where he gardened, read, and visited my sister, who lived in England with her husband and their child, my parents' first grandchild. He probably suffered from the lack of a meaningful focus

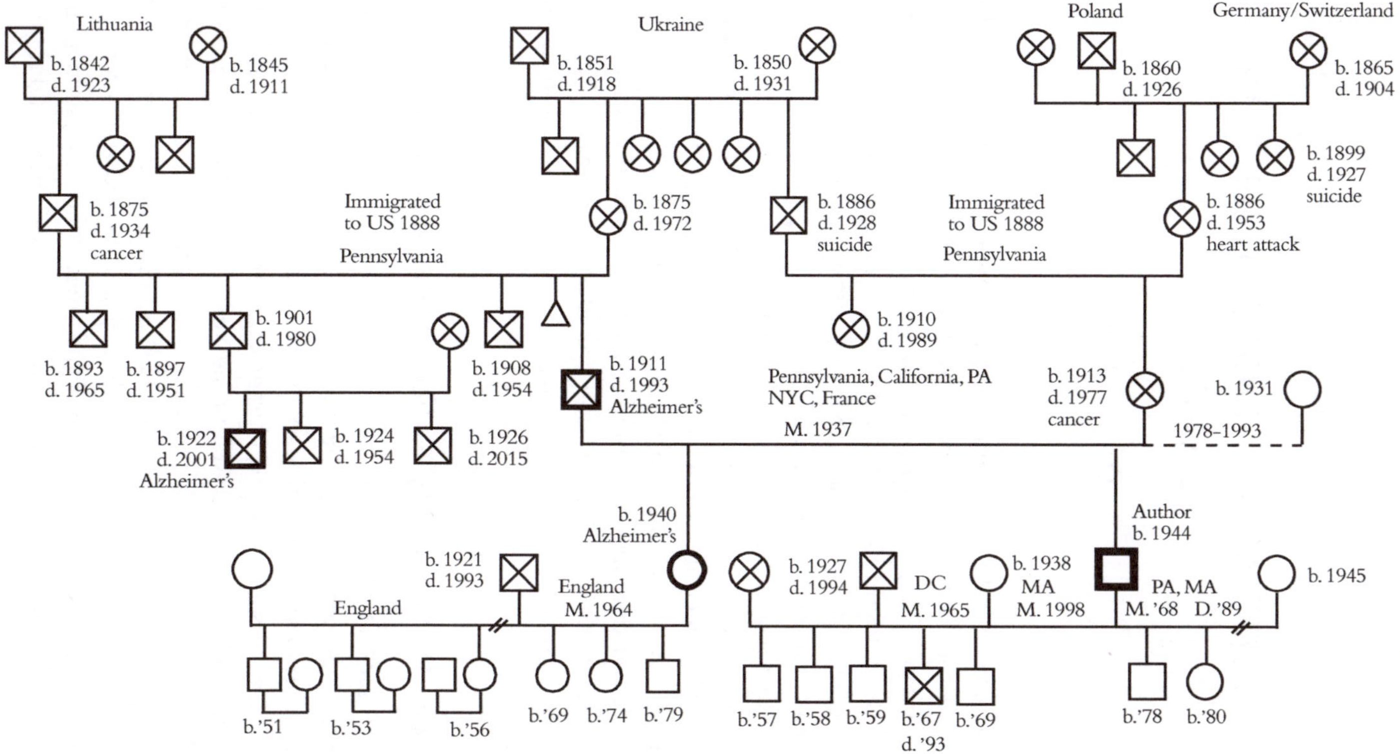

Figure 12.1 Titelman family diagram

in retirement and increased symptoms of depression that had occurred over many years.

My mother was diagnosed with ovarian cancer in 1976 and died a little over a year later in England. More than a year after my mother's death my father began a relationship with a woman who had been his French teacher in southern France. They began living together and remained intimate partners for the rest of his life. Every year my father visited me in the United States, and I visited him in France every other year. In 1979, when my father was 68, I observed that his memory was beginning to deteriorate. He had begun to lose his ability to remember numbers and some names.

In 1980 my father's last remaining brother, who also represented an authority figure for him, died in Florida. My father and I traveled there for the funeral. He was somewhat disoriented, and he confused some family names and relationships. Traveling from France to the United States was becoming difficult for him.

I noticed during the next couple of years that my father would lose his sense of direction. For example, if I dropped him off at a drugstore and told him I was waiting in the parking lot, he would get confused.

On a visit to New York City in 1983, 1 met my father and we stayed at my aunt's apartment. Sundown syndrome increases general confusion as natural light begins to fade and disorientation occurs. This took place when my father arrived following his international travel. At one point his cognitive confusion led him to go into the bathroom, walk into the shower with his clothes on, and try to get out of the apartment, as if the shower were the front door of the apartment.

At another point it was reported that my father menacingly threatened his cleaning lady, who also cooked for him, with a large kitchen knife. Fortunately, he did not attack her.

On a visit with my father at his home in France one summer, I saw him go out to his car, and though he had already stopped driving, he began twisting the gear shift and ripping at the glove compartment, as if he were attempting to drive his car.

On another visit I was doing some work in my father's yard. He became disoriented, going to the opposite side of the house and yelling to make contact with me. At first I yelled back that I was on the opposite side of the house. Soon I realized his sense of place was so fluid, unattached to objective time and space, that it seemed to me as if he were a small child. I felt terrible for having yelled back at him when I had this realization of the terror he must have been going through.

In the early to mid-1980s, my sister and my father's partner did not realize that my father was developing Alzheimer's, or some other form of dementia. Alzheimer's was almost unheard of in the region of France where my father lived. In February 1984, I suggested that he see a neurologist in France. I then sent a letter to a primary care physician, Dr. S., at Massachusetts General Hospital, whom my father had seen when he was in the United States several years before and with whom he had had a good rapport. I suggested that Dr. S. contact the French neurologist and then speak with my father on the telephone. He readily agreed to do so. In addition, I told him the symptoms and problems my father was having. I wrote the following:

> If it makes sense to you I suggest that you speak with Dr. D, the French neurologist, after his appointment with my father, and then you could speak directly to my father. At this point he has become, understandably, very upset about his loss of function, and he is hoping that there is a drug that will restore or stop further memory loss. Until this time I have not talked to him about what I think his problem might be, in order not to depress him, since there is no treatment, if he has Alzheimer's. Before he goes into a third stage of this disease perhaps a different way of dealing with him will be necessary.

I wrote Dr. S. the following letter later in May 1984:

> Dear Dr. S:
>
> I believe that your phone contact with my father, regarding his memory problem, was quite reassuring. Since I spoke with you in February my father was in the U.S. for a very brief visit. His condition continues to deteriorate as does his distrustfulness. My sister, who lives in England, is having a particularly difficult time understanding and coming to terms with his disease. In this regard, I wonder if you would write a note for me, indicating your understanding of my father's diagnosis and condition, and I could send it to my sister. I believe that would be a step for her to hear the reality. Please send me a bill for this consultation. [He never

did]. And, again, I want to thank you for your willingness to be involved with my father.
Sincerely,
Peter Titelman

A few days later Dr. S. wrote me a kind letter confirming that my father did have Alzheimer's disease:

Dear Dr. Titelman:
I write to inform you that I have talked with your father and his doctor. The information about him indicates that he has developed a disorder of his thinking that is common, one due to degeneration of brain cells termed Alzheimer's disease. This can be very slow in changing the person but invariably does produce deficits in how the brain (and mind) works. There is no treatment so the individual needs a lot of protection and sympathy from the family despite the uncontrolled difficulties that the patient has.
Give your father my best.
John S., MD

I shared the letter with my sister and my father's partner, and they finally stopped denying his cognitive dysfunction, erratic emotions, and behavior, and accepted his diagnosis when they read it.

In the summer of 1989, I took my 11-year-old son and 9-year-old daughter to visit my father. For the most part my father was in a wheelchair, and my children lovingly wheeled him around. Both children showed no fear or anxiety at being with him even though he no longer could speak. They smiled at him and he smiled back. An aunt of mine had described my father as a lady's man, saying, "All the girls ran after him, and he wasn't a very fast runner." Apropos of that comment, the only distinct words he spoke during our visit in 1989 were in response to my daughter. He said: "She's very cute." By 1992 my father was confined to his bed for the most part, unable to walk or to talk as over the last three years he had lost the ability to speak.

It was always clear that my father and his partner never wanted him to have to leave their home in southern France. Of course my sister and I, living in different countries from my father, were immensely grateful for her devotion to him. She was a schoolteacher and a loving caretaker for him. In the last several years of his life, we hired part-time caregivers to be with him in order to give her some relief when she was working. It was only in the last six months of his life that he had to go to a French nursing facility. It was near his home where his partner visited him every day until he died quietly, without speech or the ability to get out of bed, on January 28, 1993. My father was 81 and died exactly 16 years to the day after my mother had died at the age of 63.

Efforts to Define Self in Relation to My Father With Alzheimer's Disease

In this section I describe a few critically painful nodal events and my effort to be my highest-functioning self, facing situations that involved blame, suspicion, distrust, misunderstanding, and anger directed at me by my father that were generated from my perspective by his Alzheimer's disease.

In about 1981, my father had started a scholarship fund in memory of my mother at the school she had helped found and directed. He became upset because he thought that their old friends had not done enough fundraising for the scholarship, and he got into a tangle with a number of them. He was demanding and irritable with them when they asked him to come to Los Angeles to help develop a fundraising agenda and at least be a part of a couple of fundraising efforts. He said he could not come, but he was unable or unwilling to tell them that his faculties were failing. His friends were upset with him, and my father's effort to build the scholarship was thwarted. By the time I communicated my father's developing Alzheimer's to some of his friends in L.A., it was too late to mend the friendships.

In 1982, 1 decided to leave a half-time position in a clinic and go into full-time private practice. Just as I was leaving the job I had a fairly serious automobile accident in which my car overturned. It resulted in hand surgery that slowed my getting into full gear in the practice. In addition, money was tight, as my wife was just finishing her doctoral dissertation and had only a small part-time job and two little children to take care of. All this led to our not being in a good financial position.

I wrote my father in France in detail about my situation and asked him if he would be willing to provide some temporary monthly financial aid while my clinical practice, consulting, and teaching geared up. His initial response was to completely misunderstand the amount of help I was requesting by five- or ten-fold. He was angry, and at first I felt humiliated and confused. Before emotionally reacting to him out of my distress, I tried to explain the facts to him and to his partner. The situation calmed down in the short run, but over the remaining years of his life he maintained the attitude that I was taking advantage of him financially. Within a year or two, my father changed his will. He dropped me as executor and told his lawyer—someone I knew quite well—not to disclose the financial changes he had made. My feelings were of sadness and disappointment, but I could understand that this change resulted from my father being under the influence of Alzheimer's; he no longer trusted me. A few years later, when the lawyer fully understood that my father had Alzheimer's, he told me that the will had been changed to leave one-third of his assets to his partner, one-third to my sister, and one-third to me. He left the house in France to my sister and me. His decisions made sense to us.

In 1987, I visited my father in France and brought him a copy of the first book I had edited, *The Therapist's Own Family: Toward the Differentiation of Self* (Titelman, 1987). I was proud of having completed this project and wanted to share it with him. However, when I handed him the book, he took it and did not seem to know what to do with it. Of course I knew that he was no longer reading or comprehending what he saw on television. Nevertheless, I had an unrealistic expectation that he would admire the book and congratulate me for doing it. My father looked as though he was going to tear or twist the book, so I quickly removed it from his hands and handed it to his partner, who was appreciative of it. I was able to quickly respond to my father's state of mind. I knew if he had not had Alzheimer's, he would really have been proud of my work and writing efforts, as would my mother if she had been alive.

During a visit to my father and his partner in the late 1980s, in the course of dinner at a restaurant, my father became jealous and angry toward me because he felt I was being overly intimate with his partner. She and I were speaking to each other. He must have felt left out and was not participating in, or understanding, what we were saying to each other. While I certainly had known for many years that his Alzheimer's had led to serious changes, initially I was taken aback and had to think it through so that I would not express reactivity toward him. I realized the jealous behavior was an expression of his illness, not the person I knew him to have been.

During the last few years before my father died, when I would leave France to return to the United States after a visit, I would often think it was probably the last time I would see him alive. And given his severe deterioration, both physically and mentally from Alzheimer's, I would say to myself, this would be for the best; my father wouldn't want to continue to live in the condition he was in. The last time I saw him, in 1992, he was in the nursing home, and it was very difficult to help him get into his wheelchair. The condition of his teeth was bad, his general physical decline was severe, and of course verbal communication was nonexistent. Yet I found a comfort in being with him while I pushed his wheelchair outdoors in a beautiful setting. I spoke to him and felt that he was still a presence. When I left that last time, I hoped I would have another visit with him.

Several years after my father died, I fully realized how little time I had spent with him while he was suffering from Alzheimer's disease. This gave rise to pangs of sorrow that I had not done enough for him. But my parents had moved to France permanently in 1966, setting a course of great geographic distance between us when I was 22 years old, just graduating from college, and getting ready to enter graduate school. The distance was punctuated by many noteworthy visits, both in France and in the United States, usually once or twice a year, but the geographic distance was great. If my father, when ill, had come to live near me in the United States, or near my sister in England, separate from his partner and their peaceful way of life in the south of France, that would not have been what he would have wanted for himself. I really was unable to provide any other viable options for caretaking for him when he was seriously ill. My effort in relating to my father during his illness was to try to be less reactive to his attacks, fears, dysfunction, distrust, and helplessness and not to cut off emotionally or get angry toward him. My guiding principle was not to blame him, but to keep the perspective that his illness was continually running the show and that his behavior was a function of the disease. I knew that before the illness he had been a man of critical judgment, perfectionism, and mild chronic anxiety, along with having been a loving and generous father. I had to relate to my father, who, for all intents and purposes, had lost his "self." I tried to always keep in mind the "self" that my father was before he had Alzheimer's.

My Cousin's Alzheimer's Disease

My cousin D was born in 1922 and died in 2001. His daughter is the youngest of five children and has four older brothers. She told me about her father's Alzheimer's and his decline. In the 1960s the family noticed their father becoming paranoid. He often overly repeated things, and there was a great deal of arguing in restaurants and other public places. D went to a neurologist who said: "He was just tired." In the 1970s and 1980s, things continued to get worse.

In the 1990s D's paranoia became more intense. He would leave the house and walk the streets, get lost, and be picked up by the police who brought him home. At times at home, he would line up six pillows on a bed and have a board meeting, reflecting his career in business. On other occasions D would give neighbors paintings that belonged to his family, saying that he was giving them back to them. He sometimes said: "There is a woman I don't trust" when referring to his wife. During the years from 1997 until his death in 2001, he was in the hospital and then a nursing home, since his family could not manage his extreme deterioration.

Chronic Anxiety, Alzheimer's, and Me

As I watched my father live with Alzheimer's, I occasionally wondered if I would end up with that disease, thinking of the possibility of a genetic factor. It wasn't until I was 63 that my concern and anxiety emerged in response to some memory problems and some inability in finding words and names of objects. Over the next few years, night driving and my sense of direction seemed to deteriorate somewhat.

In 2007 I was visiting my stepson and his family and realized that I could not remember the name of his daughter for several hours. This was upsetting. I talked about this with my stepson and his wife, both psychiatrists, and they didn't detect any dementia that was more than an average age-related decline in cognitive functioning. They did say that if I really felt my memory was deteriorating, I might take the medications Aricept and Namenda. At some point, I started taking them, but after a week or ten days, side effects emerged and I decided to discontinue them.

A couple of years later while visiting with the same couple, I again voiced my concern about my memory and cognitive functioning. My stepson offered to give me a mental status exam with a focus on memory. I accepted, and with his wife and my wife present, I passed with flying colors.

Several years ago, I became concerned that about half the time when writing an appointment card for a client's next session, I would start to write their names in my appointment book as they were leaving my office and then forget their names. I would have to resort to looking at the names on their family diagrams or in session notes. This experience would trigger anxiety in me. My memory problem continued to worsen. Not remembering the names of people I knew happened quite frequently in many settings. But I had little trouble remembering the facts and relationship patterns of the families I was seeing in my clinical practice.

I would go through periods of feeling my cognitive functioning was fine and others where I observed lapses in memory, misuse of words, spatial relations, and uncertainty about driving directions, particularly at night.

In March 2011, I decided to have a neurological evaluation. I saw a highly recommended neurologist at Massachusetts General Hospital in Boston. After taking my history and doing a neurological evaluation, his summary was that I did not have even mild cognitive dysfunction. However, he said that with patients who were quite intelligent, sometimes it was more difficult to detect cognitive dysfunction, and therefore he recommended that I have a neuropsychological evaluation and a magnetic resonance imaging (MRI). That would give a baseline for my cognitive functioning. I did the testing in May 2011. The results of the neuropsychological evaluation showed that my cognitive functioning was in the average range of the population of my age and education cohort. I was somewhat reassured, except that the report indicated that I was functioning at a 102 IQ level on the WAIS (Wechsler Adult Intelligence Scale). Because I had been tested as having a 119 IQ as an adolescent applying to a private high school and as 129 in graduate school (taken as part of training while working in the psychology department of a state hospital), I was alarmed; 102 is just above average intelligence, and 129 is one point below superior intelligence on the WAIS. The results of my MRI were not sent to me for a few months, creating some anxiety for me. However, they showed that there were no signs of organic involvement for Alzheimer's disease or any other form of dementia. This was good news.

My effort, with mixed results, was to control my anxiety that I might have the beginnings of Alzheimer's disease in the face of some loss of memory and other cognitive problems. Was the anxiety an expression of my fusion with my father? Was my attempt to diagnose my own symptoms anxiety or honest perceptiveness, or both? Were my memory deterioration and forgetfulness related to aging, Alzheimer's, dementia, sleep apnea, or a mixture of some or all of these factors?

In January 2017, I saw the neurologist again as my memory and cognitive functioning continued to decline. The report was that there was some further atrophy of the brain, but not of significance.

While I cannot say that my anxiety that I would get Alzheimer's disease had decreased, my effort was to continue to try, still with mixed results, to lower my emotional reactivity in the following ways: 1) If I forgot a name or an idea, I tried to focus on it and allow it to come back without forcing it. I used this approach when I misplaced things. I would take a break and let my mind go back over the possible places I might have left the object. 2) I used more reminder notes for myself. 3) I tried not to complain to my wife and others too much about my memory or little events that indicated to me my failing memory or cognitive functioning. 4) I thought about plans for the future that seemed realistic but were neither overly pessimistic nor overly optimistic, in view of my perceived memory loss, cognitive functioning, and possible greater future decline. 5) I also take a course of nutritional supplements under the guidance of a researcher who specializes in new approaches to Alzheimer's disease. In addition, I exercise daily. 6) I set out to do one more edited book, with a co-editor. It was completed in 2018.

I plan for a gradual retirement, expecting to retire from my family therapy practice around 2020. These plans and goals are not set in concrete. I want to retire while I am still competent so that it can be an intentional process.

My Sister's Alzheimer's Disease

My sister had appeared to be having cognitive problems for a couple of years, starting around 2012 or before. In the summer of 2015, while visiting my wife and me, she told me that an MRI indicated she had mild to moderate Alzheimer's disease. At that time she was 75. My sister and I were able to have open, but not deep, discussions about her own reactions to being diagnosed with Alzheimer's. However, she was very straightforward regarding her diagnosis. In the summer of 2017, her Alzheimer's disease had progressed to a high-moderate level.

My sister does not have an anxious or depressed temperament. She was always, and is still, cheery and confident about her future. She remains that way even after the onset of her Alzheimer's disease and its progression.

My sister has lived in England and Italy for more than 50 years. Her much older English husband died in 1993 at age 71, leaving my sister a widow at age 52, with three children: two daughters and a son. At that time the two daughters were 24 and 18, and the son was 14.

My sister and I have had a good relationship, and she has visited me and my wife in the summer on Cape Cod for many years, and I have visited her on occasion in England and Italy.

After my sister's husband died in 1993, she became intensely focused on her three children, but they did not deal with the death of their father through open communication in the family. The first "emotional shock wave," the death of their father, who had a significant leadership position in their family, was an underlying factor in the pain of the second emotional shock wave, their mother's diagnosis of Alzheimer's and the symptoms that emerged related to "losing" their mother. In addition to the two emotional shock waves, this nuclear family has few extended family members, and they live in other countries. Also, the three siblings and their three stepsiblings from their father's first marriage have been somewhat emotionally cut off from each other since the death of their father.

Anxiety, conflict, projection, and triangles among the siblings emerged in distressed reaction to their mother's illness. These reactive patterns increased as her Alzheimer's disease moved from mild to high-moderate.

However, each of the three siblings has been taking care of her at her home in Oxford, England, or in Italy in different ways and for different periods of time. And they have coordinated the situation and their mother's needs by phone and email. They all agree that they want their mother to live at home for as long as possible.

Each sibling has had a breakup with a significant partner. The oldest daughter had two young children with an unmarried partner, and they then broke up before her mother's diagnosis for Alzheimer's. The middle daughter lived with an older male partner in the Italian mountains and ended that relationship after her mother's diagnosis. The son and his partner also ended their relationship at the time he got the news of their mother's diagnosis. The ending of the three significant relationships may likely have created more instability in their lives that added to their anxiety and reactivity in facing their mother's illness. It has been challenging for them to observe the emotional and behavioral changes in their mother resulting from her illness. The effects of losing the mother they knew before she developed Alzheimer's continue to develop.

A triangle emerged over time in which the middle daughter was in the outside position and the oldest daughter and youngest son were in the inside positions close together. However, as time has gone by the sisters have become closer again, and the three are relating positively with each other. The youngest sibling, the son, took on an overfunctioning position as family leader in dealing with their mother and her Alzheimer's condition. He figured out how to improve and rent their mother's summerhouse in Italy to generate income and also to make it possible for their mother to spend time living there. The two daughters have equally provided support to their mother. The three siblings have been engaged in researching their mother's condition and related concerns and sharing information to help their mother to the best of their abilities. It has been, and continues to be, a demanding and rewarding journey, practically and emotionally.

The relationship between the oldest daughter and middle daughter has been slowly repairing itself and is significantly less cutoff, less reactive, and more connected. The son began to move out of his overfunctioning position and put his creative work and personal life first again. He sounds a lot happier. This, of course, raises huge questions regarding how these adult children can manage their mother whose functioning is deteriorating to the point that she cannot live alone.

Poignantly, for the first time my sister is expressing a yearning to go back to America, "Where I'm from." She is becoming more able to feel and express her sadness. The younger daughter has sat and cried with her mother on various occasions. The daughter sees that her mother has a deep yearning to be somewhere that feels like home and somewhere she can feel right again and herself again. Their mother is losing her *self*, and her children are seeking to find the balance between overfunctioning and underfunctioning in order to move forward in their lives and still be responsible and accounted for with their mother and each other.

The three siblings care very much for each other, and they have the potential to not cut off from each other. Each of them shows resilience, is in the process of reaching toward a new partner, and shows a decrease in chronic anxiety.

My effort was to not get caught in their sibling triangles, to stay neutral, and to develop a greater level of one-to-one contact with my two nieces and nephew. These efforts involved occasional phone and Skype calls with the nieces who were in Italy and England and being in contact with my nephew who visited me and my wife while he works part-time in New York. Over many years I had Skype and phone calls with my sister, but she can no longer manage the video technology so we speak regularly by phone.

Reflections

In this chapter I raise questions about relating to a family member with Alzheimer's, or dementia, when his or her self is no longer present, although he or she still remains a living significant person in the family.

My effort was to relate both to my father's Alzheimer's disease and to my father as a person whose self had radically changed and diminished, but yet remained my father in the past, the present, and the future. The same is true in my relationship with my sister.

I make the distinction between the self and the person of the individual who has Alzheimer's disease. From a Bowen framework, *self* is best characterized by action. It refers not to what you say, but what you do. The concept of differentiation of self describes the self as not being an entity in itself, but rather it is always understood by its interrelationship with others, particularly with parents and the nexus of the multigenerational family that preceded them. The self is best understood in terms of the degree of separation between objective thinking and emotional reactivity. It is characterized by the I-positions and We-positions one takes in relation to significant others. It is grounded in the balance of the forces of individuality and togetherness. An individual comes into the world as a no-self and over time becomes a differentiated self, to a greater or lesser degree.

The self may be diminished and transformed through illness, but the person remains a living being with whom relationships exist. I am using the term person to describe the automatic existence of the biological and physiognomic gestalt of an individual human being from birth until death. In Alzheimer's disease, particularly when it has caused severe deterioration of the self, the person still exists in relationship with significant others through his or her functioning positions (for example, spouse, son, daughter, sister, brother, and others) and through past experiences with significant nonfamily members.

Alzheimer's disease can be a part of a mental construct triangle; for example, two living individuals—my father and I—and the disease. Although the disease is a living biological process, it functions impersonally in a triangle when one person relates to another with Alzheimer's disease as if the disease and the person are a single unit. This leads to the loss of the ability to relate one-to-one with the person who has the disease. In this situation the person and his disease are in the inside positions of the triangle, and the other person is in the outside position. For the latter to relate directly to the person with Alzheimer's, he or she must allow for the impact of the illness on the ill person's functioning, but also must seek to remain clear that the person is not the disease.

Dementia and Alzheimer's vary in intensity and rate of deterioration, as does aging. The course of Alzheimer's disease depends on genetics, possibly the level of differentiation of self to a degree, the level of intactness of one's relationship systems, environmental conditions, physical traumas, and luck. The disease varies in symptomatology, onset course of illness, the life course of the individual and the family, and the nonfamily relationship systems in which they participate.

Bowen (2017) described differentiation of self as a way of characterizing human functioning along a continuum:

> This concept provides a single dimension for understanding all people, from the lowest to the highest possible level of human functioning. People have the quality of "fusing with," or "being like" those about them. Those with the most separateness of self, and who predictably operate with this separateness under all varying degrees of stress and emotional tension, are said to be the most "differentiated." Those with the least separateness of self who either fuse into the emotional environment about them, or who bristle and fight the emotional environment are the most "undifferentiated." The most differentiated people who know what they believe and who they are, and who predictably stand on their convictions under emotional stress, are the most successful in life. They live orderly lives, they are the most productive at whatever they do, and they are free remarkably of physical, emotional, and social illness. The most undifferentiated people have the capacity of getting along in a simple, brief interpersonal situation, but this automatic tendency to compromise self to relieve the anxiety of the moment results in long-term complication. (pp. 49–50)

Alzheimer's disease appears with great variation along a continuum of human functioning. I would hypothesize that individuals at higher levels of differentiation of self are characterized by having less chronic anxiety and less emotional reactivity throughout life before the onset of Alzheimer's symptoms. The progression of Alzheimer's disease for them may likely involve less agitation, less overemotionality, less suspicion or paranoia, and fewer repetitious and obsessive behaviors than those individuals who functioned at lower levels of differentiation of self in their life course before the onset of Alzheimer's disease.

The self emerges from an undifferentiated state in infancy and evolves over an indefinite period of time. However, basic differentiation of self is usually concretized in late adolescence or early adulthood. While the self may remain intact throughout life for some individuals, some deterioration of self occurs in the aging process of most humans.

This may lead to an absence of self for those with severe Alzheimer's and severe dementia, but the person-in-relationship can continue to exist. Family members and friends can work to retain contact with the person with dementia and maintain a human connection. This was my effort with my father in his final years, and is now my effort with my sister.

Managing my anxiety about my own aging process, which may include Alzheimer's disease, is the biggest current challenge in my life. We live in an age where the average human life span is longer than at any previous time in history. There is an illusory hope that we can endlessly extend life and our mental functioning. Instead of early death, the fear many of us may now be experiencing, but are not necessarily prepared for, is that the aging process will inevitably lead to brain deterioration as well as physical deterioration.

Self-awareness, objectivity, and responsible action, all hallmarks of differentiation of self, will be increasingly difficult in the context of brain deterioration, as Alzheimer's was for my father and is for my sister, and may be for me. My effort will be to maintain a reasonable level of differentiation of self for as long as possible. I will work with determination to sustain it.

REFERENCES

Bowen, M. (2017). A systems view of the aging process. *Family Systems: A Journal of Natural Systems Thinking in Psychiatry and the Sciences*, *13*(1).

Titelman, P. (1987). *The therapist's own family: Toward the differentiation of self.* Northvale, NJ: Jason Aronson.

13

NO SYMPATHY

A Response to a Physical Disability[1]

Susan W. Graefe

Thirty years after polio's crippling assault on my seven-year-old body, I began to experience an intense need to cut through years of denial and overfunctioning, to look squarely at the facts, and to allow my feelings about that most painful part of my life to take their rightful place.

I needed to make peace with the years of silence, denial, intellectual and emotional overfunctioning, and compensations for physical incapacities. I needed to explore what that illness meant for my family and friends, and then for colleagues and clients as I moved from the dependency of a child on crutches to marriage, motherhood, and a successful career as a clinical social worker. I needed to start to listen more carefully to my inner thoughts and to observe my life patterns in broad and open ways. The key to the process has been, and is, the sorting of facts from emotions in this highly charged area.

As I near the 33rd anniversary of polio's intrusion into my world, the pieces of the puzzle are coming together. I am freer of the need to overfunction as a way of proving to myself, and the rest of the world, that I am a capable human being. I am aware of my nuclear and extended families in new ways and of their patterns of functioning in response to crises and to family illnesses. In addition, I can recognize a connection between my choice of a career as a clinical social worker specializing in the treatment of elderly people and their families and my responses to illness and family systems, both conscious and subconscious.

At the time of my graduation from high school, 22 years ago, a local newspaper interviewed my mother and me about the impact of polio on the family. My mother said that no one can estimate the endless effort parents put forth during a child's long illness, as well as the worry, constant care, and draining financial expense. She credited the success of my struggle to the fact that my family gave me "lots and lots of love and no sympathy." That clearly stated philosophy became a permanent part of the basic fabric of my being.

Family Systems Under Stress

As one begins to look at the effects of a major illness, several major areas emerge immediately: 1) the patient's and the family's emotional system at the time illness begins, 2) subsequent development of both as the illness continues, 3) response of the patient to the physical limitations imposed by a crippling illness, and 4) response of both the nuclear and extended families to the needs imposed by these limitations.

With respect to both my needs and my limitations, denial was the cornerstone of my nuclear family's behavior. My extended family, however, provided some sympathy and indulgence as a balance to this. My maternal grandmother and maternal aunt relieved me of general housekeeping tasks when I was in their presence, and they chided my mother for involving me in too many activities in addition to housekeeping chores. However, I was continually reminded by my mother that if I allowed myself to be "pampered," I might never regain my strength or walk again. My mother's prescription was powerful, and she enforced it vigorously. I believed her fearsome assessment, but it was difficult to concentrate only on the sheer drive she demanded when, within me, I often wanted to be pampered and taken care of. This anguish always intruded.

Cheered on by my parents, I pursued life with a vengeance. I did not allow my two Canadian crutches to get in the way of being an avid softball player. Although I could not run, I could hit a line drive, and one of my friends ran bases for me. Football and basketball were a little more difficult, but no matter what the sport or activity, I found a way to adapt. In high school I was known as the "nonjumping" cheerleader and never missed a game in three years.

In all, these achievements contributed to the illusion that I had few, if any, limitations. My family and I defined, by our own attitudes and actions, the view we wished others to accept.

Achieving this projection of competency despite adversity was a triumph over the initial facts of my case. At the onset of my illness I lived for two weeks in the terrible loneliness of an isolation hospital. I was completely paralyzed from the waist down and also in my left arm. It was a crucially traumatic experience for a seven-year-old.

The next three months were spent in a chronic care hospital. I remember my mother's words as I was being put in the ambulance for the trip to that hospital: "You have been very ill, but now you are going to be fine." At the time, I thought being "fine" meant running and jumping with the rest of the children. These hopes were dashed by three months in a ward with 40 other polio victims in various stages of affliction, living out their lives in iron lungs, rocking beds, wheelchairs, walkers, and crutches.

I remember feeling very frightened, as well as experiencing indescribable physical pain. My limbs were immobilized for a time by sandbags weighted to keep the muscles stretched. Many times a day my body was covered with wet wool hot packs; I never was told the purpose of this treatment (even now, the odor of wet wool stimulates body aches and nausea). I was among the youngest patients on that polio ward. Many of the patients were adults, and several of them died while I was there. There were a number of high school and college students, and also some very young children who were unable to express their feelings in words. I was shy and timid, fearful of asking for help, and frightened by the atrophying bodies surrounding me. How could I ever be "just fine"?

I discovered the radio. Its soap operas and adventure stories were my bedside companions. Every day there were visitors, usually one or both of my parents, a family friend, or a neighbor. I have little or no memory of the presence of extended family—my parents were the key figures.

Mother's Determination

My mother pushed constantly for the best possible treatment for me. She worked hard to convince me that I would walk again if I would do even more than what I was told to do. If I was told to exercise for 10 minutes, she encouraged 15 or 20. If I was supposed to walk one length of the hall in my walker, then she pushed me to do two lengths.

In a recent conversation, I asked my mother what this period was like for her. She focused on two words: fear and determination. Her fear was of "the dreaded disease" and her sense of lack of control over its crippling effects on my body. My mother, an overly responsible eldest child, was always in control of everything, or so she and we believed.

Her determination was the cornerstone for overcoming my illness, and she went to great lengths to help me recover. I was awed by her persistence in knocking down barriers to good treatment. She confronted complacent doctors with demands for answers to her many questions. She worked on my body for hours, following carefully the instructions of the physical therapist she had searched out; I became my mother's project.

During the first year of my illness she quite neglected herself. That self-deprivation created a kind of backlash in me, keenly felt over the years. I always assumed that her pent-up anger was caused by my failure to live up to her expectations for coping with adversity.

While my mother and I were on a trip alone four years ago, she asked what it was like for me during that first year and the subsequent dealing with the effects of polio. I had waited for her to ask that question for almost 30 years.

It was a year before I could respond effectively. I was then able to share my feelings of physical and emotional pain that I had always believed she did not want to hear. I also shared my perception that she felt that my illness had nearly ruined her life. This open and direct conversation was a turning point in my relationship with my mother. We were able to share long-overdue tears.

During my childhood she had finally accepted the fact that my recovery would be long and slow, but she did not share that fact with me until these conversations several years ago. As we finally discussed our perceptions of my childhood years, she related having experienced an immense sense of loneliness in not having any help, either physically or emotionally, from her family or from my father's family.

They were present for visits and for giving gifts to me, but not for pitching in and helping with respite care and to relieve her and my father. My grandparents, aunts, and uncles tended, instead, to be quite critical of the extent to which my parents "pushed" me into the normal activities of daily living. The determination of my parents to see me succeed in overcoming my illness and their sense of denial kept them nonreactive to criticism and to the anxiety of others. This, in turn, enabled me to engage in many activities, which were both healing to my body and effective in helping me develop a sense of self in which I viewed myself as more normal than disabled.

Recently my mother acknowledged that although she allowed me a great deal of freedom and independence, internally she had experienced tremendous anxiety over my safety and my vulnerability. I had been totally unaware of her anxiety, as well as of the physical risks involved in many of my activities and adventures. I am thankful that she kept her anxieties hidden, for this allowed me to take risks. And while I admire her ability to conceal her fears, I know the costliness of such a gift.

I am now aware of the extent of the trusting bond that actually existed between my parents and me, an extremely crucial trust for someone as physically dependent as I was. Learning about my mother's anger and disappointment in her family's response to my illness was helpful. I had always believed that all of her anger stemmed from me and my illness, that through my illness I had been responsible for "messing up" her life. Now I know that at least some of her anger belonged elsewhere—with her family. With these new realizations, I feel a lessened need to maintain the superhuman stance I always felt necessary to make her happy with me.

Father: Steady and Dependable

My father's steady presence, as the nonaggressive parent, brought a balance of quiet and levity to my mother's intense, action-oriented reactivity. He provided much actual physical care in the early stages of my illness. My need to be carried in his arms, I now realize, was emotionally and physically difficult for him. He never complained and never shared his emotional pain. Looking back, I recall feeling that he always appeared unhappy, as if he were carrying heavy burdens. He had to work hard for the financial support of the family.

His time with me was often spent in just talking about things unrelated to my illness. He introduced me to sports, and I became a New York Yankees fan, endlessly reciting statistics on American League players and important games. He pitched balls for me to hit and shot baskets with me in front of the garage.

His quiet, unwavering support was always there. If he saw me struggling with a physical task, he intervened with possible adaptations, but not with discouragement. He encouraged new interests: cheerleading; rifle matches, in which I proudly won target shooting prizes; swimming; fishing; sailing—he taught me to fish, I taught him to sail. His interests extended to my academic pursuits, particularly mathematics, which was his strength and my downfall.

The message from my father, though not verbalized, was clear: I was capable of doing anything. Even though this was my mother's message also, my father conveyed it in more expansive terms.

Over the past nine years, in a reversal of roles, I have spent considerable time visiting my father during his several hospitalizations. Typically, he protested the necessity of my traveling a considerable distance to visit him. Once, in 1977, when he was close to death following the removal of a kidney, we had a very quietly significant visit together. I was able to reminisce about the importance and meaningfulness of his hospital visits to me as I went through polio and a series of rehabilitative surgeries. I was able to share my sadness over his illness, and we both struggled to hold back our tears. Gently I suggested that it was important for us to be able to shed our tears together. In those few moments of blended tears, we felt permission to thank each other for our mutual presence and support over the years. We were able, in the usual quiet and understanding ways in which we lived our lives together, to grieve over his illness and to speak of the possible loss of his life.

My father recovered from his kidney surgery, but is currently in declining health. I have yet to ask him exactly how my illness affected him. I think, however, that we can now share verbally this particular bond.

Siblings and Peers

My brother, who is three years younger than I, was too young to understand events during the early years of my illness. Very caring neighbors and friends took care of him when my parents visited me in the hospital. He became my primary friend and companion during those early years when I could not keep pace physically with peers who were running around and riding bicycles. We shared an emotional closeness even though his interests developed in very different directions from mine. Neither academically nor athletically oriented, he was encouraged to pursue his artistic, and later his entrepreneurial, talents. Despite our closeness, he and I have yet to be able to talk about what it was like for him to grow up with a handicapped sister or about its effect on our continuing relationship. Breaching that particular silence is part of my continuing work of healing.

Peer relationships became difficult for me, beginning with the loneliness and isolation of the months of hospitalization. There, the gnawing fact that our bodies were different from those of other people was something none of the polio victims on my ward could talk about; it was easier to stay in touch with the inner persons who had existed before the illness and to ignore or deny the existence of the distorted and atrophied bodies we inhabited. For all of us, there was one vital deprivation: the permission to grieve the loss of physical functioning that each of us had experienced.

I made a promise at that time that someday I would help people who were sick to talk about what they were going through. For me, however, there was no one to acknowledge and listen to my physical and emotional pain. When I cried, I was told I should not, because other people were worse off than I, even dying. In my own quiet way, I began observing and listening to the pain of others at that early age. Listening to them speaking about their feelings was a comfortable way of relating to people and, of course, a way to circumvent acknowledging my own. In the hospital I was always the friendly visitor for other patients. I know now that I was defining a sense of purpose for myself that was beyond my own physical rehabilitation.

Relating to my peers was a different matter. They were not sick, and my crippled body was outside their experience and comprehension. How could they relate to a peer who could not run and jump and ride bicycles? Occasionally they came to visit and played games or watched television with me, but I could sense that they did not really want my slow, awkward, ugly body in their active seven-year-old lives. Later, at school and in the community, efforts were made to integrate me into normal activities, but my embarrassment about the way I looked and walked made these efforts difficult for me to accept. Returning to school was not easy after being away for a full year and being taught by a teacher for the home-bound. I had missed socialization, and third grade went badly. I felt very conspicuous dragging my weakened body with two Canadian crutches.

However, in the fourth grade I had the first of a series of teachers who took a special interest in me. My fourth-grade teacher took me aside one day after I had sat for an hour wistfully watching my classmates learn to square dance. "It must be hard for you to watch the other kids do things that you cannot do," she said. I cried. She was the first person to acknowledge and address my feelings. I thought no one would ever recognize the depth of my anguish, the deep hurt I could not allow myself to voice. Then she expressed her admiration for my courage and the strength of my family. She was very specific in identifying the number of intellectual and creative talents she observed in me. Unfortunately, she was only one person. No one else gave me permission to feel sad and grieve, and I could not allow myself these essential feelings.

Family Patterns

Looking back into those years is still painful. Today, as a therapist based firmly in a family systems orientation, I must consider the compelling issues involved. Of particular interest to me is the history of illness and loss in my extended family system and the way in which illnesses and deaths have been dealt with over time. The maternal side of my family furnishes many examples (Figure 13.1).

My maternal great-grandmother died at age 40, leaving four children, aged 16, 13, 11, and 6. She is described as a model mother, attractive, hard working, and mild mannered. The story goes that several days before her death she was struck by lightning, which left her feeling ill. Several years ago I learned from her death certificate that she died having a miscarriage. As far as I know, her own children either did not know this or simply never talked about it.

After her death, my maternal great-grandfather provided well for his family, even hiring a live-in housekeeper to help with childcare. He became the patriarch; everyone turned to him for answers to life's problems and for financial and emotional security. He built a summer home for his adult children to "keep the family together"—a successful effort.

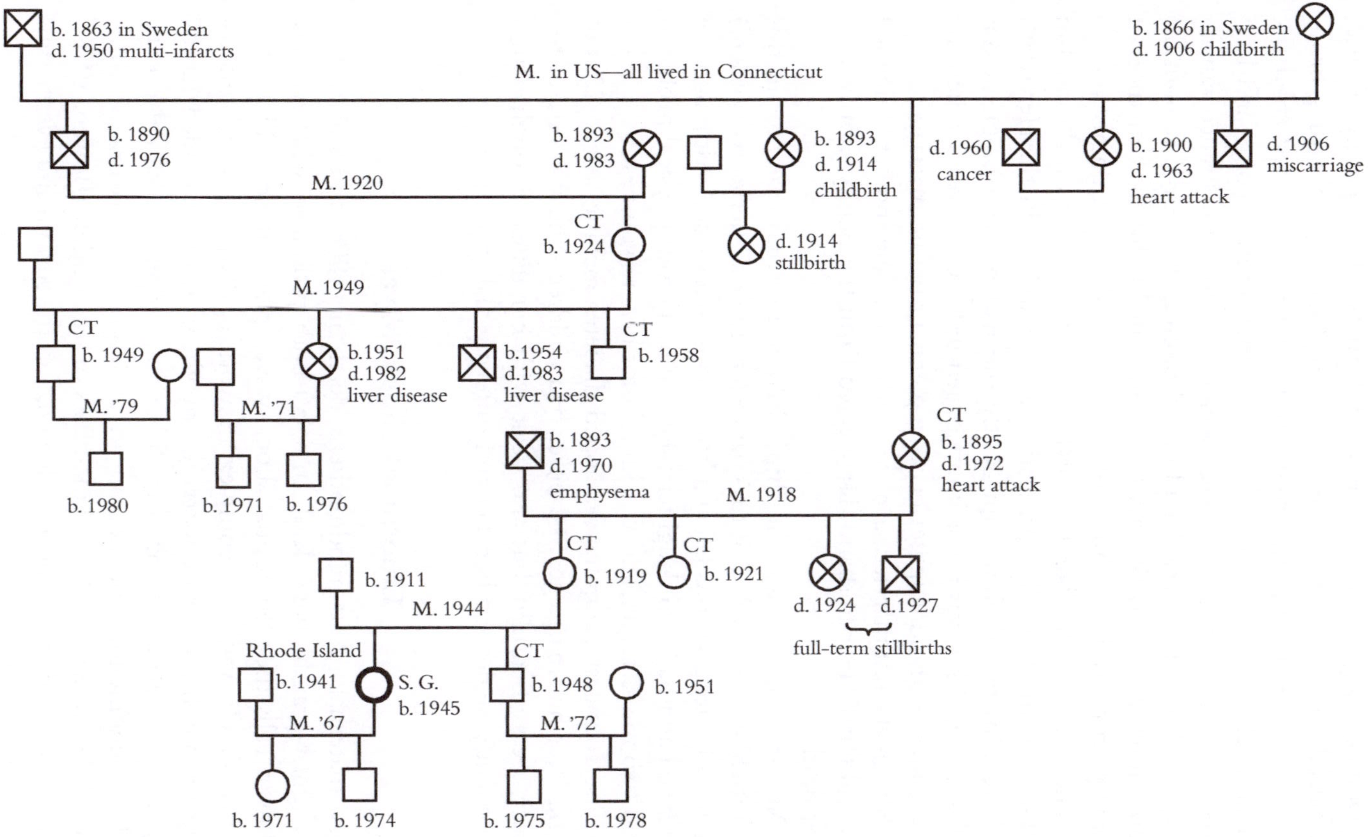

Figure 13.1 The maternal family diagram

Despite my great-grandfather's efforts to normalize family life after the death of his wife, all of his children had serious, continuing problems with coping with the stresses of their lives. The oldest child, my great-uncle, went to work to augment the family income and later went into the U.S. Army, with which he served in France during World War I. He married, had one daughter, and held a responsible job. However, he drank heavily throughout his life as a method of coping with his demanding father, difficult wife, and arduous job.

The oldest of the daughters, who was described as the "most fun loving" of the four siblings, died at age 21 in childbirth. Her death was seldom talked about; apparently she had become pregnant out of wedlock. This was not acknowledged until recent years, when my great-uncle's granddaughter became pregnant before marriage.

My great-aunt married several months before she and her child died in childbirth. Her husband disappeared from the family shortly after her death.

My grandmother was the third child and second daughter in this family. She developed St. Vitus's dance (chorea—a "nervous disorder") at age 11 after a serious fall at a house construction site. Although she married and had two daughters, she had numerous physical problems and two miscarriages, and was known for her nervousness.

The youngest daughter developed diabetes mellitus at age 23, not long after her marriage. She never had children. She was one of the early users of insulin, but also dealt with her illness through denial, frequently neglecting her diet and suffering diabetic comas.

Emotional Shock Waves

My maternal great-grandmother's death in 1906 and my maternal great-grandfather's death in 1950 both produced what Murray Bowen calls the "emotional shock wave" phenomenon. The emotional shock wave is a complex network of "after-shocks" following serious life events occurring anywhere in the extended family system in the months or years following serious emotional events. The phenomenon operates on an underground network of emotional dependence of family members on each other (Bowen, 1976). The emotional dependence is denied, and the serious life events thus appear unrelated.

Although the shock wave phenomenon occurs most often in families with a significant degree of denied emotional fusion, it also may occur in families that are closed to discussing sensitive issues, such as death and illness. The closed communication system is an automatic emotional reflex to protect self from anxiety, although most people will say they "avoid taboo subjects to keep from upsetting the other person" (Bowen, 1976, p. 336). It is as if the shock wave triggers the physical process into activity.

Following the deaths of key family members, a pattern of physical and/or emotional dysfunction often emerges. In my own family I have explored this as far back as the deaths of my maternal great-grandparents. As noted earlier, there was a high degree of dependence on my maternal great-grandfather. His adult children and their families cared for his physical needs in later years, but all were emotionally dependent on his presence. As long as he was alive no one else had to take much responsibility for family life.

Following my great-grandfather's death, there were many instances of physical and emotional dysfunction within the family. Both my mother and my maternal grandfather developed serious asthma, which was the beginning of lifelong chronic bronchial disorders. My great-uncle and his wife began a pattern of heavy drinking, which has continued into the next two generations: Their daughter is an alcohol abuser, and two adult grandchildren have died from alcohol abuse. My great-aunt's diabetes worsened and she suffered several diabetic comas. Although my grandmother became the clan leader, she developed myriad chronic physical problems, including leg ulcers, stomach ulcers, breast cancer, and heart disease. She also became somewhat reclusive and was, perhaps, phobic. She died in my presence on December 23, 1972, of a sudden, massive heart attack while entertaining the family for dinner. I contracted polio just two years after the death of my maternal great-grandfather.

My illness was contained in a matrix of anxiety about polio from a national perspective. People actually bought polio insurance out of fear of the summer epidemics of the disease.

Throughout the continuing shock waves of illness, denial was the prevalent pattern. It is important to understand that the loss of significant family members did not cause the subsequent illnesses; rather, the illnesses were part of the response to anxiety as the family tried to realign itself.

Replications

In Bowen theory, the nuclear family emotional system is described as having patterns that replicate past generations as they repeat in future generations (Bowen, 1976, p. 78). Bowen also says that in every family system there is emotional fusion, and the greater the fusion, the more likely the family is to become symptomatic in periods of high anxiety. He notes that there are several important ways in which a family handles high anxiety: emotional distance between spouses, marital conflicts, dysfunction in one spouse, and impairment of one or more children. I was a likely candidate for absorbing a large dose of family anxiety. I had been seriously ill with measles several months before contracting polio and had had a tonsillectomy the previous spring. I believe that as the oldest and highly valued grandchild in a very enmeshed family, which also worked hard to deny grief and crisis, I lived out the role my parents covertly assigned me—that of an extremely competent child without limitations.

This family environment of illness was perfect for compounding the emotional effects of polio, whose victims were often so glad to have survived, or to be able to walk, that they felt guilty about complaining or being concerned about symptoms or residual effects. Polio victims often denied their disabilities and were encouraged to "count their blessings."

In reexamining my own history, I have observed two models of reaction to illness and disability in my family: 1) denial and 2) the use of illness or disability as an excuse for not functioning. I learned denial from my parents, who persisted in all efforts, no matter how they felt or how many obstacles were inherent in the illness and in its rehabilitative aftermath. From my maternal grandmother and my mother's sister, who both suffered from multiple physical maladies, I learned the "convenience" of illness. That is, if no one was available, my grandmother got around well, took care of herself, and even met the needs of others. However, if someone was there to wait on her, she took advantage of the fact. It was therefore hard to assess a way to do anything I really wanted to do; however, at times I like to be dependent, although I still have difficulty communicating my desire for help. How much of "functioning" is actually function, and how much is really dysfunction? What are my physical capabilities, and what are my actual limitations? Never having been allowed to recognize limitations, it is difficult to concede that there are barriers of any kind. My mother's "no sympathy" was a challenge, indeed a command, to do my best. However, since my mother never allowed any limits, how could I learn them?

The Continuing Effects of Polio

The specter of polio is again in the news in 1985 as the post-polio syndrome (or post-polio sequelae) begins an insidious debilitation of an estimated one-fourth of polio survivors and strikes dread in all who have a history of polio. Symptoms of the post-polio syndrome include fatigue, muscle weakness and pain, debilitating joint pain, breathing difficulties, and intolerance of cold. I now have an additional reason to examine using all my resources, both the facts and the feelings inherent in the painful legacies of this illness.

In a *New York Times Magazine* article (1985, July 7) regarding polio's legacy, Dr. Jaquelin Perry notes:

> These people push themselves more than most of us. They've put up with signs of strain to live a normal life. I always say that people who have had polio are over-achievers, because so many of them are out to prove they can do as well as those who didn't have it.

In the same article, Susan S. Turner, a social worker, confirms that many post-polio patients "view themselves as super-achievers or workaholics." Turner wrote: "Part of the panic people are feeling is the nightmare of not feeling self-sufficient" (Horowitz, 1985).

Whether I become a post-polio syndrome victim or not, the manner in which I deal with function and dysfunction is important: By adopting my family's denial, I was enabled to lead an essentially active life, and it was not until my junior year in college, while seeing a therapist, that I finally acknowledged and began to mourn the fact that I could not run or jump or walk long distances. Even more telling, it was only three years ago that I showed a long-hidden photograph to a group of social work colleagues as we worked on family systems issues in our own families. I am shown seated in a wheelchair, accepting a plant from my Brownie Scout troop. Sharing this photograph was a major breakthrough in facing the many years of denial and embarrassment about that part of my life. I had never wanted people to feel sorry for me any more than I would have wished them to make fun of me. I wanted to be treated as a normal human being. While symbolic of many things, the photograph primarily serves to dramatize my differences from others rather than my similarities to them.

The central issue in recounting my experience with polio concerns limits and the awareness that physical limits and emotional limits are not always effective partners. Indeed, they are often at odds with each other. My inability to allow myself to recognize physical limitations is frequently counterproductive, resulting in serious fatigue and pain in my limbs. As a result, I do not always perform well in my roles as wife, mother, and daughter; community organization volunteer; or clinical social worker. My super-functioning sometimes makes the other people in my family and work systems less functional, which is not helpful for them or me.

I do not want to help replicate the pattern of past generations, in which one or two super-functioners (overfunctioners) in each generation carried along the family members who functioned minimally, or underfunctioned. I try to achieve a delicate balance which allows me to be less functional at times, knowing that I am a solid enough self to return to normal functioning again, and further allows other family members and my clients to develop as normal functioners.

Professional Determinations

In the process of training to become a clinical social worker, I realized that there were many areas in my own life where I was stuck. This realization in turn revealed impasses in similar areas of my clinical work with individuals and families. In view of this difficulty, I began additional training in family systems thinking. In 1974, I participated for a full year in a group with other therapists, facilitated by Paulina McCullough at the Family Institute at Western Psychiatric Institute and Clinic in Pittsburgh. We studied our own extended families as a way of learning more about family systems. As I worked on the process of differentiation in my own family, I realized that I was already manifesting the behavioral characteristics of an overfunctioning oldest daughter, just as my mother had done before me. I also saw the extent to which I was overfunctioning in both my nuclear family and work systems. In addition, I experienced severe panic attacks for six months, beginning within a month of my grandmother's death (at which I was present). I gasped for breath, just as she had done. I did not realize fully the impact of her loss on the unresolved anger that I had directed toward her passive domination of the family system. My mother now moved to the position of being the clan leader, and the message became clear that as the oldest daughter I would be the next in line.

The differentiation process has continued over the past 11 years with ongoing efforts to remain detriangled. Though difficult, this work has been invaluable in my personal life and professional growth and development, and in my clinical work with families. Work on one's family issues is clearly a birth-to-death process, with new developments at each stage of the life cycle. Every year I uncover new information, which, although helpful in understanding patterns, rarely brings immediate gratification or a sense of useful direction. Instead, it usually surfaces in unexpected ways and at unexpected times.

During this past year I took a risk in my relationship with my parents and several of my friends and colleagues by showing them a videotape of a consultation done by Murray Bowen with me at a conference for professionals in March 1984 in Northampton, Massachusetts, sponsored by the Family Living Consultants of the Pioneer Valley.

Dr. Bowen interviewed me about the work I had been doing on my extended family during the preceding ten years. In addition, I decided to show my initial drafts of this chapter to the same individuals.

Taking such risks is dangerous, in that family members, friends, and colleagues are often negatively reactive to spoken and written perceptions of family events and interactions. They may become defensive, may attack, or even withdraw from contact. There is also the risk of having the viewer or reader become fused with any emotions expressed and thus be unable to view the material objectively. This can lead to overidentification with the writer and lack of separateness.

My experience with both the tape and the writing has been very positive. I believe that it has provided a new level of understanding with my parents and has opened conversation about topics we had been unable to address. They have both expressed appreciation for my sharing and have said that it added something to their lives. The effect on my friends and colleagues has been much more varied. Their questions and comments have been helpful in enabling me to think more clearly and in broader terms about my family and the experience of illness. Through sharing, I have also learned a great deal about their families, which speaks to the universality of coping with human suffering and trauma.

In view of my family history and life experiences, it is no accident that I chose to become a family therapist. The awareness of my capacity for observation and listening to people's pain began when I was a seven-year-old patient in the polio ward trying to make sense of what had happened to my body and those of my fellow patients. I was puzzled and frustrated at the time by the fact that there was no one who would acknowledge my physical and emotional pain, extreme fear, and loss of function. Such an experience of illness often results in a particular sensitiveness, which may become evident in a number of ways. I developed "antennae" that are particularly sensitive to people experiencing physical and emotional trauma from external circumstances beyond their control. I experienced the effects of living in a closed family system that perpetuated the myth that I had no physical limitations from the polio. It was not until psychotherapy during my college years that I realized the fact, and the extent, of my unresolved grieving. With the nurturance and acceptance of a listening therapist who herself had experienced an incapacitating physical trauma as a young person, I became aware of my own capacity for listening and reflecting as well as the value of my experience as a strength in helping others.

Any vocation coming out of a strong life experience should be followed with caution, lest personal factors override professional performance. As a family therapist, my personal inclination to overfunction must not be allowed to deter my clients from reaching their maximum levels of functioning. On the other hand, personal awareness of the potential for emotional shock wave patterns can, indeed, be helpful in encouraging clients to be more open and communicative at the time of loss or serious stress and to avoid harmful denial. When shock waves are evident, my experience allows me to be less reactive to them and to understand the natural cause of their existence.

A "given" in my life is that my extended family remains locked into shock wave patterns. I continue to try to facilitate communication with and among extended family members by stressing the facts of any given situation and seeking to allow the release of feelings, both of which bring healing. I realize that my own differentiation is not easy for my extended family to accept and will not necessarily change their life patterns.

My professional orientation and experience influence and inform my personal family systems, promoting the continuing growth and challenge that lead to more personal integration. I can see also that my personal experience with family systems under continuing stress is an enabling force in my work with clients.

The interplay between the professional and the personal aspects of my life brings a particular kind of balance and perspective. My hope is that it serves to free my nuclear family and provide increasing liberation from replicating harmful patterns of the past.

The value of the past is the perspective it brings to the work of the present and to the hope for the future.

Epilogue

Thirty years after writing "No Sympathy: A Response to a Physical Disability," I remain in awe at the wisdom of my parents in adopting this approach to our family experience with my polio in 1952. They were able to assume a firm position of providing me with support and encouragement, enabling me to maximize my potential as a relatively well-functioning human being despite criticism from extended family members.

My father died in September 1990 following several aneurysm surgeries and three years on renal dialysis. During that time I was stretched thin trying to maintain my private practice, manage involvement in volunteer organizations, be present to my nuclear family, and be with my parents in Connecticut on a weekly basis.

Several months before my father died, my nephew made a serious suicide attempt on his 15th birthday. He spent several months in a psychiatric program. My father was very reactive to his grandson's near death and seemed to become frailer in reaction. He made the decision to stop his dialysis and was able to die at home using hospice services. A year after his death I became seriously depressed, a delayed reaction to how much of a mainstay he was in my life.

My maternal aunt went into a deep depression following my father's death, as she had become very dependent on him for help as her health had declined. She eventually was unable to live on her own and spent the last several years of her life in a nursing home, dying in June 1994 of metastatic breast cancer.

My mother remained independent despite encroaching chronic obstructive pulmonary disease (COPD) and serious ulcerated legs. She moved to an assisted living facility in 1999 and died in September 2001. My brother and I were able to work as a team in the care of our parents. He lived closer to them so was present for the hospital emergencies, while I was present on a weekly basis to help with tasks of daily living.

In the fall of 2012 about the same time I was diagnosed with stage 2 breast cancer, my brother was diagnosed with serious esophageal cancer. I was fortunate to be treated with a lumpectomy and radiation with no recurrence.

My brother was less fortunate, having extensive chemotherapy, radiation, and tube feeding until his death in April 2014. While my brother was ill he was also caring for his wife, who had become seriously impaired by alcoholism and severe arthritis in her spine. She was hospitalized for a month before her death of cirrhosis of the liver in May 2013. My brother moved to an independent living facility at the time of his wife's death. He decided to stop his tube feeding and go on hospice care much as my father had 23 years earlier. I was able to be present with him throughout his last six weeks of life. This was an extremely meaningful period for my brother and myself and his son.

In 2002 I began to have increasing symptoms of post-polio syndrome and had to begin using Canadian crutches and a leg brace to walk. Although this was discouraging, my determination has never wavered, and I have continued to stay as active as possible with sailing, swimming, and frequent travel both in the United States and abroad.

I attribute my ability to basically stay on course in both my personal and professional life to my ongoing contact with the Georgetown Family Center, Western Pennsylvania Family Center, and the New England Seminar on Bowen Theory.

NOTE

1 This modified chapter was first published in *The Therapist's Own Family: Toward the Differentiation of Self*, edited by Peter Titelman, PhD, 1987. Northvale, NJ: Jason Aronson. (Reprinted with permission from Rowman & Littlefield Publishing Group.)

REFERENCES

Bowen, M. (1976). Family reaction to death. In P. Guerin (Ed.), *Family therapy: Theory and practice* (pp. 42–90). New York, NY: Gardner Press.

Horowitz, J. (1985, July 7). Polio's painful legacy. *The New York Times Magazine*.

IV

DEATH IN CLINICAL PRACTICE

14

FAMILY REACTION TO DEATH IN CLINICAL PRACTICE

An Approach Based on Bowen Theory

Laura Havstad

The Clinical Hypothesis From Bowen Theory

Family relationships profoundly affect the emotional adjustment of family members to death and loss. Over time, the effects of death on one family member can be intensified by the reactions of others in the family and lead to emotional chain reactions. These emotional chain reactions in family relationships can create serious difficulty, and symptoms in a family member can follow. Bowen referred to as this as the "emotional shock wave" (1976). Several predictions from Bowen theory organize clinical observations when an increase in chronic symptoms in a family member follows a death. First, family relationship patterns may shift and intensify after a death. Second, the shifts in relationship patterns affect family members differently and lead to their different trajectories of impairment or resilience following a death. Third, Bowen theory predicts that if a family leader is coached to differentiate a self from the family emotional system, the patterns of the family emotional system can shift and moderate. As the reactive patterns of the relationship system moderate, the symptoms of family members impaired in the family reaction to death will moderate as well.

This chapter will focus on a clinical approach to observing the impact of death on individuals in the multigenerational context of the family emotional system. In individually oriented clinical practice, symptomatic responses to the death of a family member are typically conceptualized in terms of the individual's psychology in direct relationship to the lost person. Widening the lens to the family unit shifts the focus to how a death affects the group of individuals who are bound together in an emotional system. It is in the context of the dynamic interplay of family relationships that individual symptoms are understood and addressed here.

The clinical formulation is this: In reaction to death the patterns of the family emotional system that impair or improve the functioning of some of its members can be set in motion or intensified. This can become the most important factor governing the course of either preexisting symptoms or those that emerge following death and loss and whether they persist or resolve. The family patterns of the emotional system and associated individual symptoms can be moderated and relationships strengthened, without cutoff, when a family leader can take themselves out of the patterns while maintaining active relationships with all involved. In this way, a death in the family offers significant opportunities for working on differentiation of self from the family emotional system for a family member willing to lead for the benefit of all in the family.

Trajectories of Loss and Resilience and the Family Emotional System

Research by George Bonanno and his associates on individual adjustment following death and loss (Bonanno, Westphal, & Mancini, 2011; Bonanno, 2005) has demonstrated individual variation in reaction to loss and the frequency with which emotional trajectories following loss result in symptomatic adjustments in the overall population. When symptoms occur in the individual, this reaction to death in the family might be short-term or long-term. Individuals might suffer depression, anxiety, or various illnesses as well as prolonged and complicated grief. While recommendations for mental health intervention have increased for almost anyone who expresses grief, the normal course of adjustment shows that most people are resilient.

Figure 14.1 illustrates the adjustment or failure to adjust back to the baseline level of well-being after death or a potentially traumatic event. Most people follow a trajectory of resilience after loss and do not experience more than short disruptions in normal functioning. A smaller percentage is symptomatic for longer but will recover

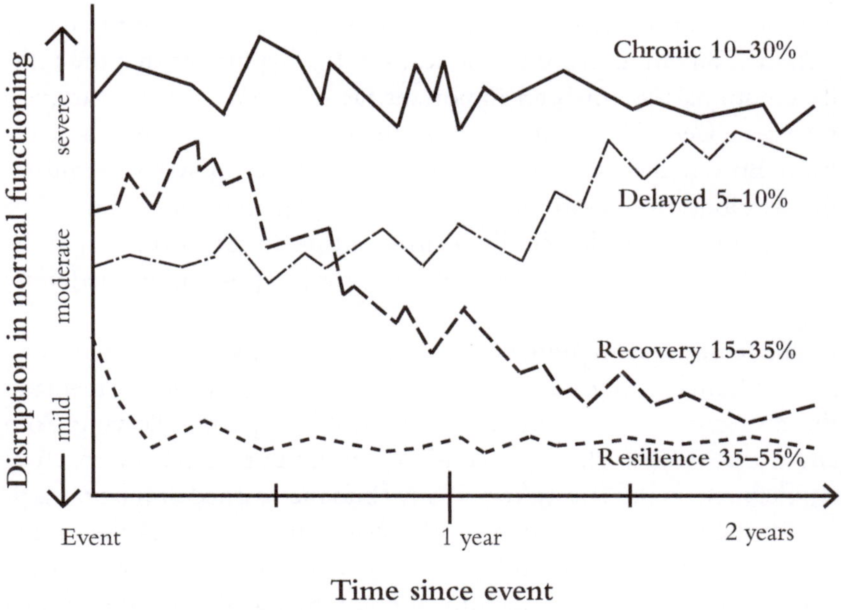

Figure 14.1 Prototypical trajectories of disruption in normal functioning during the two-year period following a loss or potential trauma (Bonanno, G. A. [2005]. Resilience in the face of potential trauma. *Current Directions in Psychological Science, 14*(3), 135–138).

over time. The least frequent outcome of loss is a delayed reaction in individuals who become chronically impaired following a death or potentially traumatic loss.

It is possible to draw a graph similar to Figure 14.1 to depict differences in trajectories following loss *within the family* (see Figure 14.3). Predictions based on Bowen theory are that 1) most family members are resilient and adapt well following loss, 2) a smaller number of individuals in the family will have symptoms and recover over time, and 3) sometimes a family member will adjust with the development of chronic symptoms in reaction to a death and fail to recover. Based on Bowen theory, the expected distribution of resilience and chronic difficulty within the family adapting to death result from preexisting differences in the adaptiveness of individuals in the family to nodal life events. This variation is a function of the dynamics of the family system as an emotional unit and leads to the hypothesis that the family emotional system is an important factor producing the variation in trajectories of loss that occurs in the overall population. The view from Bowen theory is that the family relationship system regulates the distribution of emotional impacts after disruptive life events. The variation in how well a family member adapts to the disruption in the death of a family member will reflect his or her position in the family system.

The family system influences the trajectories of loss and resilience in line with preexisting relationship patterns in the same way it mediates the distribution of chronic anxiety and the impacts following from any nodal event. When the family is calm, the patterns are inactive. Anxiety enters the family system any time the balance of relationships is disturbed, as happens after death. When anxiety enters the family system, it activates relationship patterns that then determine who, if anyone, ends up with an additional emotional load. This determines the distribution of trajectories of adjustment for family members following death. Because of the way the family emotional system works, adaptive flexibility falls to some who are freer from the system to adjust for self, while others in the emotional unit are left to carry the emotional load. This process is profoundly automatic, almost entirely outside of awareness, and usually unintentional. The system provides for the resilience and recovery of most family members, while few may have prolonged symptomatic adjustments in reaction to loss.

The prediction here, based on Bowen theory, is that variation in trajectories of adaptation following loss is a product of relationship patterns in the family emotional system. Percentages of resilience and impairment in one direction or another will shift depending on a family's level of differentiation and the degree of its cutoff from extended family. There will be more instances of prolonged impairments in families with lower levels of self. A cut-off nuclear family unit has fewer extended family relationships to manage anxiety and will have more instances of prolonged difficulty. In any given family, shifts in the active family relationship patterns, or in their intensity, determine both whether one or more family members move into a symptomatic position and which family members are vulnerable following a death in the family.

Family Reaction to Death and Clinical Practice Based on Bowen Theory

Conventional clinical approaches to prolonged reactions to death aim to work through grief and resolve the relationship to the lost one in individual or group treatment. Research suggests that when this approach addresses normal expressions of emotion in the early stages of loss, it has little value and can lead to complications (Schut, Stroebe, van den Bout, & Terheggen, 2001). More current research-based clinical approaches focus on fostering emotional flexibility in the expression of emotion and engagement with goals, enabling the individual to re-engage with life in a way that restores identity and meaning (Mancini & Bonanno, 2006; Papa, Sewell, Garrison-Diehn, & Rummel, 2013). These approaches are congruent with Bowen theory. The most important difference of the clinical approach based on Bowen theory, with long-term adjustment in mind, makes use of the fact that the family emotional process mediates the intensity of the impact of the loss. By coaching a family leader toward increased differentiation of self in the family emotional system, the intensity of the patterns that organize the automatic emotional functioning of the family is moderated. This reduces pressure on the most impinged family members and leaves them freer to function for self.

The four patterns of the nuclear family emotional system that operate when differentiation breaks down under pressures for togetherness that increase with anxiety are conflict, emotional distance, adaptation of a spouse to pressures from the dominant one, and parental projection of distress to a child. Real and imagined threats instinctively trigger these patterns, which stabilize the family and its members. These relationship patterns have evolutionary roots in the behavioral repertoires of threatened animals—*fight, flight, dominant and subordinate posturing*, and *coalitions* that occur in animals down the social hierarchy. Each human family has its mix of how they use the four patterns. Some families use mostly one pattern and other families use a mix of all four. Marital conflict occurs when two spouses fight to hold onto self—neither one giving in to the other—while remaining intensely engaged with one another. Children are unaffected by conflict between the parents as long as they are not triangled into the parents' relationship. *Flight*, or emotional distance between spouses, enables them to avoid conflict and the fight to hold on to self. Two other patterns require that someone give up some self to the system. A subordinate spouse gives in to the emotionally dominant spouse and maintains relationship harmony at the expense of their autonomy. In this interaction, the adaptive spouse is said to "lose self," while the other spouse gains a higher level of functional self. If the adaptive one quits giving in, the relationship becomes conflictual. The one who repeatedly gives up self to the other is vulnerable to developing clinical symptoms. In the fourth pattern, the family projection process, it is the focused-on child who loses self.

In the family projection process, the emotional focus on a child preserves marital harmony at the expense of the development of the child's independent self. The child is conditioned to function for his parents' emotional needs and will often rebel in protest. In the family projection process, the child is triangled into the parental relationship when they together focus on the child and unwittingly constrain the development of emotional autonomy in the child. It is this pattern that is most characteristic of the family in the clinical example presented here. In this family, the projection process worked, as Bowen described it, as a process that "begins with anxiety in the mother. The child responds anxiously to the mother, which she misperceives as a problem in the child" (Bowen, 1978, p. 381). "The father usually plays a support role to the projection process. He is sensitive to the mother's anxiety, and he tends to support her view and help her implement her anxious efforts at mothering" (Bowen, 1978, p. 381). "The anxious parental effort goes into sympathetic, solicitous, overprotective energy, which is directed more by the mother's anxiety than the reality needs of the child. It establishes a pattern of infantilizing the child, who gradually becomes more impaired" (Bowen, 1978, p. 381). "People impaired by the projection process . . . do less well with life" and "have lower levels of differentiation than their siblings" (Bowen, 1978, p. 381).

The family system produces different trajectories of adaptation to loss for different members of the same family by way of these relationship patterns. Following death, the way the patterns shift determines who in the family will have the most emotional difficulty. When the emotional reaction to death is not overly intense and anxiety-driven, it can be fairly easy to coach someone, underfunctioning and feeling helpless, to pick up their functioning and to connect with others who can provide what is needed to accomplish the tasks ahead. Bowen's chapter, "Family Reaction to Death" (1976), lays out principles of intervention in the immediate aftermath of death designed to prevent the potential shock wave going forward. The clinical example described next focuses on an example of a cascade of symptoms in a family following the death of a young adult child. A longer-term problem emerged out of intensified family patterns of emotional distance between spouses and the family projection process. This case illustrates family therapy based on Bowen theory in which the therapist coaches a motivated family member who is willing to take responsibility for self in working toward differentiation of self.

Differentiation of Self in a Family After the Death of a Young Adult Child

The clinical hypothesis for therapy based on Bowen theory is that coaching a family leader toward increased differentiation moderates the intensity of the patterns that organize the automatic emotional functioning of the family system. This reduces the emotional pressure on an impinged family member with a prolonged symptomatic adjustment. The clinical case presented here illustrates this approach.

In this example, the mother embarked on a long-term effort toward differentiation following the accidental death of her oldest son, who died at age 28 in an auto accident. Following the death of the oldest child, a younger brother did not experience symptomatic disruption of his functioning, whereas the youngest sister suffered increasing emotional difficulties. The daughter's severe difficulty occurred as part of the family reaction to death and the increased pressure of her position in her family's emotional system following her brother's death. The functioning of the family members was disrupted to different degrees based on their position in the family patterns. The mother worked to separate herself over and over from the impairing family patterns, sometimes when levels of anxiety were very challenging. Her success led to a shift that moderated the family projection process in which the daughter absorbed the largest share of anxiety in the nuclear family.

The family had three young adult children, including their oldest son who died in August 1988 (Figure 14.2). Their second son was 25

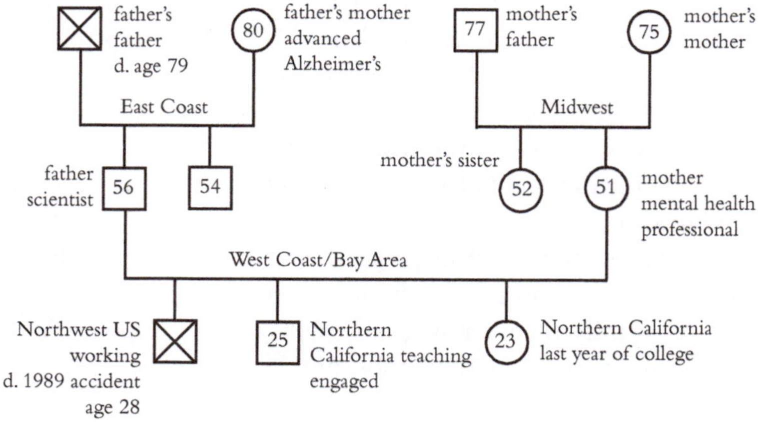

Figure 14.2 The family at the time of the oldest son's death

and their daughter was 23. The son who died had traveled a somewhat rocky path as a young adult. The father was a highly educated scientist, and the oldest son was very bright and full of promise. His parents' expectations for their son were high, but he started and quit college several times and did not finish. His parents were disappointed, but at the time of the accident, the son was finding his direction building a small business while doing industrial labor in a geographically distant state.

The trajectory of adjustment following the oldest son's sudden death was different for each member of the family. The second son, the middle child of this family, was engaged to be married and was beginning his teaching career at the time of his brother's death. He was upset, yet he continued on his course. This son had been the child most free of the family projection process. He responded with emotional maturity to his brother's death. He increased his contact with his parents and opened up with them, letting them know how he was doing in a way he hadn't before his brother's death. The middle son was on a resilient trajectory following the sudden death of his oldest brother.

For the parents, their son's death intensified a pattern of emotional distance, and each of them functioned poorly for some time. The father was devastated and very depressed. Years later he said that he had wished he could cry because he hoped it would give him some relief, but he didn't know how. The husband and wife were very respectful of the pain they knew their spouse was suffering, but they were unable to help one another. They did not want to upset one another talking about their son or their reactions to his death. So the emotional distance grew. The father just tried to find a way to keep going. He did not have any support network outside the nuclear family. His own mother had died right after his son. This provoked minor reactions in him and the family because she had been severely diminished with losses of functioning and self, following years of decline with Alzheimer's disease. The father continued to work. The mother was involved with her sister and parents and was in more contact with others outside the family. She continued to study for her license exam in counseling. She began consultation with this author, a Bowen theory coach, in the fall of 1989 just a few months after the son died. The parents' trajectory after their son's death was that of initial disruption of their functioning and some prolonged symptoms, followed by recovery.

When her brother died, the daughter was in her last year of college. She had a prolonged disruption of her functioning and some severe symptoms that lasted for about five years following her brother's death, as she increasingly became the focus of the family projection process. The third child and only girl, she had been special to her mother. At the same time, having three children stressed the mother. The daughter felt like one child too many. The mother saw her daughter as more needy than her sons and requiring protection from emotional upsets. She counseled her husband on how to talk to their daughter without upsetting her, a common pattern in the parental triangle of a focused-on child. The daughter began to have some significant emotional difficulties by the time she was 12 or 13.

The family's reaction to the oldest son's death intensified their emotional patterns; namely, distance in the parents' marriage and the family projection process. In the year after the death, the anxious focus that had been on the deceased son shifted to the daughter, who had been the primary object of parental anxiety for most of her development.

The daughter was doing relatively well when her brother died. She was moving along in college and was in a relationship. However, she had been quite close to her oldest brother and she had a huge reaction to his death. They had been buddies and confidantes growing up. The oldest brother looked after her when he knew she was keeping secrets

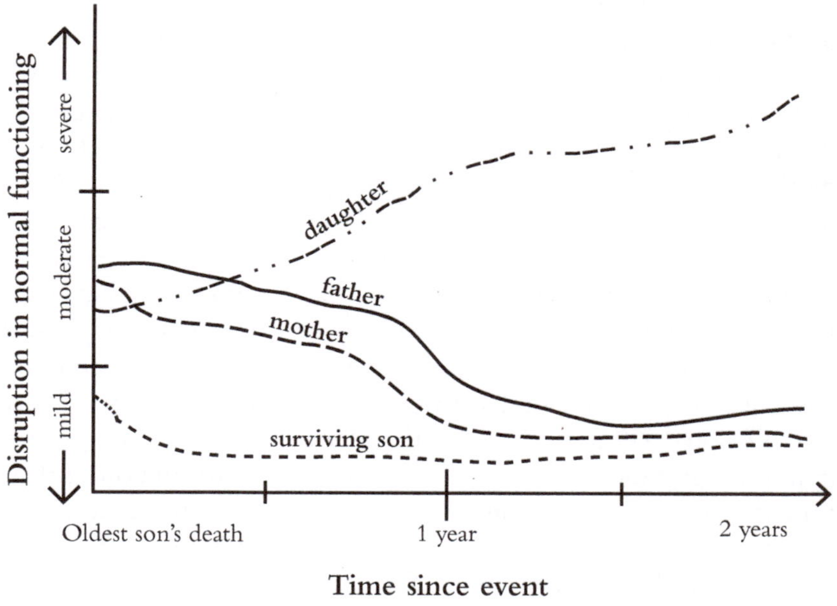

Figure 14.3 Trajectories of disruption in normal functioning in family members during the two-year period following the oldest son's death

from their parents. Despite his own use of pot, when he caught her trying it, he warned her off of it and said if she ever used it again, he would tell their parents. She never used it again. They liked to talk, and her brother's death left a tremendous hole in her life. The daughter was also shaken by unfinished business about their past sexual involvement. She had mentioned it in her last letter to him, and in his last letter to her, he had said, "We'll have to talk about that some time." But they never had that talk.

The mother's anxious focus began to shift from her own problems to her daughter when the daughter began having panic attacks in the spring of 1989, eight months after her brother died. At that time the mother took her counselor's licensing exam for the second time. Having failed it the first time, the mother was filled with her own anxiety but she went on to pass the exam. About the same time, the daughter started therapy. Living six hours from her parents and near her surviving brother, she became more isolated when her brother moved across the country for his career at the end of that summer. A couple of months later the daughter was depressed enough to see a psychiatrist and she began antidepressant medication that fall of 1990, but her depression continued to intensify.

In July 1991 her surviving brother married, separating her more from him. At her therapist's suggestion, she entered a support group for women sexually abused by their fathers. The therapist, who had become very important to the daughter, recommended the group because of her sexual experience with her brother who died. There were no groups for women whose brothers abused them. The support group thought that if a brother abused you, then the father must have also abused you, and they pushed the daughter to remember what the father had done to her. The daughter accused her father of sexual abuse in the fall of 1991, three years after her brother's death. The therapist believed the daughter when she accused her father. Her father totally denied her accusations. He was angry and kept to himself to avoid upsetting his wife. No one in the nuclear or extended family believed the daughter's accusation against the father. The family was upset, and apart from the mother, they blamed the daughter for accusing their father. They believed something was very wrong with her.

The mother believed that her son could have abused her daughter when he was intoxicated; however, she did not believe that her husband had sexually abused their daughter. The daughter became distant with her family for a while. In May 1992, the mother attended a therapy session with her daughter. At the therapy session, the mother maintained her position that she did not believe the father had sexually abused the daughter.

One of the central principles of differentiation of self is the ability to be in emotional contact with everyone in the system without taking sides when the family polarizes around an emotional issue. The father, the surviving son and his wife, and the mother's parents and older sister focused on what was wrong with the daughter. They blamed her and felt sorry for her. The mother's goal was to step outside of the family projection process. The rejection and pathologizing of the daughter *automatically* put her alone in an outside position while everyone in the family emotionally banded together. The mother *deliberately chose* an outside position by separating herself from the family's view that the problem was in the daughter. This is not easy to do, especially when the togetherness of the family system is activated by an emotional event as inflammatory as accusations of sexual abuse. The strategy worked. The mother believed that seeing her daughter's condition as a family problem and not blaming the daughter would make it possible to stay connected to her, and the daughter did stay connected to her mother even though her mother did not believe the father had abused her. At the same time, the mother believed that her daughter really believed her father had abused her, so she did not believe her daughter was lying or making it up. The mother was open with her daughter and with everyone in the family about what she believed.

The daughter's relationship with her therapist became tense before the therapist was to leave for a long vacation. In July 1992 the daughter made a suicidal gesture in the therapist's bathroom. Later that month while her therapist was away and her parents were out of contact on a hiking trip, the daughter made a serious suicide attempt. She was fortunate to have been found in time for her life to be saved. She remained suicidal and unstable for about 18 months.

After her daughter's suicide attempt, the mother really intensified her effort to work toward differentiation of self in the family. She worked at staying out of the family projection process and tried to avoid focusing anxiously on her daughter. She continued to communicate to everyone in the family her belief that the daughter's emotional difficulties were symptomatic of a family problem. In her family of origin, the mother objected to a pattern of anxious focus and feeling sorry for others. The anxious focus on her daughter repeated the anxious focus her parents had on her older sister. The mother took the position that her parents' treatment of her sister and her daughter as poor things made them feel and act like poor things.

Here are some examples of what the mother did to not go along with the family projection process in her family of origin, starting with a phone conversation after a visit with her parents (Figure 14.4). She said to both her parents on the phone:

> I've been thinking about my sister and what I said about her being such a whiner. I don't think you guys get it. What's with her? When is she ever going to grow up? Sometimes I think I was born feeling sorry for her. Do you guys realize that the time Dad spanked both of us for what she did, I felt sorry for

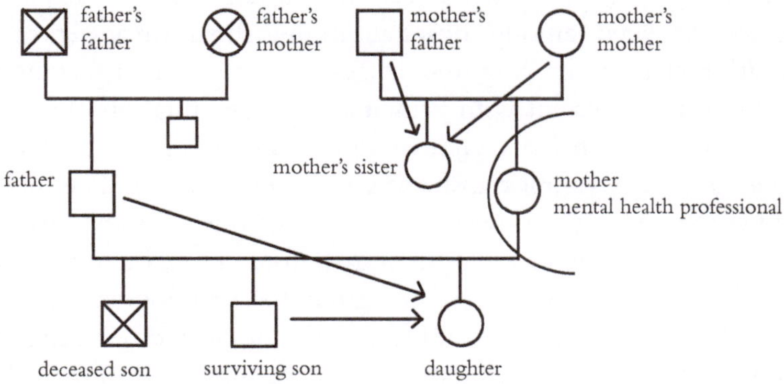

Figure 14.4 Mother separates self from the family projection process

> her? Well, I'm through feeling sorry for her. What good has it ever done? It just makes her worse. Then she becomes a poor thing, a wreck, someone who can't take it. And she looks to everyone else to fix it. Well, I'm tired of being responsible for her happiness.

Predictably, her parents were baffled. She followed up by writing to her mom:

> What I am upset about is the way you and dad cater to my sister's weakness and the way I cater to my daughter's weakness, and the way dad caters to yours. I'm not mad at my sister or my daughter, I'm just fed up with this whole family process that we all play a part in. Look at the price. Look at my sister. Look at my daughter.

Then, to her father she wrote:

> You say some people are just born to be difficult. I would say some people are born into a difficult position. That's where I see my daughter and my sister. Their positions are so similar that I keep mixing up their names. And they both have told me how much alike they think they are. I just don't buy the bad seed theory however much of a relief it would be.

Meanwhile, the mother herself was often in an anxious state, as her daughter careened among hospitalizations, shock treatments, and medication changes, making suicidal gestures and another serious suicide attempt. Consistent with principles of differentiation of self, she kept in contact with her daughter while also attempting to manage her own anxiety without transferring it to her daughter. The mother would use an idea from Bowen theory to hold onto, and then use that to relate to her daughter rather than give in to automatic impulses to anxiously overfunction by trying to guide her or impose answers, or pressure her about what she should do. She supported her daughter's decisions for herself. At the same time, it became necessary to draw limits when she received panicked middle-of-the-night calls from her daughter. These seemed to be an abdication of any effort by the daughter to manage her feelings by herself. Part of the projection process is functioning for the child when the child can function for self; that is, overfunctioning. It was not easy for the mother to make the judgment call when it was important to not answer the daughter's phone calls.

The total effort paid off and gradually the daughter stabilized. In the relationship with her distraught daughter, the mother worked thoughtfully to respect her daughter's struggles and to refrain as much as she could from indulging her immaturity. The daughter stabilized and gained self-control.

Over several years after the daughter stabilized in early 1994, a few more important shifts in the family system occurred. One was that the father came to an understanding and acceptance of what led to his daughter's accusation of sexual abuse. He heard a story on public radio about recovered memory therapy and how patients could have false memories planted by suggestions that abuse had occurred. The therapy would push patients to uncover their "repressed" memories. Often the "recovered memory" of sexual abuse had not actually occurred (Loftus & Davis, 2006). Understanding his daughter's accusations as false memories produced by suggestion in a recovered memory therapy session gone wrong made it possible for the father to resume his relationship with his daughter. Eventually, they even became close.

The surviving son, however, remained angry and rejecting of his sister. This brother and his wife did not want the daughter to be at family holidays. If she was present, they acted as if she did not exist. The mother persisted in her efforts in applying the principle of differentiation of self. After initially giving in to keep the peace, she no longer went along with them. When she was with her son and his wife, she would bring up her daughter in conversation. She declared that holidays were for everyone in the family. In 2007 she decided to make the daughter and son co-trustees of the parents' estate. Estate professionals had advised against this arrangement because the siblings were not getting along. The actual impact of the mother's trustee decision was that it motivated the son and his wife to get along with the daughter. Over time, contact and goodwill were restored to a significant degree in the sibling relationship. The family was then intact, it included everyone, and the daughter moved forward in her life. Maybe it goes without saying that the mother found these results very gratifying.

Through her effort the mother had successfully separated herself from the family projection process enough to make a profound difference. Her actions moderated the family's blame and rejection of the daughter, thereby shifting the projection process. The mother did not go along with the blaming or cutoffs, the daughter recovered, and the family emerged fully intact without cutoff by the end of 2008. This was 20 years after the oldest son's death in 1988. The mother continued to work on differentiation of self in the family. She tackled the emotional distance with her husband, her overly positive relationship with her surviving son, and the family projection process with his children.

This family's reaction to death is an example of how a family will use existing patterns until they are overloaded and symptoms emerge. The challenge of loss in a family triggers acute anxiety and intensifies patterns that manage the family's chronic anxiety. This increases the risk of symptom development. In this example the mother uses Bowen theory, with the help of coaching, to achieve greater differentiation of self from the family patterns of managing anxiety. This kind of effort moderates such patterns and frees the impaired members to function with less pressure from family relationships. Action taken by a family member in this way interrupts the transfer of family anxiety to the one who becomes symptomatic, giving them more room to recover.

Discussion and Conclusion

This chapter describes a clinical approach to coaching a family member when chronic symptoms emerge in the family shock wave triggered by a death in a family. This unique approach is based on principles of Bowen theory, with the goal of long-term change in the family system. The primary principle is to identify a family leader who is interested in understanding their part and is willing to change their behavior in patterns that impair family members. The family leader contains their own anxiety-driven automatic reactions in order to shift their functioning in the direction of differentiation of self from the family emotional system. Progress depends on someone who will act independently of the old, familiar, anxiety-driven emotional patterns. A family leader gains in her own level of differentiation when she takes action based on her independent assessment of the family patterns rather than acting as part of them. When a family leader can sustain this kind of effort, the family changes to the long-term benefit of all of its members.

In the recent history of mental health, it has become common practice to refer almost anyone who has suffered loss to individual or group therapy for grief work. Meanwhile, the principles of therapy based on Bowen theory are consistent with what the research is showing, that these referrals can complicate adjustment for the recently bereaved (Bonanno & Kaltman, 1999; Schut et al., 2001; Wortman & Silver, 1989, 2001). The drive for unnecessary intervention may be based on the same emotional forces that drive anxious overreactions in the family when it pathologizes intense emotional reactions like those that often follow death. In his chapter, "Family Reaction to Death," Dr. Bowen wrote about principles to address the immediate aftermath of a death in the family. His clinical goal was to fend off the shock wave phenomenon in which anxiety travels through the family, creating an emotional chain reaction with the potential of triggering serious complications for vulnerable family members. Dr. Bowen recommended that the family and community come together around the bereaved in the social rituals that recognize the reality of death, such as the funeral. He stressed the importance of supporting the individuality of family members surviving the loss and encouraged them to function, make decisions, and connect with others. This approach focuses on the strengths of the person and not their deficits. It encourages coping and not helplessness. The research supports confidence in the probability of resilience after loss as the likely trajectory for most people. It does not support the position of treating deficits in the bereaved. This is consistent with the approach devised by Dr. Bowen based on family systems theory (Bonanno & Burton, 2013; Papa et al., 2013). Whether in the family or in the helping professions, the process of recovery can be complicated and resilience suppressed when helpers overfunction. The perspectives of the research and of Bowen theory seem to converge on this point.

A potential point of contact between the predictions of Bowen theory and the findings from the resilience research is that variation in trajectories of adjustment to loss in the research populations is likely to be, in significant measure, a product of the family emotional system. It is hoped that the clinical example here shows how the family system creates this variation in how its members adjust to death and loss, for the working benefit of the clinical practitioner and researcher alike.

REFERENCES

Bonanno, G. A. (2005). Resilience in the face of potential trauma. *Current Directions in Psychological Science, 14*(3), 135–138.

Bonanno, G. A., & Burton, C. L. (2013). Regulatory flexibility: An individual differences perspective on coping and emotion regulation. *Perspectives on Psychological Science, 8*(6), 591–612.

Bonanno, G. A., & Kaltman, S. (1999). Toward an integrative perspective on bereavement. *Psychological Bulletin, 125*, 760–776.

Bonanno, G. A., Westphal, M., & Mancini, A. D. (2011). Resilience to loss and potential trauma. *Annual Review of Clinical Psychology*, 7, 511–535.

Bowen, M. (1976). Family reaction to death. In M. Bowen (Ed.), *Family therapy in clinical practice* (pp. 321–335). New York, NY: Jason Aronson.

Bowen, M. (1978). *Family therapy in clinical practice.* New York, NY: Jason Aronson.

Hansson, W. Stroebe, & Schut, H. (Eds.) (2001). *Handbook of bereavement research: Consequences, coping, and care* (pp. 705–737). Washington, DC: American Psychological Association.

Loftus, E. F., & Davis, D. (2006). Recovered memories. *Annual Review of Clinical Psychology, 2*, 469–498.

Mancini, A. D., & Bonanno, G. A. (2006). Resilience in the face of potential trauma: Clinical practices and illustrations. *Journal of Clinical Psychology, 62*(8), 971–986.

Papa, A., Sewell, M. T., Garrison-Diehn, C., & Rummel, C. (2013). A randomized open trial assessing the feasibility of behavioral activation for pathological grief. *Behavior Therapy*, *44*, 639–650.

Schut, H., Stroebe, M. S., van den Bout, J., & Terheggen, M. (2001). The efficacy of bereavement interventions: Determining who benefits. In M. S. Stroebe, R. O. Hansson, O., Stroebe, W., & Schut, H. (Eds.). *Handbook of bereavement research: Consequences, coping, and care* (pp. 405–429). Washington, DC: American Psychological Association.

Wortman, C. B., & Silver, R. C. (1989). The myths of coping with loss. *Journal of Consulting and Clinical Psychology*, *57*, 349–357.

Wortman, C. B., & Silver, R. C. (2001). The myths of coping with loss revisited. In M. S. Stroebe, R. O. Hansson, O., Stroebe, W., & Schut, H. (Eds.). *Handbook of bereavement research: Consequences, coping, and care* (pp. 405–429). Washington, DC: American Psychological Association.

15

FAMILY REACTION TO DEATH

Variation in Differentiation of Self

Michael J. Sullivan

Introduction

Families vary in how they adapt and realign after a death in the family. This variation occurs within and between families. In some families functional regression follows a significant death, with cascading social, emotional, and physical symptoms; explosive relationship conflict; and cutoff. Much like an avalanche careening down the mountainside, once the snow load exceeds the strength of the snow pack, it gains in speed and volume, stopping only after it reaches the run-out zone. This process has been described as the "emotional shock wave" (Bowen, 1978, pp. 324–328), with anxiety transmitted throughout the relationship network. "After-shocks" generate anxiety that exceeds the adaptive capacity of the family, contributing to chronic impairments. Several decades might be required to achieve a stable realignment. In the extreme this can end with extinction. In other families, a significant death can be followed by the emergence of acute symptoms and relationship disruption across the family network. A new equilibrium is often achieved only with the addition of new members. Some members thrive, whereas others develop impairments. Over several generations these differences become more pronounced.

Finally, there are families who experience bereavement, realign, and move forward. For these families, death, usually in later life, is recognized as a natural process, anticipated with the family realignment thoughtfully planned. Often followed by a sense of relief, family members maintain a reasonable level of emotional independence with minimal symptoms. This chapter will examine the variation in how families adapt to a significant death.

Differentiation of self (Bowen, 1978, p. 424), the cornerstone concept of Bowen theory, accounts for the variation in how families adapt to the death of a significant member. The concept of differentiation of self describes the integration of the emotional, feeling, and intellectual systems within the individual and the intensity of emotional reciprocity in relationship with others. At low levels of differentiation, little discrimination exists between these internal systems. The intellectual system functions as a weak appendage in service of the dominant emotional and feeling systems. At higher levels more autonomy develops between these systems with an increasing potential for observation, direction, regulation, and appraisal.

Relationships play an important role in reciprocal emotional regulation. Internal regulation occurs through relationship fusion. The emotional intensity of relationship fusion is greater at lower levels of differentiation. This emotional give-and-take is expressed in a variety of forms. Bowen theory proposes five basic patterns: distance, conflict, overfunctioning/underfunctioning reciprocity, projection, and cutoff. In periods of calm these automatic patterns manage the emotional intensity between people. However, a disturbance in relationship fusion generates anxiety, and these patterns become more pronounced.

Death represents one of the most profound disturbances to relationship fusion, as it involves both the loss of the person and the role they played in maintaining the family emotional equilibrium. The family's level of differentiation influences both the method and timing of death and the adaptation and realignment afterward.

This chapter will present examples of three different patterns of adaptation to death of a significant family member. The Allen family represents a regressive spiral that follows the unexpected death of a mother with young children in a chronically anxious family. With the Booth family, the background emotional process drives a variety of acute symptoms and exaggerated relationship patterns following the death of the grandmother. Functional stability is achieved only after new members are added. The final example reflects the benefits of maintaining personal contact and "working on self" when participating in the death process. The death of Mr. David's brother and mother are followed by a sense of relief and enhanced emotional and social functioning.

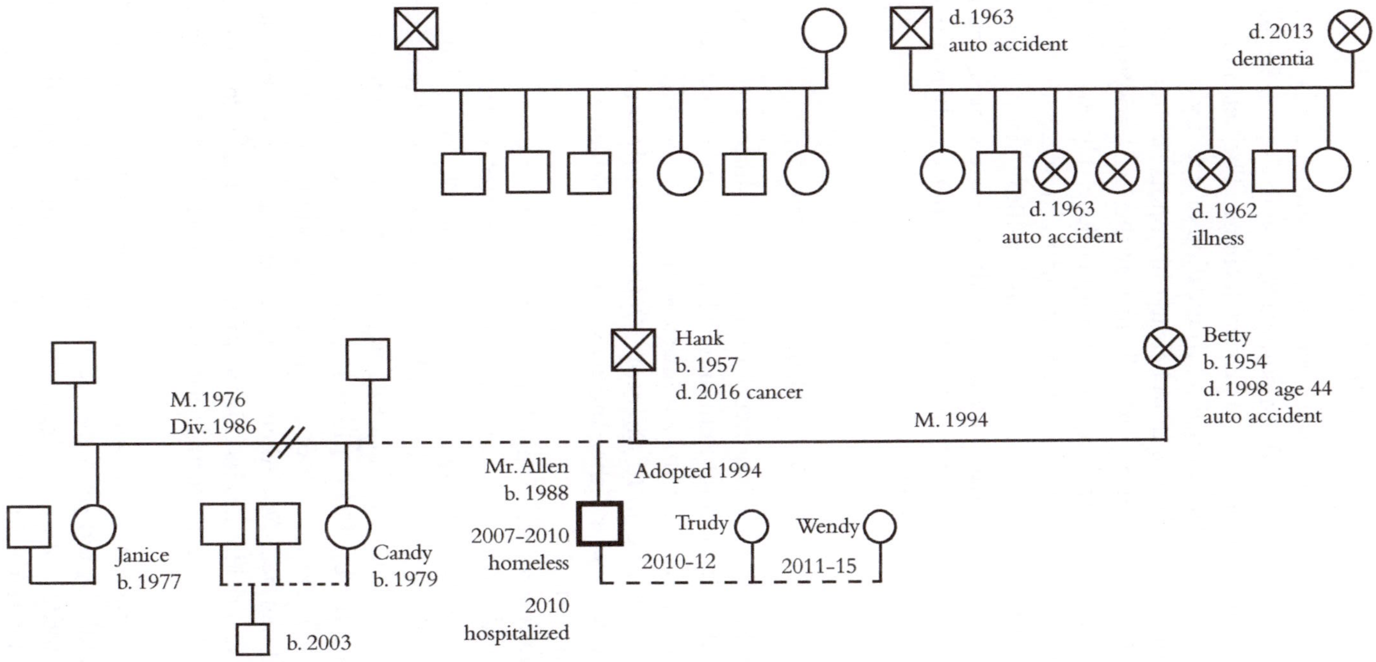

Figure 15.1 Allen family diagram

Clinical Profiles

Mr. Allen sought psychotherapy following the breakup of a two-and-a-half-year relationship. Mr. Allen complained of an overwhelming sense of hopelessness, fatigue, and depressed feelings. The relationship had given him a sense of direction and a foundation of stability (Figure 15.1). He considered the relationship to be the "high point of my life."

At age 27, he was employed full time at the local hospital, had an apartment, and was attending community college. This was significant progress from the earlier years of couch surfing, homelessness, and psychiatric hospitalization. Cut off from his family, with only occasional contact with his older half-sibling, Mr. Allen saw few prospects in his future. His relationship with his girlfriend and her family had become his primary social contact.

History

Mr. Allen knew only fragments of his family history. His mother, Betty, was the fifth of eight children. His grandparents had converted a chicken coop on the family homestead into a home, adding a room as each child was born. In the early 1960s the family was involved in a traffic accident. Her father and two sisters were killed and Betty was severely burned.

Betty graduated high school, married, and had two daughters: Janice and Candy. This first marriage ended in divorce some time before Mr. Allen was born. Betty had a relationship with Mr. Allen's father, but they broke up before he was born. He never met his father and had little information about his father or his parents' relationship.

Following his birth, his mother returned to the family homestead and built a home next door to his grandmother. His mother began dating and married. Mr. Allen was adopted at age six by his mother's second husband, Hank. His middle sister, Candy, began to act out and was sent to live with maternal relatives. She never returned to live with the family.

Mr. Allen recalls childhood to be a "high point in my life." The youngest child by ten years, he had a "special and playful" relationship with his mother. She ran a daycare in the home. With the addition of Hank, the standard of living improved. His mother finished her degree, began a career as a security guard, and was active in numerous community projects.

Death

At age ten, Mr. Allen's life suddenly changed. His mother was killed in an automobile accident. It was a freak accident, a result of careless driving of a local teenager. The village mourned. The local newspaper wrote a story about her civic contributions. Over 500 people attended her funeral. The following spring a memorial plaque was installed in her honor at a local park.

Mr. Allen describes the next eight years as the "worst time in my life; everything became muffled." Hank quit working and just sat there. Mr. Allen's social contact was limited to visits with his grandmother who lived next door, his eldest sister Janice, and a neighborhood friend of his mother. Mr. Allen was constantly grounded for poor school performance. One day he returned from school to discover his dog had been given away. Later Hank burnt his childhood toys because "I was having too much fun." His grandmother suddenly left when he was 14. She moved to Wyoming to live with her eldest daughter. Mr. Allen later learned that his grandmother had been diagnosed with "dementia." Mr. Allen felt more hopeless. Twice he ran away. He grew more resentful toward Hank. At 18, he said he was "kicked out" following an argument over his spending habits with the settlement from his mother's accident. He severed all contact with Hank and his adopted extended family.

Mr. Allen enlisted in the Marines. Within the first month, he was hospitalized due to an allergic reaction. He was discharged and spent the next several months recovering at the home of his eldest half-sister.

Over the next three years, Mr. Allen lived a nomadic lifestyle, couch-surfing with friends, living in shelters, and living homeless. Self-described as addicted to video games, Mr. Allen played for hours and developed great skill locating venues that provided free Wi-Fi. He became a fixture at the public library. His poor self-care and overwhelming feelings of hopelessness led to a hospitalization for major depression. Not welcome to live with Janice, he was discharged to a homeless shelter that provided outpatient counseling and employment assistance. He was placed in a retail store. There he met an older female coworker, Trudy, who befriended him. She invited him to move in with her, and within weeks they were living together because "she felt sorry for me." They became constant companions. They found togetherness criticizing others, particularly their work supervisor. He said, "I helped her stand up for herself." One day they walked out of work because of "unfair treatment" and never went back.

Mr. Allen found work in a restaurant with a family atmosphere. He quickly mastered job skills and soon offered unsolicited suggestions to coworkers and supervisors about how they could improve their efficiencies. He became smitten with an 18-year-old coworker, Wendy. They began to date, taking long walks and planning a life together. When Trudy discovered he was seeing someone else, she threatened him and abruptly ended their living arrangement. Mr. Allen refers to Trudy as "alcoholic, psycho, and a liar and thief."

As he pursued this new relationship with Wendy, Mr. Allen began to make life plans. He moved into a new apartment, enrolled in the local community college, found a better-paying job, and bought an automobile. He planned to follow his girlfriend and transfer to a state university. His life circumstance had improved. Despite their seven-year age difference, Mr. Allen said he was "adopted" by Wendy's family.

Wendy excelled in school. She was accepted to a university and offered an internship that required she relocate several hundred miles away. Mr. Allen struggled academically and failed to complete the required prerequisites to transfer. After two-and-a-half years Wendy broke off the relationship as she had no interest in a long-distance relationship.

Consultation

In the early consultation sessions, Mr. Allen focused on managing disturbing feeling states activated by the breakup. When he learned Wendy had moved he said, "I decided to write her off as dead." He detailed recurrent disappointments in relationships and the many times he was let down by those he trusted. He recounted how his family "collapsed" after his mother's death. He still felt bitterness toward Hank with whom he hadn't spoken in nine years.

He learned via social media Hank had stage IV colon cancer. He was living 75 miles away at the home of his mother. Mr. Allen weighed the risks and benefits of making contact and finally decided to do so, first by email and then by phone. Regular visits followed. Mr. Allen helped with work projects and car repairs. Hank bought him snow tires. Corresponding with this reconnection, he began to actively date via the social media site, Tinder. He encountered three short-lived romances with women in complicated life circumstances. He said he became infatuated and involved in helping them "deal with their problems" only to have the relationship suddenly end. He resumed contact with old friends and began to go to music concerts. He started to regularly exercise, moved into the home of a coworker, and worked three jobs for several months to retire debt and establish savings.

Hank died that winter. Mr. Allen participated in Hank's end of life and the funeral process. He was present and accounted for, serving as a pallbearer. He later reflected, "His intentions were ok, I just disagreed with the way he went about it." The funeral also provided an opportunity to resume contact with several extended family members. He began to acknowledge some benefit from his upbringing.

Mr. Allen experienced a setback when he was not included in the estate settlement. The family home was left to his uncle, Hank's younger brother. Mr. Allen had hoped the house might be left to him and his sisters. Negative feeling states resurfaced. His physician referred him to a cognitive behavioral therapist.

That spring, Mr. Allen attended an open house at his elementary school. Several teachers and counselors remembered him and his mother. They reminisced about his elementary school days. Afterward, Mr. Allen visited the family homestead and his grandmother's house. The next week he stopped by the local animal shelter and adopted two rescue dogs, a mother and son that had been neglected by their owner. Both dogs were on medication for anxiety. There was a reciprocal calming effect between Mr. Allen and his dogs. His mood was significantly improved with this strong attachment. The dogs were calmer in his presence.

Summary

This is an example of functional regression at a low level of differentiation following unexpected loss of a parent during a vulnerable period—when there are dependent children. In the few years prior to Betty's death, a functional niche of stability had been achieved, preceded by a life pattern of intense relationship fusion, chronic anxiety, projection, and cutoff. With her death this niche was lost and never recovered. For Mr. Allen, this unresolved loss generated chronic anxiety and contributed to a lifelong pursuit of emotional stability through intense togetherness with others. The emotional intensity of these relationships would eventually end in cutoff. Mr. Allen's social functioning reflected this pattern: reasonably stable social functioning when in a relationship, regressed functioning when in cutoff. Increased emotional flexibility and social engagement occurred shortly after he reestablished contact with Hank and his extended family. How well Mr. Allen remains in contact will determine whether these gains are temporary or sustained.

The Booth Family: Background Emotional Process

Mrs. Booth originally sought consultation about her 17-year-old son, Jack. A high school senior and successful multisport athlete, Jack had changed in recent months from outgoing and cheerful to sullen, oppositional, and irritable. He pushed away from his mother. She managed and directed the administration of his life with the justification "he tends to be easily distracted and forgetful." This change corresponded with the development of Jack's romance with a classmate. They started dating a year earlier, and over time the intensity of the relationship noticeably increased. They were in constant contact. Theirs was a passionate relationship punctuated by bitter arguments and dramatic break-ups followed by euphoric make-ups.

Jack's academic performance declined, placing his athletic career in jeopardy. As Mrs. Booth became alarmed, Mr. Booth, in response, forbade Jack from having further contact with his girlfriend. Explosive father and son conflict followed and prompted the request for consultation.

The emotional intensity continued over the next year. Jack felt he was in an emotional no-man's land, conflicted by his desire for approval and support from his parents, yet feeling the strong pull of attachment to his girlfriend. She criticized his parents, complained he didn't care enough, and threatened suicide. His mother worried that

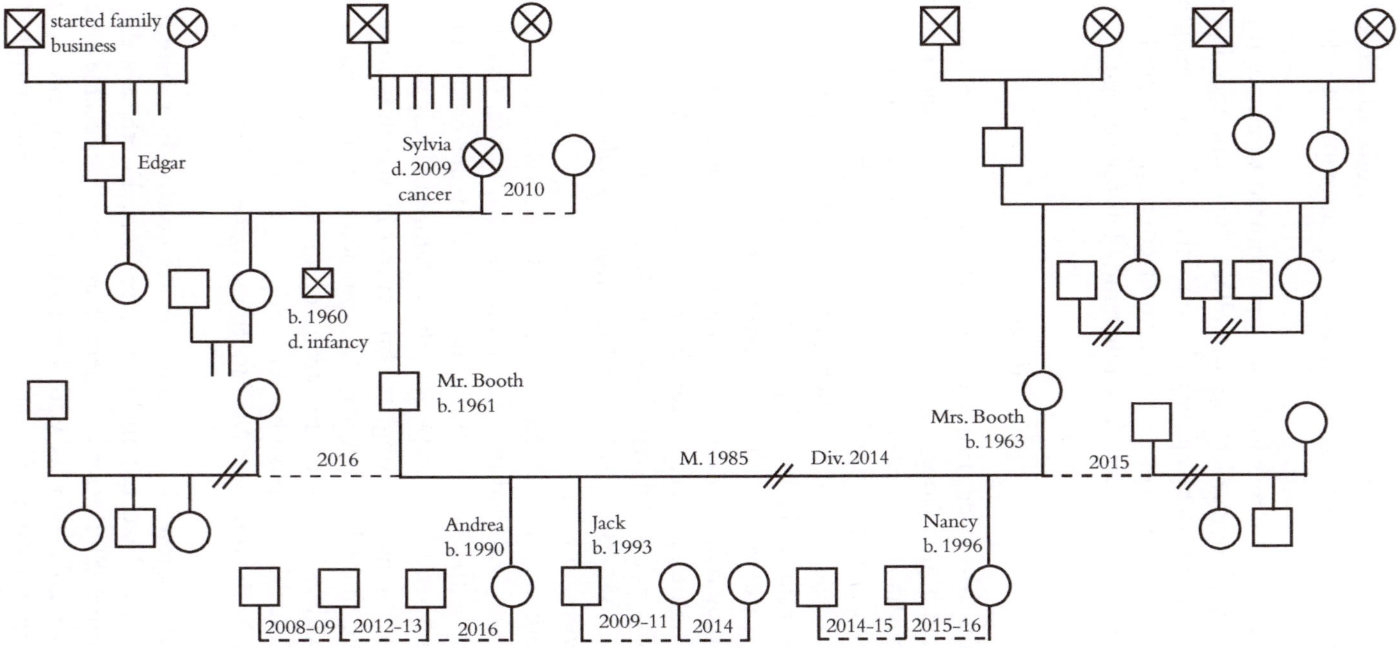

Figure 15.2 Booth family diagram

he would "ruin his life." She complained her husband needed to be more involved, yet criticized him when he attempted to do so. Mr. Booth withdrew.

Jack graduated high school and was admitted to a state university. However, a week before leaving for college Jack announced he would not attend in order to be closer to his girlfriend. Conflict erupted. His parents took the position he could either go away to school or move out without their support. Jack reluctantly left for college.

History

The Booths had been married 25 years (Figure 15.2). They met shortly after high school, courted through college, and married in 1985 once Mrs. Booth graduated. Both went to work in Mr. Booth's family business started by his paternal grandfather. He worked in operations while Mrs. Booth helped his parents manage the business. Her business skills filled an important niche in the family enterprise. She would later reflect, "I was recruited by this family." In the first five years, they built a house on the family property and had their first child, a daughter, Andrea. Over the next six years, Mrs. Booth gave birth to two more children, Jack and Nancy. As she became more absorbed in Mr. Booth's family, Mrs. Booth gradually became less involved with her own.

Mr. Booth was the youngest of four. He had two older sisters and a brother who had died in infancy. His mother, Sylvia, was the emotional hub of the family. Well known within the community as a cheerful and kind-hearted person, she organized family and community events. She had a strong attachment to Mr. Booth who was born after the death of her first son. She yielded to her husband, Edgar, who was widely known for his strong opinions, explosive temper, and distrust of outsiders. Unlike his wife, Edgar was frequently critical and dismissive. As the only son, Mr. Booth was expected to join the family enterprise.

Mrs. Booth grew up in a small town nearby. Her parents were retired. Both had worked in health care. Mrs. Booth was the eldest of three sisters. She described herself as "the responsible one." She maintained regular contact with her parents but had only occasional contact with her sisters. She said, "We have different lifestyles." Mrs.

Booth had a closer relationship with her father. She would help him with work projects around the house. She tended to become more "annoyed" with her mother. Although her parents had been married many years, they incessantly bickered.

Over time Mrs. Booth recognized the income from the family enterprise would not be sufficient to meet the needs of their growing family. She took outside employment and left the family business. The following year, Mr. Booth took full-time work as a consultant but continued work in the family business at night. A marital pattern of distance and conflict emerged accompanied by feelings of loneliness and resentment.

Three years later, Mr. Booth's mother, Sylvia, was diagnosed with breast cancer. His eldest sister moved back to town to assist in her treatment. Her return altered the family equilibrium. As Mr. Booth began to confide in his sister, Mrs. Booth increasingly felt on the outside. His mother's cancer went into remission.

Death

Eighteen months later Sylvia was diagnosed with colon cancer. This time she refused treatment. Andrea had started her freshman year at a prestigious East Coast college. She became involved in an intense romance that ended poorly and left her in extreme emotional distress. Her distress became Mrs. Booth's primary focus. Jack's romance began at the same time.

That summer, Sylvia died. Within three months, Mr. Booth's father began to date. Six months after his wife's death, his new companion moved into the family home. This new relationship was seen as a threat by the family. Mr. Booth and his sister worried how this would affect their inheritance. Considerable family discussion focused on what to do about this threat. As Mr. Booth increasingly leaned on his sister, the marital conflict between the Booths became more frequent.

Following Jack's departure for college, the relationship patterns became more pronounced. Mr. Booth became more reactive. He criticized Mrs. Booth for failing to "act properly." He began to carry a handgun and became preoccupied with fundamental religious beliefs. He installed a tracking device on Mrs. Booth's car and monitored her cell phone use. Andrea challenged her father, resulting in conflict and cutoff. Jack was placed on probation after his first year in college. He struggled to balance the conflicting demands of academic and fraternity life.

One night Mr. Booth returned home after Mrs. Booth had gone to bed. He woke her and spoke for several hours describing a new spiritual insight punctuated by wild laughter. The Booths separated afterward, and Mr. Booth moved in with his sister. Nancy began treatment for anxiety. Mrs. Booth filed for divorce.

Consultation

Emotional reactivity remained high throughout the divorce process. The family polarized. Jack dropped out of college, moved in with his grandfather, and cut off from his mother. Nancy cut off from her father. Andrea began dating an unemployed musician with a drug habit and cut off from the entire family. A variety of attorneys and therapists were engaged as the family emotional process was externalized. The family social network splintered. Mr. and Mrs. Booth's cutoff included their extended families.

As the divorce process concluded, the emotional reactivity decreased. Mrs. Booth recognized the similarities in the relationship patterns of her children, her mother-in-law, and her marriage. She began a sustained effort at defining a self. She reconnected with her family of origin and extended family, began to regularly exercise, and started home remodeling projects. She eventually bridged the cutoff with Andrea and Jack. She demonstrated more assertiveness and confidence in self. In her work system, she engaged conflict rather than retreated from it. She rekindled a romance with a childhood friend, now a successful entrepreneur. When an anxious family member questioned her judgment, she responded: "I'll pick and choose the disappointments I will participate in."

Jack eventually made a thoughtful decision to forego college and pursue his long-standing interest in agriculture. He has rapidly advanced in this career. He moved into an apartment with his girlfriend of three years. He maintains contact with both parents and extended families. Andrea's romance was short-lived. It ended shortly after her boyfriend met her family. She applied and was accepted into graduate school, and eventually resumed regular contact with her parents and both extended families.

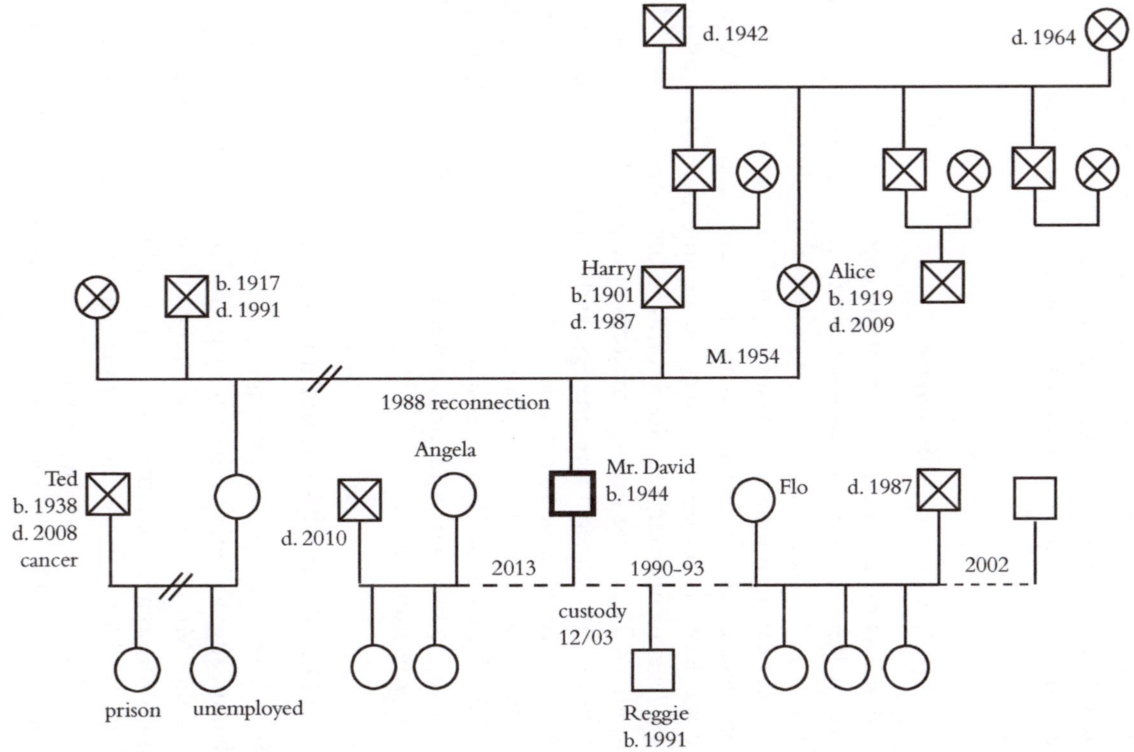

Figure 15.3 David family diagram

Nancy graduated from high school with honors and now attends college. She remains in cutoff with her father and has superficial contact with the parental extended family. She remains strongly attached to her mother and remains in therapy for anxiety. She has struggled with social relationships. Mr. Booth lives with his fiancée and her three children on the property shared with his father and sister.

Summary

This case illustrates the phenomenon of the emotional shock wave as described by Bowen. The grandmother's death was followed by a variety of social and emotional symptoms in several family members and exaggerated relationship patterns resulting in divorce and cutoff. Each symptom became the focus rather than the force that drove it. When anxiety was low, the relationships were stable and there was a reasonably high level of functioning. However, as anxiety increased with the grandmother's illness and death, symptoms emerged. The reaction to each symptom generated more anxiety, and other symptoms developed. Eventually, the process extended into the social network. Anxiety gradually subsided with Mrs. Booth's effort to define a direction for her life. This was followed by similar efforts by her ex-husband, son, and daughter. A new equilibrium was achieved when each developed a new relationship.

David Family—Relief and Enhancement

Mr. David, a 60-year-old retired manufacturing representative, sought consultation after assuming full custody of his 13-year-old son, Reggie (Figure 15.3). Mr. David said he was "raised by women" and felt insecure in his role as a single father. Mr. David had three cancer surgeries in two years. Although the cancer treatment had been successful, he experienced anxiety about mortality.

Reggie's mother, Flo, had recently relocated to Idaho with her boyfriend to open a ranch. To do so she relinquished her parental rights to Mr. David. He and Flo had met at a self-awareness retreat in California. Their short but intense relationship ended amicably after Reggie's birth. They actively co-parented and remained close friends.

With a lifelong interest in self-development, Mr. David had a variety of therapeutic and personal growth experiences. He spent several years active with a well-known West Coast retreat center dedicated to a deeper understanding of self and society, where he studied with many of the pioneers in the personal growth movement of the 1970s. He held a leadership position in a global self-improvement network. His expectations of consultation were clear. He stated he wanted to "do some work" and find a new direction for his life.

History

Mr. David was born in Massachusetts, but his parents separated shortly before his birth. He grew up with his mother, Alice, and grandmother in a working-class neighborhood. Mr. David rarely saw his father, who remarried and moved away. His older brother, Ted, six years his senior, lived with the family for only brief periods. Ted spent several years in psychiatric and medical facilities. Mr. David remembered his mother as fun loving, playful, and spontaneous when he was young. He also had a close attachment to his grandmother, "I was her pet," he said, but remembered that she often "criticized my mother" and "required a lot of attention."

When Mr. David was ten years old, his mother met and married Harry, a 53-year-old bachelor. A veteran, attorney, successful businessman, and politician, Mr. David described Harry as a "straight arrow" who "knew what he wanted." He treated "my mom like a queen" and she, in turn, devoted herself to him. Her anxious concern about Harry's approval replaced her fun-loving playfulness.

She yielded decision making to him, reflected in the often-repeated phrase "We'll have to see what Harry thinks." Family life became structured with a focus on appearances and etiquette. Ted attended boarding school. His occasional home visits were unpleasant occasions with explosive conflict, frequently ending with his early return to school.

Mr. David graduated from a small, conservative, private college and moved to the West Coast, where he was employed as a manufacturing representative. He was introduced to the personal growth movement and embraced the emphasis on self-expression and discovery. He maintained regular nonpersonal contact with his mother and rarely spoke to her about the insight he gained from his self-discovery experiences. When he attempted to get personal, his mother would typically redirect the focus to her relationship with Harry.

In 1987, Harry died. Later that year Mr. David felt a sudden interest to find his biological father. He began a search. His father, in poor health, was living in Connecticut, retired from a career as a college history professor. He was receptive to meeting with Mr. David. Over the next three years, they maintained active and regular contact until his death. Reggie was born that same year.

Consultation

When Mr. David began consultation, his mother resided in an assisted living facility. Ted, disabled for several years, was living in poverty in a low-income neighborhood in New Jersey. Mr. David started to make more frequent contact with each. His brother was divorced and estranged from his family. His adult children had marginal life adjustments. One daughter was in prison on a felony drug charge, the other was unemployed and living with her mother.

Ted was diagnosed with cancer shortly after Mr. David resumed contact. Over the next few years, Mr. David made regular visits. They developed a new openness. He helped organize home health care and handled his brother's affairs at the end of life. Mr. David also made contact with his brother's ex-wife and daughters.

A pattern of conflict characterized the relationship between Alice and Ted. When they had contact, Ted would ask for money. If his mother refused, Ted would demand, she would criticize; they would argue and then stop talking for long periods of time. They were not in contact when Ted died. Mr. David never told his mother about her son's death.

Alice's health quickly deteriorated after Ted's death. She increasingly expressed fear about dying in poverty despite her considerable wealth. She often complained about the staff and was suspicious of others. She questioned whether she could trust Mr. David and threatened on more than one occasion to remove him from her will. She was demanding and rarely appreciative.

Mr. David continued to oversee her care. Reggie accompanied his father on several of the visits. She died a year after Ted's death. She left her entire estate to Mr. David. He established a trust for Reggie, gave his nieces money, and established a college fund for each. They felt they were entitled to half the estate. They filed a lawsuit again Mr. David but their case was dismissed.

Mr. David consciously worked at managing a balance between his sense of duty to his mother and brother and his responsibility to himself and his son. After his mother's death, he felt relief with periodic feelings of loneliness. Six months after her death, he arranged to leave 40% of his estate to charity. After 15 months he felt a sudden deep appreciation for his mother, "I am thankful [that] while she wasn't emotionally demonstrative she took care of me financially."

Mr. David has become a well-renowned artist and developed several unique art projects that have increased public awareness about social issues. His work presents a background context and an objective reflection, promoting a deeper understanding of those who struggle with chronic impairment.

Since 2013 Mr. David has been in his first deeply committed relationship, with Angela. He has reflected, "I never thought I would find such true love at this stage of my life." Reggie excelled through high school and college. He travels internationally and works in the entertainment production industry. He and Mr. David remain in regular contact.

Summary

This case example reflects a moderate level of differentiation with an orderly realignment following the deaths of a sibling and parent. Although relationship patterns indicative of chronic anxiety, cutoff, and significant impairment are present, thoughtful long-term planning and a sustained effort at maintaining engaged contact resulted in a nonsymptomatic bereavement and a forward focus.

Conclusion

The three case examples presented in this chapter reflected three distinct patterns of adaptation and realignment following a significant death. The level of differentiation for each family is reflected in the pre-death family organization, the death process, and the level of reactiveness following the death. At lower levels of differentiation, chronic impairment and exaggerated relationship patterns compromise functioning following a significant death. Replacement, the addition of a new relationship, is the most common form of realignment. At moderate levels, acute symptoms emerge, generally contained within the child most involved in the parents' marriage. At higher levels of differentiation of self, death by senescence is more common. Death is followed by a sense of relief and manageable bereavement.

Families seen in a clinical practice typically present with concerns regarding a disruption in relationship equilibrium, a breakup, an acting-out teenager, or distance in an important relationship and the associated distressed feeling states: heartbreak, sadness, fear, and anxiety. In general, consultation is sought for the symptoms that emerge following death—a network of underground emotional "after-shocks." The connection between the symptom and the death is often minimized or denied. Anxiety generated by the symptom often contributes to a narrow view and cause-and-effect thinking. The focus centers on symptom relief, in other words, "fixing" the identified problem with the reduction of the distressed feeling states and associated anxiety the goal.

While there are countless methods of temporarily reducing anxiety, the triangle is the most common. Most techniques of managing anxiety involve the distressed person, the disturbed relationship, and the helper. The presence of a less anxious third person can contribute to a reduction in anxiety. With the slight reduction of anxiety, a perspective change occurs and with it an awareness of options that allow access to problem-solving abilities and enhanced cognitive flexibility. When seen in a broader context, the problem seems manageable, anxiety decreases, the distressed feeling state(s) subsides, and the symptom dissipates. Most people terminate a clinical effort once the relationship equilibrium is restored or a new relationship develops.

However, the presenting problem is an expression of a broader background emotional process—the degree of unresolved emotional attachment each person carries from the past. The level of unresolved emotional attachment determines the emotional intensity of relationship fusion, the extent people "lean on each other," how much "self" a person can develop, and how much self is absorbed in the give and take with others. Said another way, the degree of emotional independence one experiences in life is determined by the extent the emotional attachment to the past is resolved and the degree one can be a self in relationship to important others.

REFERENCE

Bowen, M. (1978). *Family therapy in clinical practice.* New York, NY: Jason Aronson.

16

EMOTIONAL PROCESS AND THE MANAGEMENT OF CHRONIC ILLNESS AND DEATH

David S. Hargrove and Elizabeth Grady

Clinical and administrative practice indicates that family development heavily influences the manner in which families experience and manage chronic illness and the last days of life of specific family members, particularly parents of adult children. As death approaches, families typically gather when possible. Anxiety that has been a part of the family emotional process intensifies and can exacerbate the behavior of one or more of the members. As Bowen pointed out in his chapter on death, "No life event can stir more emotionally directed thinking in the individual and more emotional reactiveness in those about him" (Bowen, pp. 321–322). Further, this anxiety inevitably will transmit to members of professional health care teams that are charged with the care and comfort of dying patients and, as a result, the health care team becomes part of the emotional system.

Bowen family systems theory offers a framework within which to understand the development and transmission of this anxiety. This theoretical perspective suggests strategies for managing the dying process for both family members and teams of health care professionals involved. It is at once both intensely personal and, yet, relies on the ability of a family and the individuals within it to work toward more reasonable and less emotional involvement in the process. This chapter addresses chronic illness and death within families and how the family's ability to adapt may influence the type of care and the satisfaction in the care that they receive. This will be considered from the perspective of Bowen theory.

First, we briefly outline a theoretical perspective grounded in Bowen theory for understanding the anxiety associated with chronic illness and death of a family member. A significant aspect of this discussion relates to the transmission of anxiety both among family members and to persons in the health professions charged with the care of chronically ill and dying patients. It is important to emphasize the anxiety of the family and the means by which it is transmitted to the health care team. The amount of anxiety influences the ability of each group to be effective in adapting to the situation. Second, we provide an extensive clinical example of how the emotional process of a particular family influences the expression of anxiety within the family and the team of health professionals.

Bowen (1978) postulates that death in families is described by "open" and "closed" relationship systems (p. 322). Open systems are characterized by greater freedom in communication with others, whereas closed systems are characterized by less freedom to communicate anxiety-laden material with each other. The specific concepts of Bowen theory that most directly bear on this process are the family projection process, triangles, and the multigenerational transmission of anxiety. It should be clear, however, that since Bowen theory consists of concepts that interlock with each other, all eight principles of the theory likely will be highly relevant to a given case. Within Bowen theory, it is important to see how each of the concepts is connected and typically is relevant to understanding case information.

As families develop, patterns of behavior emerge that influence the functioning of the individuals within the family and the family itself. As Bowen pointed out, several variables contribute to the emotional process that regulates the life of the family. This is particularly true in times of stress and intensified anxiety. For example, as parents realize that relationships outside the home influence their children, the perception of loss of control can create distress. This may result in parents' attempt to overcontrol or be more involved in the lives of their children. The father who becomes a "Little League dad" or the frequently discussed "helicopter parents" exemplifies this effort.

As children move toward adulthood, complete education, and enter the workforce, the parental triangle shifts further as parents attempt to manage their own anxiety without children on which to focus. Sometimes this focus can shift to grandchildren. Sometimes it can focus on other relationships.

As parents age and become vulnerable, strength and power in the family shift. The anxiety that parents projected onto children is complicated by the concern that children project onto parents as they become elderly and more fragile. The greater reality of approaching death enhances that anxiety.

Both individual and family development occurs within the context of these shifting triangles. Adult children, attempting to manage their own relationships, experience the parental triangle from a different perspective: one of being the stronger, more able persons in the system.

The onset of chronic illness and pending death enhances the intensity of the anxiety in the family, leading to more or less functional means of managing themselves. Responsibilities of both parents and children are easily overlooked in this intensity.

An important determinant of the family's response to chronic illness and death is the level of differentiation of self in the family. Upon the onset of chronic illness and pending death, lower levels of differentiation of self within a family system will likely result in higher anxiety. That increase, in turn, influences the behavior of the family and its relationship with the ill and dying person as well as with the professionals involved in care. Persons who typically manage anxiety with cutoff will absent themselves from the process. Persons who typically become dominant in managing stressful situations may become assertive in this situation.

Bowen points out that "some well-functioning families are able to adapt to approaching death before it occurs" (1978, p. 328). He cautions that there is not a universally held definition of "well-functioning" but that families vary in adaptive responses to the process of dying and death.

This theoretical perspective provides a means of understanding the experience of a family in the difficult time of chronic illness and death and the fragile dimensions of the relationship with the physicians and other health care professionals who provide essential care at that time, whether it is critical care, palliative care, or hospice care.

Case Study

The following case study is an amalgamation of cases in which each of the authors have been involved in various capacities. It demonstrates the power of the emotional process of a family to influence the adjustment to chronic illness and death.

Several themes emerge in this particular family's experience of death and its repercussions. First is the power of health-related beliefs that revolved around toughness and denial that influence the reactivity of the family to death and loss (Rolland, 1994, p. 138ff). Second is a culturally based suspicion of the motives and integrity of health professionals that shapes both help-seeking behavior and the assumption of personal responsibility for one's own health. Third is the impact of the experience of health care providers, family, and friends involved in the clinical care of critically ill and dying persons.

Clinical Presentation

John was a 71-year-old Caucasian male living in rural Kentucky with his wife, Ellen, 68 (Figure 16.1). Both have retired from teaching careers, electing to stay in the same town in which they have lived for 42 years. John presents with chronic heart disease, complaining of increased difficulty breathing and swelling of the ankles. After he neglected his health for 30 years, his wife insisted he see a physician. John was overweight, a heavy smoker, and drank alcohol, almost to excess.

After canceling two appointments with the physician in their small town, he reluctantly kept an appointment. He expressed resentment about seeing a young female physician. The physician, Jeanne Mayhew, MD, was a 32-year-old Caucasian female in the small, rural community. She took the position because of having grown up in a similar small town. She had no children.

John's first appointment with Dr. Mayhew did not go well. First, the receptionist immediately requested that he complete paperwork describing his health. Included in this form was a family history questionnaire. Second, the nurse, a former student of John's, sought information about why he sought medical assistance. Third, John was told to disrobe and put on a gown. John felt his privacy was violated by people he did not know and with whom he had no history.

Dr. Mayhew greeted John upon entering the room, and John immediately indicated why he should not be there and that he made the appointment to please Ellen, "who had a thing about seeing doctors for one thing or another." As he got up to leave, Dr. Mayhew

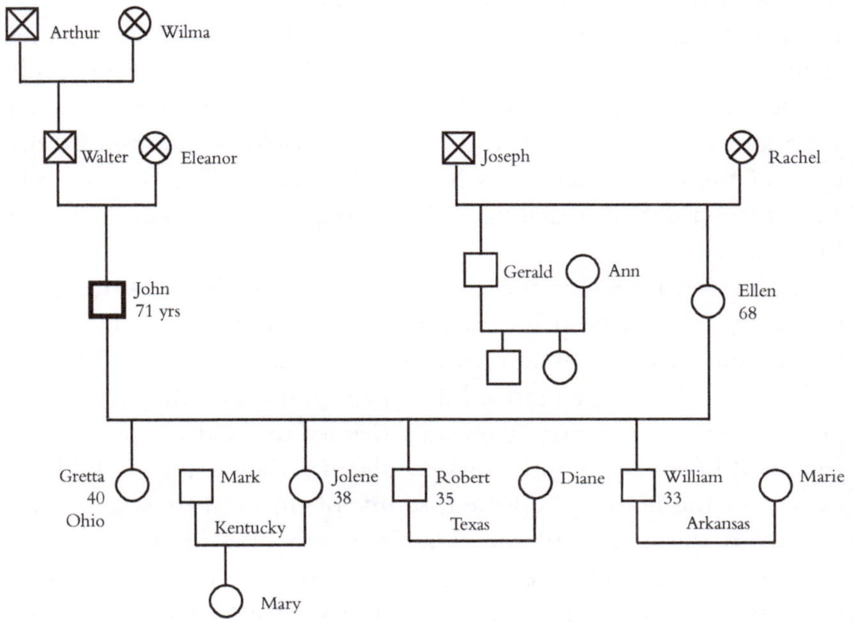

Figure 16.1 Family diagram

engaged him in conversation about his family. As he relaxed, John told of his four children and grandchildren, giving hints of the interpersonal distance between himself and his offspring. After her physical examination, Dr. Mayhew believed that a psychosocial intervention plan was necessary. She ordered new medications and a referral to a visiting social worker.

Social History

John and Ellen were natives of Kentucky, children of parents who worked in coal mines. They both had sought to escape the seemingly inevitable work in the mines and met at college. After completing their training in education, they settled in John's hometown to "give back."

The new couple rented a house in town and began their teaching careers. Unexpectedly, soon after their new start, Ellen became pregnant. This created a different focus for the couple, who were trying to make ends meet on paltry teachers' salaries and there was a significant struggle to adapt. John took on additional coaching duties at the school to supplement their income. These added responsibilities demanded time away from home, and tension developed between John and Ellen. They hoped this tension would be resolved by the birth of the child. Gretta was born and became Ellen's focus while John maintained his teaching and coaching duties as they struggled financially.

In somewhat regular succession, the other children were born, requiring John to keep his teaching and coaching duties and Ellen to continue working. The births of the additional children, Jolene, Robert, and William, continued the financial stress on the family and, presumably, underlay marital tensions that led to the distance between John and Ellen. Since both worked full-time, they required childcare outside of the home, a consistent source of financial stress and worries about the quality of the care. Over time, the focus continued to be on the firstborn, Gretta. Both parents were concerned about her development and, later, her inability to make friends and engage in age-appropriate activities. The other children appeared to develop without difficulties apart from their resentment of Gretta's apparent "special place" in the family.

At the time of John's medical difficulties, Gretta was 40, Jolene was 38, Robert was 35, and William was 33. Gretta was single; the others were married. Gretta was employed as a teacher in Cincinnati, Ohio; Jolene and her husband resided in the same community as her parents. Both sons had married and moved to Texas and Arkansas, respectively. The family rarely gathered except Jolene and her husband, parents of one child. They frequently visited with her parents and it was a source of tension in their marriage.

Gretta's relationship with her parents was a tense one, characterized by distance, approaching cutoff. While Gretta was the oldest, she was the child of focus in the family, and both Ellen and John pinned their hopes for reproduction and material success on her.

Although Gretta had a number of suitors in both high school and college and in her young adult years, no relationship ever moved toward marriage or stability. She asserted that she was not interested in having children, that her teaching responsibilities fulfilled those needs.

The social worker to whom John was referred, Jim Blassengane, was able to develop a positive relationship with John after just a few visits. They both came from small Kentucky towns and shared the experience of having been high school athletes at similar times. Blassengane hypothesized that John's experience of managing loss was an important factor in the distance from his wife and his children. He inquired of John's earliest experiences of loss. John cautiously discussed his mother's death when he was 12 years old. The following paragraphs are taken from that story:

> The Rev. Haskell Williams had a sense of self-importance as he approached the junior high school on a September morning. His task was to tell a 12-year-old boy that his mother had died. Immediately following the death, the boy's father asked the minister to fetch the boy to tell him of his mother's death. The unexpected death of Eleanor, the mother, followed a two-week hospitalization for an emergency hysterectomy after which peritonitis had set in.
>
> "I recall hearing my name called over the intercommunications system, directing me to go to the principal's office. The minister took me out of the building without explanation. Outside a band played a military march and the minister said, 'You are going to be a tough soldier, aren't you? Your mother just died,' the minister told me."

John recalled the disbelieving numbness of hearing this announcement. His father, Walter, a 35-year old salesman, was at the house along with his mother, Wilma, John's grandmother, who had arrived from rural Virginia. Eleanor had entered the hospital prior to her death for a hysterectomy, and in the early morning hours she appeared to go into shock and died. John's recall of that experience was characterized as one of distance, a lack of connection with his father or others who were around at that time.

Upon leaving Dr. Mayhew's office following the initial visit, John reluctantly agreed to use the prescribed regimen that he was told would improve his breathing. John initially mistrusted that these would work but at the encouragement of his wife, he agreed to try them for a week or so. John was surprised at the great relief this new regimen brought him. His breathing became easier and his legs were less swollen. For the next six months, John felt better and even took up a volunteer coaching job. Relationships with the children and with Ellen improved, and John even felt well enough that he and Ellen hosted Christmas dinner at their house. All four children and their individual families attended. Even Gretta initially seemed relaxed.

One month after Christmas, John was on his way to the store when he noticed chest pressure while walking. He had to stop and sit down to catch his breath. When he got home Ellen remarked, "John, you look ill." She decided to call Dr. Mayhew, against John's request.

Dr. Mayhew instructed them to go to the ER for workup. Once there, John underwent a series of tests revealing that he was in the midst of a heart attack and a chronic obstructive pulmonary disease (COPD) flare. He was taken to the cardiac lab where it was determined that he would need cardiac surgery. Ellen notified all four of their children with the update in John's health. By that evening, Jolene had arrived at the hospital and had declared that she would be staying overnight, telling her mom "go home and rest, Mom, you need it." Robert had not yet called back (he was away on a trip with his family), and William requested Ellen call with updates. Gretta, crying, seemed irritated with Ellen for not seeing the warning signs sooner. After hearing that Jolene was already at his bedside, she told her mother, "Well it seems it's under control so call me if you need something," and she ended the call. Overnight unexpectedly a code blue was called when John suffered a cardiac arrest. The house officer physician who first arrived at bedside asked for John's health care wishes paperwork.

Unfortunately, John had never discussed his health care wishes with Ellen when he was healthy and therefore the family, namely Ellen, would now be looked to as surrogate decision makers. Over the years Ellen attempted to discuss issues like living wills with John but this triggered in John a strong reaction, always replying, "Why do you always have to bring this up when everything is fine?!" In truth, John may have been even more confused than Ellen. He felt that it was a sign of weakness to discuss these things. John did not fear death per se as much as he feared a "bad death," which he imagined involving a great deal of suffering. The idea of "losing control" over his body and surroundings was uncomfortable for him. John was not able to articulate his feelings and he avoided the topic, hoping that one day he would die peacefully in his sleep. Without a document reflecting health care wishes, the house officer turned to Ellen for interaction. In a panicked state, she asked that all efforts be made to resuscitate John. The code blue team successfully regained a pulse and John was intubated, sedated, and taken to the intensive care unit (ICU).

Ellen and Jolene called the other children immediately notifying them of the events. William, now back from his trip, requested he be given regular updates just as Robert had been getting. Over the next two weeks, John's condition remained the same. The medical team attempted multiple times to trial him off the ventilator machine but this repeatedly failed.

The ICU physician, Dr. Bailey, was the doctor caring for John. Dr. Bailey came from a large Irish family with seven siblings. Her father was an alcoholic, and everyone knew her mother as "a saint." Dr. Bailey's siblings were scattered across America. She was the first in her family to attend medical school and regularly sends money home. Dr. Bailey suspects that her brothers (who are still living at home) take some of the money she sends. This angers her but she doesn't bring it up. She feels this would only add more stress to her mother. Dr. Bailey is 37 years old, single, has no children, but dates "when she can find the time." She is a marathon runner who eats only vegan and stays on a strict schedule. Dr. Bailey rarely sees her family and only goes home, which is over 500 miles away in New England, on holidays. Her last romantic relationship, which lasted two years, ended after her boyfriend had an affair. She is one of five members of an ICU physician group. At her last evaluation, Dr. Bailey scored poorly on her communication skills with patients and families. Based on data and staff reporting, the head physician in her group suspects that Dr. Bailey is not effectively discussing end of life with families.

After 14 days under Dr. Bailey's care, John has made no significant improvement. Dr. Bailey requested a family meeting. Gretta, who had been visiting only at night, agreed to come only after 8:00 p.m., which required Dr. Bailey to change her running schedule. The hospital staff saw Gretta as being "difficult" and "critical." Nurses avoided Gretta as much as possible because they felt her constant remarks were a problem. Gretta believed that Jolene and Ellen were incapable of grasping the severity of the situation and that she should be more appreciated.

She told her brothers: "Nothing would be getting done if I weren't speaking up!"

Dr. Bailey learned that Jolene and Ellen were available to meet for a family meeting at any time and that both sons agreed to be present by telephone on a conference call. Dr. Bailey decided to change her running time to early morning so Gretta could be present.

This family meeting did not go well. This was the first time that Ellen and all four children were present (sons present by phone) since Christmas dinner months ago. Jolene and Ellen sat next to Dr. Bailey with the conference phone on a table. Gretta stood by the door saying, "I sit all day."

Dr. Bailey began the conversation inquiring what the family understood about John's condition. Before anyone could speak, Gretta interrupted Dr. Bailey, saying: "Well, if anyone ever gave us an update maybe we would know." Dr. Bailey reminded Gretta that she had been spending at least 40 minutes a day in conversation with her mother and sister. This seemed to irritate Gretta who replied: "Well, fine, I guess, but you people just don't seem to know what you're doing is what I understand." Robert interjected, "Let the doctor talk, Gretta, for God's sake, that's enough!" At this, Gretta left, slamming the door behind her. Ellen stood silent, staring at Dr. Bailey, hoping she would take control. Gretta did not return.

Dr. Bailey continued with the family meeting without Gretta's input. With Gretta's abrupt departure, Dr. Bailey felt angry, thinking to herself, "It is just as well she left." Dr. Bailey knew she "was not alone" in her frustration with Gretta. Since John's admission, the family had gained a reputation around the ICU. Gretta believed that John had been the sickest patient in the ICU. Many times she said: "Someone needs to be the squeaky wheel if he's going to get the attention he needs!" Jolene apologized on behalf of their family and tried to explain "how difficult Gretta is" by telling stories of their childhood to the nurses. The staff began to keep interactions as minimal as possible to avoid conflict. Gretta's interpretation of their avoidance was that the staff was incompetent and that this demanded even more attentiveness on her part.

Dr. Bailey continued the family meeting giving her updates. Over the previous day, John's kidneys failed and, due to the side effects of medications, his fingers and toes were losing circulation. Dialysis and amputation were indicated. Earlier that morning, Dr. Bailey had two other patients die on her service after prolonged ICU stays, both with a high level of physical discomfort. Dr. Bailey believed John was headed down this same path, and she hoped that this meeting would lead to John's family deciding to focus on comfort. She delivered her updates using a serious tone of voice and pressured speech. Dr. Bailey strongly believed that John was not going to survive his current illness given his poor response to the treatments. Her recommendation would be to prioritize comfort and stop the machines. She felt uncomfortable telling this to the family. Dr. Bailey received little training in talking about death and dying in medical school and she lacked the confidence in having these conversations. In her own family, Dr. Bailey was raised not to confront difficult topics such as her father's drinking or his death from alcoholism. In general, when it came to topics in which feelings of sadness could be triggered, Dr. Bailey tended to create distance. While she feared a prolonged dying process for John, as well as another "sit down" with her boss, she hoped that the family would come to the conclusion on their own that John wasn't going to survive. Ellen, now questioning herself as John's proxy, expressed a feeling of paralysis by Dr. Bailey's news. Ellen thought to herself, "Well, we've done so much already, would stopping now make none of it worth it?" Ellen noted emotion in Dr. Bailey's tone of voice and posture. Not knowing how to interpret this body language she assumed Dr. Bailey was still hoping John might improve. She concluded, but kept it to herself, "I don't want to let her (Dr. Bailey) down by giving up."

Following the family meeting, and after a long conversation with each other, Ellen, Robert, and William concluded that John "wouldn't want this" and that the machines should be stopped. Jolene, crying, repeatedly said, "I can't be ok with this," which caused the others to waver. Ellen, now worried about both Gretta and Jolene, went to Dr. Bailey to request that John start hemodialysis and undergo amputation. Dr. Bailey, frustrated with their indecisiveness, thought, "They just don't get it." She asked that they reconvene in another 48 hours and reminded them of the issue of timeliness in making such decisions.

That evening John suffered another cardiac arrest. Cardiopulmonary resuscitation (CPR) was performed, again at Ellen's request. Ellen and Jolene called to notify William and Robert. Ellen asked that Dr. Bailey call Gretta "since she won't answer the family's calls."

Dr. Bailey reached Gretta and informed her of John's status. Gretta replied, "You're killing my dad and wait until you hear from my lawyer." This again triggered Dr. Bailey's resentment toward the family. She angrily reflected on how she had sacrificed her running commitments to meet with them. This reaction was clearly tied to her own feelings within her family's lack of appreciation for what she was doing for them by sending money and maintaining contact.

Dr. Bailey met with Ellen and Jolene the next day. Ellen tearfully decided that the machines should be stopped after 24 more hours. This sudden change in decision making came after Ellen had a conversation with a nursing technician during routine care who made a passing comment: "Wow. He looks really sick. Seems like he might not make it. Hope your family is ok." This statement prompted Ellen to take the position: "We need to be realistic and let him go." Everyone except Gretta, who was still not answering the phone, agreed with the sentiment, and John died immediately after the breathing tube was removed.

William, the youngest, offered to be the one to deliver the news in person to Gretta. In a rage, Gretta claimed to be the only one who "really understood dad" and "he would have never given up." She threatened never to speak to her mother or sister "ever again." In response, Ellen called and left more voicemail messages, but Jolene decided, "Well, fine, this makes my life easier."

Gretta and her siblings with their respective families attended the funeral. Gretta did not make eye contact with her mother or sister. Over the next few years, the family infrequently made contact. Jolene, during the week of the funeral, discovered to her surprise that she was pregnant. She thought, sarcastically, that this new baby "is just what my marriage needs." She decided to distance from her "toxic family" to spend her energy on her new child and husband.

Four years later, Ellen, living with Jolene, became depressed after she learned through a neighbor that Gretta had cancer. Ellen and Gretta's relationship never recovered following John's death. The family supported this distance after Ellen was diagnosed with the beginnings of dementia two years after John's death. Jolene "had enough on her plate" after her youngest child was diagnosed with behavioral issues. The boys felt that they "would help more but had their own lives to worry about."

Interpretation, Theoretical Points, and Conclusion

The emotional process of this family influenced the behavior of the individuals throughout the treatment, hospitalization, and death of the husband and father. Several factors evident in the case description demonstrate the high level of anxiety in the family over time and how it influenced the family's experience in the last days prior to the death and the death itself.

First, John's reluctance to seek medical assistance for clearly remarkable symptoms was consistent with his father, and with many other lower/middle-class males (Addis & Mahelik, 2003). The fact that the physician with whom he had an appointment was female likely further influenced his hesitation.

Second, the recommendation that John get physical and psychosocial help likely also complicated his perceptions of Dr. Mayhew's plans for further care. His discomfort with initially seeking help for the medical difficulties likely was associated with getting help for problems that are "all in your mind."

Third, John and Ellen resided in their town over a long period of time, and both had visible occupations as schoolteachers and John was also a coach. This longevity likely led to sensitivity about illness and disability, which frequently in many Appalachian communities is thought to be "weakness."

Fourth, Ellen's early and unexpected pregnancy heightened the stress that the family experienced, leading to the formation of triangles with the health care system and, eventually, the childcare system. It also changed the nature of Ellen's relationship with the school system and its personnel, showing that anxiety experienced in one context can be demonstrated in another.

Fifth, the birth of Gretta, the firstborn, identified her as the likely child of focus, which apparently turned out to be the case. Their focus on her appeared to have led to overintensity in the relationship between her and her parents. Her inability to form other sustainable relationships is an indicator of that fusion and tension. Her behavior in the context of the hospital room and eventual cutoff from the parents and siblings were further evidence of the fusion.

Sixth, when a patient or family is less adaptive to a health crisis, they are more likely to react in haste that puts them at risk of gaining a reputation among hospital staff as "overreactive" or "difficult." Gretta's criticisms made the staff want to distance from her. Without proper communication from the staff, a family member is left speculating if their loved one is receiving adequate care, as suspected by Gretta, or if they are being labeled, as suspected by Jolene.

Seventh, if the patient and the family are not able to adapt, medical decisions are avoided or based in emotion as opposed to fact or thoughtfulness. This family faced unavoidable decisions such as CPR and dialysis. Since John did not express his health care wishes during times of better health, the family was put in a position to make decisions for him. The chaos that occurred during the last days of John's life reflected this family's inability to adapt to these circumstances. Surrogate decision making can repeatedly reactivate a low-functioning family system with each decline in health, as it did in the case of John.

Eighth, the intensity of the family's anxiety is reflected in the relationships with the health care team. Not only the patient and the family are part of the emotional process—so is the hospital staff. The interruptions provoked in the lives of the physicians were evidence of this transfer of anxiety. Dr. Bailey's anger that she changed her running schedule to accommodate Gretta is an example of these interruptions. Nursing staff avoided this family instead of managing their own emotions, which resulted in less focus on the patient. Gretta detected a distancing staff and misinterpreted this behavior as incompetence. Dr. Bailey's difficulty with direct communication and her fear of a poor evaluation prevented her from remaining calm during the family meetings. Finally, Ellen made choices based on Dr. Bailey's demeanor and out of fear of disappointing Dr. Bailey.

Ninth, when a patient's and family's anxiety results in conflict in response to a health crisis, they are less likely to be satisfied and more likely to find fault with caregivers and their plans. They also may be more likely to threaten legal action that typically has the opposite of its intended effect. Unfortunately, their dissatisfaction detracts from time spent with their loved one, and this lost opportunity can have lasting consequences. Gretta spent the majority of her time focusing on the competency of the ever more distancing staff. Jolene used her time engaging with nurses about issues with her sister Gretta. Both sons remained geographically distant, and Ellen stayed more or less "paralyzed." These poorly adaptive reactions to John's illness resulted in less time spent with their husband and father in the final days of his life and had consequences for family relationships years after his death.

Tenth, the ability of the patient, family, and the treating provider to stand apart from emotion and anxiety, without becoming reactive, is proportional to the likelihood of reaching a successful plan. This case also is an example of how a person outside of the emotional system can sometimes be more effective in communicating with families in crisis. It was the technician who unknowingly changed the outcome by speaking clearly and calmly.

From the perspective of Bowen theory, efforts toward differentiation of self may be reflected in a diligent approach to preparation for death, both on the part of one or more family members and the dying person. In this family, as in many families, preparation was not done and both the process and event of death were denied.

Bowen theory asserts that when one or more family members become more responsible by engaging in the process of differentiation, with a Bowen coach, the family has a better chance to deal with chronic illness or death in the family without denial. Efforts to stand apart from the system while being within it are met with resistance or "pushback." The case study presented several instances of efforts to take stands, particularly with regard to the choice of utilizing extreme measures for maintaining life along with the anticipated resistance.

The process of dying reaches beyond each family and the individuals within it and is influenced by a variety of institutional values that characterize culture and a way of life. With regard to death, defining self requires a focus on the emotional processes of larger social institutions that have a stake in the ways people's lives end. As a result, differentiation of self in the process of dying or involvement with a dying family member is complex and subject to the range of "pushback" from multiple contexts, including, but not limited to, the family. Social institutions, professions, and business enterprises have a distinct investment in the process of dying.

Death and the Medical Profession

Among the first institutions encountered in the process of death is the medical profession. As Gawande (2014) pointed out, medicine exists essentially to keep people alive. He rather differently expands the mission of medicine to think about, plan for, and eventually accept death. He differentiated between medical care to prolong life and medical care to prolong death. Butler (2013) supports this point in her account of her father's death by affirming that the struggle to be a self in the face of medical care is a difficult, arduous task that takes an enormous toll on both individuals and families. Kevorkian (1991) provoked enormous controversy with his recommendations for physician-assisted suicide, proclaiming that a patient had a right to die.

Gawande (2014) and Butler (2013), among other medical practitioners, have introduced other points of view that differ from traditional thinking and practice. The medical specialties palliative care and hospice care aim to improve communication between staff and family. Both anticipate the high level of emotions associated with the death of a loved one. Professionals in these specialties are trained to remain nonanxious and effective in their communication with patients and families facing a terminal illness.

Just as a person cannot redo the birth of a child, we also have just one opportunity to experience and cope with the death of a family member. Family patterns are passed down through generations, and the adaptive mechanisms made by individuals in the context of death and dying are no different. These behaviors are commonly repeated by future generations over time.

Bowen family systems theory offers a breadth of perspective to understand the functioning of family units in which a member is suffering from chronic illness, likely to result in death. Additionally, the theory helps to understand the reciprocal relationship between the anxiety of the family itself and the functioning of the health care team as a unit. Further, as demonstrated by the case study, each member of the health care team is involved in a family, bringing additional anxiety into the mix. The operative concept of Bowen theory, differentiation of self, becomes an important concept for members of the family and the health care team, as families and professionals strive for the most adaptive experience for the dying person, the family of that person, and the effectiveness of the team.

REFERENCES

Addis, M., & Mahelik, J. (2003). Men, masculinity, and the contexts of help seeking. *American Psychologist, 58*(1), 5–14.

Bowen, M. (1978). *Family therapy in clinical practice.* New York, NY: Jason Aronson.

Butler, K. (2013). *Knocking on heaven's door: The path to a better way of death.* New York, NY: Scribner.

Gawande, A. (2014). *Being mortal: Medicine and what matters in the end.* New York, NY: Holt.

Kevorkian, J. (1991). *Prescription: Medicide: The goodness of planned death.* Amherst, NY: Prometheus.

Rolland, J. (1994). *Families, illness, and disability: An integrative treatment model* (pp. 141–143). New York, NY: Basic Books.

17

DEATH AND AIDS

Families and Society

Andrea Maloney Schara

In the beginning of 1981, five men had been diagnosed with severe immune deficiency. By the end of the year, there were 270 cases among gay men. Of these cases 121 people died in a cruel and lingering way. Death from AIDS continues to be miserable for all concerned (Avert.org, 2017). Fear erupted. An unknown contagion was killing people. The cause and method of transmission were a mystery. Emotional beliefs spread as fast as the virus. A popular belief spread through the population was that a plague was punishing gay people. A few who could be more objective were able to observe the emotional processes. Anxiety and fears increased. There was more scapegoating of individuals in families and groups in society. People were projecting fears onto one another, decreasing the ability to relate well. Questions: Could individuals resist this social contagion and think for self? Would decreasing fear improve relationships with others and increase immune functioning? Research indicates that altering one's coping style can affect the immune system (Koolhaas, de Boer, Buwalda, & van Reenen, 2007). The effort to understanding how any social system functions around an illness like AIDS is of significant value today. Currently 36.7 million live with HIV infection. Since the early 1980s, more than 70 million people have been infected with the HIV virus and about 35 million people have died (Global Health Observatory, 2017).

A pilot study was formed to demonstrate that by coaching those with HIV/AIDS to alter reactive family relationships their health would improve. People at the Georgetown University Family Center were resistant, but Murray Bowen, MD, the director of the center, saw the potential. Bowen encouraged the study. Possible correlations between improving relationships and improvement in immune functioning existed theoretically. AIDS provided a way to measure the T-cell count regarding the changes in behavior. The T-cell count was the gold standard of immune functioning (Crowe, 1990). If relationships improved and the T-cell count went up, this might be an indicator for a larger trial. Participants for the study were recruited from the Whitman Walker Clinic in Washington, DC (Whitman Walker, 2017). Due to the resistance to family ideas, this researcher/coach volunteered to lead a support group at the clinic for those who had HIV or AIDS. Most were distant from their families. The hypothesis: People could increase their health by having the courage to forge more open family relationships. It seemed counterintuitive to those in the support group. One explanation was that if there was fear in the relationships system, and a fear response activated cortisol, and cortisol damaged the immune system, then whatever one could do to lower arousal in the face of a real or imagined threat would be positive (Stoecklein, Osuka, & Lederer, 2012). Entering challenging relationships to alter one's immune system required belief plus courage. In society AIDS forced individuals to take on issues like discrimination, increasing research funding, drug availability, costs of treatment, prevention, long-term medical care, respect, and legalization for the partnerships between gay men, and, lastly, the impact of one's death on family and friends. Many that lead society to think differently included Ryan White (d.1990), who contracted AIDS as a child and was banned from school; Magic Johnson (who came out in 1999); and Randy Shilts, (1986) who wrote *And the Band Played On*. This kind of courageous openness forced the public to see AIDS as a disease, not an evil; a disease that might be affected by open relationships.

Hypothesis Based on Bowen Family Systems Theory

The hypothesis: *Those individuals willing to have more open relationships with important individuals in their families of origin would alter how anxiety was automatically managed in relationships.* Despite the stress involved in forging more open relationships, the overall result would be that engaging family members would be protective (Olsen, Olsen, Gunner-Svensson, & Waldstrøm, 1991; Seeman, 1996). Over evolutionary time four automatic mechanisms absorbed anxiety in social groups: 1) distance, 2) conflict, 3) reciprocity, and 4) projection. The fifth way was to be more open and to solve problems or to alter the way the social group communicated, known as differentiation of self. When individuals are more open in relationships, eventually, there is less fear and anxiety to activate the four mechanisms (Stoecklein et al., 2012). The family unit itself becomes more "intelligent" in regard to problem solving. Individuals are challenged to take actions based on principles. The urge to think and act for self is always opposed by a demand for conformity. The togetherness urge, to go along with the group's beliefs, often blindsides people (Nickerson, 1998).

Those in the pilot program became better observers of the pressure to conform and the emotional reactivity opposing acting more for self, based on one's principles. To the degree that fear cannot be handled in relationships the four mechanisms are activated. No thought needed. Just as a person draws his or her hand away from a hot stove, withdrawal from intense relationships works to lower anxiety. However, problems are not solved. There is little cooperation or support in the family unit. The initial challenge was how to tell family members the uncomfortable truth: "I am gay and soon to die."

As people could be more open, the original hypothesis had to be expanded to account for the reports of an increase in symptoms throughout the family unit. One explanation: The openness regarding an impending death in the family unit created an "emotional shock wave" (Bowen, 1976). The anxiety spread out to other relationships. This decreased the anxiety in the diagnosed individual. In mature families, we saw an increase in cooperation, whereas in lower-functioning families they continued to cut off relationships, leaving the diagnosed individuals more vulnerable. The implication: More mature families could manage more anxiety as a function of being involved in an emotional family unit. This may have enabled HIV/AIDS individuals to live longer than predicted.

HIV and the Immune System

William Chris Woodward wrote in *Scientific American* the following clear description of the T cells and how they change as HIV becomes AIDS:

> An HIV infection begins with a sharp rise of virus in the blood stream and a consequent drop in CD4 T cells. The HIV hides in the CD4 cells and replicates. The immune system can keep HIV levels steady for several years. Eventually, though, the virus gains the upper hand. AIDS is diagnosed when the CD4 T cell level drops below 200 cells per cubic millimeter of blood or when opportunistic infections arise. (Normal is 500 to 1,000 cells per milliliter). Stage 1: HIV infection. Stage 2: AIDS—T cells below 200.
>
> (Woodward, 1999)

The Whitman Walker Clinic and Family Systems Research

The Whitman Walker Clinic in Washington, DC, is the place where motivated people go to find the latest ways to improve health. In 1985 one option was to join a research group. The Management of AIDS by Understanding the Family as an Emotional Unit was one such group. Those initially recruited were members of an empowerment group for individuals diagnosed with HIV/AIDS. This researcher/coach volunteered for two years (1985–1987) as an empowerment group leader. Time was needed to explain the usefulness of reconnecting with one's family and biofeedback training for the mind–body connection. Initially, there was little interest. The effort was at odds with the prevailing mental health focus on the importance of trauma, for more supportive caregivers, for expressing feelings, and for drug treatment (Whetten, Reif, Whetten, & Murphy-McMillan, 2008; Blank, Himelhoch, Walkup, & Eisenberg, 2013). Encouraging individuals to move toward difficult family relationships involved asking people to alter their coping style from disengagement to engagement. It took a year for one person to volunteer to join the pilot study. Over the next ten years, 35 people volunteered to participate in the study.

The Usefulness of Biofeedback With Family Systems Coaching

A three-generation family diagram enabled a basic understanding of the automatic nature of the four basic mechanisms described earlier. Confirmation bias leads us to seek confirmation for our ideas, beliefs, and grudges, increasing our sensitivity to others (Plous, 1993). Being able to identify automatic reactions and bias increases the ability to think rather than to react. A new idea to be in better contact with family members often took weeks to consider.

Biofeedback training (as taught by Lillian Rosenbaum, PhD, Georgetown University Family Center) enables people to relax, entertain new ideas, and integrate feelings and thinking. Using biofeedback instruments, people could see the impact of talking about relationships in relation to their physiology. As they talked about relationships, they could use the feedback to exert more conscious control over their physiology and become less reactive and emotional. Biofeedback rewards efforts to increase hand temperature and lower EEG and EDR by hearing a positive tone. In a few sessions, most people could learn to warm their hands while imagining talking to important others. After an upset, they would notice their cold hands and could then recover by warming their hands. People would train by saying: "I feel my body as warm and relaxed" (Benson, 1975). They were gaining more conscious control over physiology and psychology, resulting in calmer mental states and more openness to others.

Changes in a Support Group

The first couple from the Whitman Walker support group volunteered in 1986. Mr. G was the outspoken leader in the support group, and Mr. C was his long-term partner. Mr. G's health was precarious. His T-cell count was 17. Since being diagnosed he had been distant from his family but now he was motivated to talk openly with his family to make amends, to prepare them for his death, and to hopefully be close again. As he made better contact with his parents, he reported to the empowerment group what happened. Mr. G's stories made family systems theory and biofeedback a believable approach. The group members began to ask questions as to how Mr. G told his parents about his diagnosis (see clinical case next). What people heard was that despite his parents having issues, it was worth it to be close to family again, and yet to remember and be careful when talking about your HIV or AIDS diagnosis. As a result, people in the group would say things like: "I am going to ask my dad if I can talk to him alone." "I am going to ask my mom if she is sitting down." "I might ask my mom out to a public place for lunch so she will manage herself." Members of the group were looking for ways to keep from scaring others to death due to the hysteria about AIDS. The fact was that during the first nine years of the epidemic, the life expectancy was only 8 to 22 months (France, 2016).

Learning From Mr. G and Mr. C: The Relationship System and AIDS

Mr. G was a financially successful 40-year-old gay man diagnosed with AIDS. Mr. C was his 47-year-old partner who was HIV positive, and who saw himself as the caretaker for Mr. G. They had been together for 14 years. Emotionally, both were very distant from their families. Both had relatively high socioeconomic performance. Mr. G had been written up in *Time* magazine for his work. In his emotional life with his peers, Mr. G noted that his sexual orientation toward same-sex partners had originated in his teenage years, primarily to release sexual tension. He had a very distant relationship with his religious mother and his father, who had a mostly "go along with my wife to get along" attitude. When Mr. G was 25, he met Mr. C for the first time. Mr. C wanted to have a more long-term relationship. Both men agreed that they would have an open relationship. They were primarily invested in maintaining their relationship and did not put demands on one another for a monogamous relationship. In the 1970s, this open status was very common in the gay community, long before AIDS was a threat. Neither Mr. G nor Mr. C was open to their families as to their relationship. Both were fearful of being looked down upon in society and fearful about being gay, much less being HIV positive or having AIDS.

Mr. G had been diagnosed with AIDS in January 1987. In February, he had pneumonia and was hospitalized for 35 days. In addition to pneumonia, Mr. G had lesions of Kaposi's sarcoma. One was on his chest and one on his nose. One of the drugs he had taken damaged his pancreas, and he took insulin for the side effects of the drug. Mr. G's initial hope was to live until August and go on a vacation with Mr. C to Providence, Rhode Island. Mr. G somehow lived until 1988—another year and a half—with a T-cell count fluctuating from over 100 to 17. His partner, Mr. C, had an initial T-cell count over 600, giving him an average of three more years to live, but he lived until 1993. Both men believed that their immune systems could respond to improvements in relationships and that it would take courage to learn how to be more open in relationships, especially with family members. They both used biofeedback to monitor and manage anxiety and found it useful in planning for, and in the recovery from, relationship stress.

Mr. G.'s Nuclear Family

Mr. G, at 44, was the oldest of his three siblings: a younger sister, a brother, and finally a much younger sister (Figure 17.1). Mr. G's parents were alive. His mother had been diagnosed with lung cancer several years ago and was currently in remission. When he was a teenager, Mr. G became aware of the pressure and responsibility to live up to the family tradition and to be an oldest caretaker. His response was to run away. Part of this reaction was the fear he would act out his sexual fantasies and get caught, thereby bringing shame to the family. He found himself wishing that he could die, as his fantasy life was so at odds with his family values. Being homosexual would bring shame to the family. These tensions were resolved, to some extent, by quitting college in his junior year and joining the Navy. His father had served in the Navy. This was a way that he could run away, live a hidden life, and bring no shame to the family. On the surface, the relationships with his family members were positive, just very distant.

The Maternal Side of the G Family

There were early deaths and a considerable number of physical, social, and psychological symptoms in Mr. G.'s maternal extended family during the 1980s. This was about the time he was infected with the HIV virus. Most of the maternal side lived close to each other. Mr.

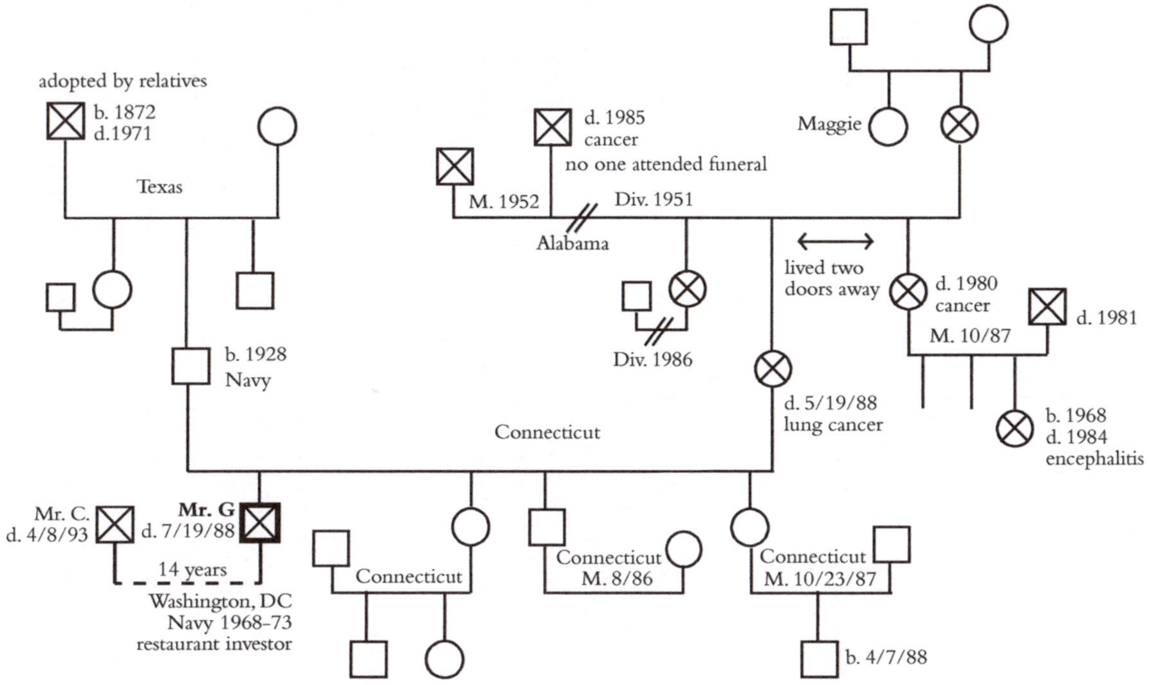

Figure 17.1 Mr. G's family diagram

G.'s mother had an older and a younger sister. Not much was known about the maternal grandfather, as the grandparents had divorced years earlier. No one in the family had kept contact with him. When the grandfather died in 1985, none of his children went to his funeral. Intense emotional cutoff persisted, influencing Mr. G's feelings that if he did anything "wrong" the tentative nature of relationships was such that he would be cut off. The grandmother, at 87, lived two blocks away from Mr. G's mother. In 1980 Mr. G.'s aunt, his mother's youngest sister, died of cancer. The following year her husband died, Mr. G was not sure from what. They had three children, the youngest of whom died in 1984 at the age of 16 from encephalitis. His mother's oldest sister was married with no children. Rumor noted that she and her husband had drinking problems. Their marriage fell apart in 1986. Mr. G said that no one in the family saw a connection between the increasing stress, drinking, and the divorce. Following the divorce, the aunt moved in with her mother. This upset Mr. G's mother, as she was fearful that her mother tended to worry and rescue this older sister. Caretaking for her older sister would put too much of a strain on her mother's health and this was the reason she did not like her sister.

Mr. G. thought about how to interrupt the intensity of his mother's worry. Listening to his mother talk about her mother's problems made him feel paralyzed as to what to say.

Reflecting on this multigenerational problem, Mr. G. decided he could tease his mother and said: "In our family, we have a merry-go-round full of people to worry about and fall off the merry-go-round." His goal was to describe the family worry humorously in a way that allowed him some degree of detachment and some degree of saying his "truth" despite the social pressure to say nothing. Later, in talking with his mother about the symptoms and deaths around his illness, he describes the impact people have on one another as being like a house of cards. When one card fell out, the others better be strong.

The Paternal Side of the G Family

Mr. G's father was the middle of three siblings, the oldest a female and the youngest a male. His father was 64 years old, and Mr. G was 44. Mr. G had been named after his paternal grandfather who had died in 1971. Partially because he was named after this grandfather, he felt an identification with him. The family story was that the paternal grandfather had lost his own family to early death and was adopted when he was a youngster by his cousins. Therefore, caretaking had been very important to him. Seeing the family history gave him more insight into how social pressure and the tendency to cut off had affected him. Being more himself was the antidote.

Mr. G's Effort to Defining Self in His Family

Mr. G wanted to be more open with his family about his life with Mr. C. He knew that his mother, being very religious, would find it hard to accept his sexuality. Because his lifestyle and sexual orientation had been hidden for a long time, it was hard to predict how upset family members might be. Clearly, the most important person to tell was his mother. If he could be more open and honest with her, then he could do it with anybody. In the coaching biofeedback sessions, he would think about the best approach and how to manage fears. His purpose was to be ready for whatever happened. The day Mr. G re-entered the family to tell his parents about his diagnosis, they immediately knew his health was in jeopardy. There were tears in this emotional exchange, after which they both said they had missed him and were relieved to be told why he had been so distant. After they settled down, he explained how important it was to tell them in person and that he planned to tell his siblings too. His youngest sister was getting married soon. It was important to tell her and his older sister, who had teenagers. The parents, predictably, strongly objected. They explained how worried they were about telling his youngest sister and spoiling her wedding plans. Mr. G noted that it might spoil more of her plans to have to go to a funeral that she was totally unprepared for. After all this openness, Mr. G felt closer to his parents.

The challenge remained to talk with his oldest sister, who had protected him from his mother's anger when they were growing up. Her loyalty and approval were particularly important to him. The niece and nephew, who were 17 and 16, had become strangers to him and he wanted to have a more real relationship with them. When he told his sister, she got upset and recovered enough to beg him not to tell her children. His position was that they needed to know for the same reasons that she needed to know. People do better preparing for death. That was his position.

There was to be a family reunion to celebrate his grandmother's and his father's birthdays. By using the biofeedback time, he could imagine being able to take his niece and nephew apart from the family group and tell them he had AIDS. When the time came, he was spontaneous and had little fear. The younger ones were pleased that he had such confidence in them and were not frightened of him or his disease. They hugged him, grateful to know the truth. Mr. G told them he was not going to participate in pretending that nothing was wrong and he said he was also not afraid to live or to die. In his mind, this was going to be an example of a new family tradition: honest talk. Mr. G returned to his parents' home and told them he was planning his funeral and had picked out some things for his mom to read at his funeral. She said, "If you died before I do, I will refuse to go to your funeral, do readings, or sing nice songs." Mr. G was shocked, and then he began to realize the position he had put her in. Honest talk was not all there was. By assuming she should do this and that for him, he was controlling her. Amazingly, he had tried to control his mother. Mostly he had thought: "She is controlling me and I do not like that." So he took a deep breath, calmed down, and said that he respected her wishes. In fact, he could see how he had been controlling her instead of offering her freedom and options. Another opportunity to change his part in the relationships came about when Mr. G's father asked his son if he should leave his Episcopal church to join his mother's Catholic church. Mr. G told his father, "I know you're trying to make Mom happy but I hope you will realize, as I did, that, she would like you to follow your own beliefs, rather than changing yourself to go along with her." After these exchanges, Mr. G experienced more tolerance and an understanding of the importance of differences between people and developed a greater awareness of the fragile nature of the boundaries between people. How easy it was to get too involved or too distant. Mr. G's overall effort was to be less automatic: pleasing, cutting off, getting mad, blaming, and/or fighting. Over time he increased his level of awareness, seeing the family more as an emotional unit programming members to react instead of acting thoughtfully to achieve a better outcome.

Relationships Shifts and Physiology

The degree to which Mr. G could respect others for who they were while defining more clearly what he would and would not do appeared to have a positive short-term influence on physiological functioning. It may be a coincidence that there was a connection in time between changes in the family relationships and the functioning of the immune system. One example is Mr. G's correlations between perceived positive and negative family events and his white blood cell count. On January 29, 1988, Mr. G talked with his sister and told her about his diagnosis. His white blood cell count went up. On February 29, 1988, his mother had a recurrence of her cancer and died on May 19, 1988. A month prior, on April 7, his youngest sister's son was born. Two months after her death and three months after his new nephew's birth, July 19, 1988, Mr. G died from complications of a liver biopsy. The assumption is that greater openness with his sister positively affected his immune system.

Preparing for Death

After his mother died, Mr. G lost his "go" power. Physicians suggested that Mr. G have a liver biopsy, and this procedure, which was not necessary, ended his life. Mr. G said he did not seem to have the will to fight. His partner, Mr. C, was against the biopsy and yet could not persuade his partner to say no. Mr. C was clear that no matter what they discovered, no positive results could occur from a biopsy because of his overall health, so why risk it? Mr. G communicated to his siblings so they were aware of the high-risk nature of the surgery, and they and his father came down to be with him. Mr. G had an orderly and peaceful death. Perhaps this was a better death than the one he might have had at home. After Mr. G's death, his partner, Mr. C, continued to be involved with Mr. G's family. He became a godfather to Mr. G's nephew, the son of Mr. G's youngest sister, who was born April 7, 1988, three months before Mr. G died.

Mr. C continued to participate in the pilot program until he died on April 8, 1993. The following is a brief family history of Mr. C.

Mr. C's Nuclear Family

Mr. C was a 40-year-old younger brother with two older brothers (Figure 17.2). He functioned as an only, as he was born eight years

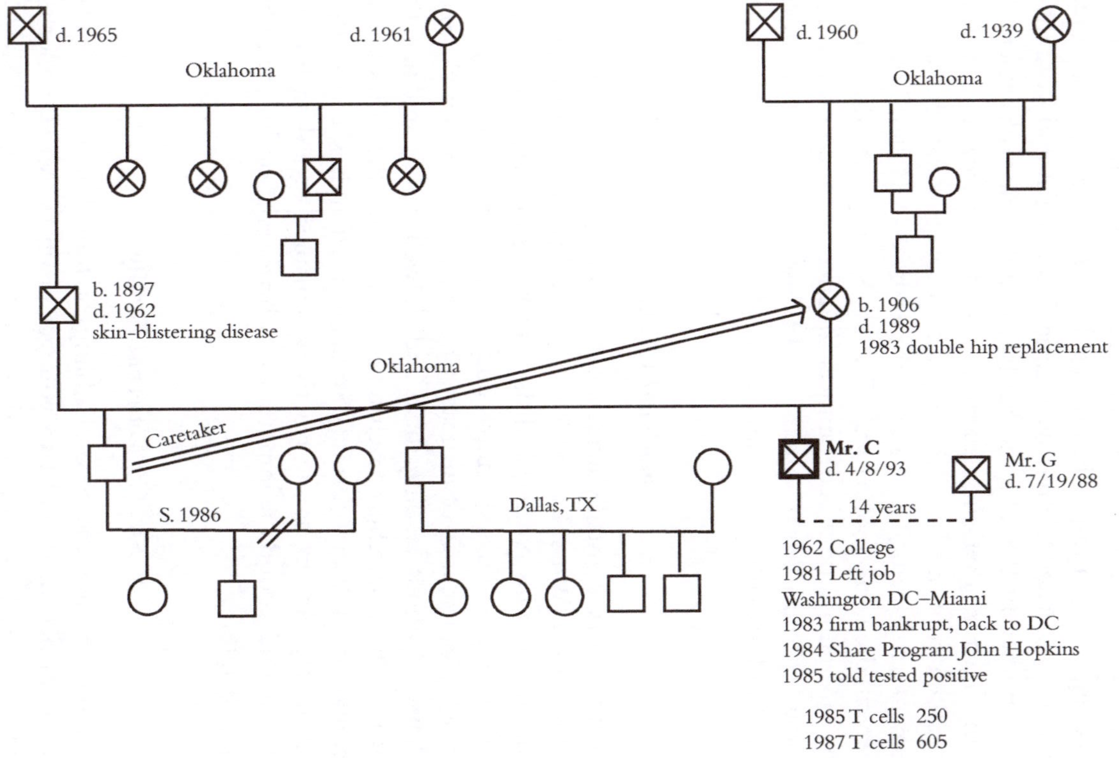

Figure 17.2 Mr. C's family diagram

after his middle brother. They were all raised in Oklahoma. The nuclear family oriented around Mr. C's mother, who had been the strong one carrying the family through all kinds of difficulties. She took care of her husband, who died the year that Mr. C graduated from college. The family talked of his death as a blessing. The older brother had inherited the relatively large family farm and lived there with his mother. In 1983, his mother had a double hip replacement. In 1986, the older brother's first marriage ended in divorce. The ex-wife and children continued to live nearby. Shortly after the divorce, this brother married again. The middle brother lived in Dallas, Texas, and had five children. His mother was 87 when Mr. C joined the research group. This family used geographical distance and emotional cutoff to handle problems. Mr. C often found himself agreeing with others without thinking about the consequences.

Emotional Cutoff

A sketchy history is usually evidence of a long-term emotional cutoff in the family. When I asked Mr. C about his family of origin, he told me he asked his mother and she sent him four pages of detailed notes. This response made it more difficult for him to learn anything for himself. As evidence of his reactivity, he put all his mother's notes in a drawer, without reading them and showed no interest in family history. The researcher/coach teased him about the notes saying they contained the secret formula for being a self and, of course, they needed to stay hidden. Polite reactivity remained regarding his history, but he understood the importance of better relationships with his family of origin.

Mr. C's Maternal Family

Mr. C's mother was the second sibling of four. She had an older brother, who had died, and two younger brothers. Mr. C's mother was the closest to the younger brother next to her and his son. Mr. C's maternal grandmother had died early in 1939, and her husband, Mr. C's grandfather, had died in 1960. He did not have a relationship with anyone in either extended family until he began the coaching.

Mr. C's Paternal Family

Mr. C's father died in 1962 from an unusual skin-blistering disease. His father had been the oldest of five children, all of whom were now dead. The paternal grandmother had died in 1961, and his paternal grandfather in 1965. There were several deaths in the 1960s on his father's side of the family. Then his father died a year after his mother. The emotional distance may have had a lot to do with these deaths around the time Mr. C graduated from college. It appeared that the emotional cutoff with the paternal side was greater than the one in the maternal side.

Defining a Self in the Family

After Mr. C found out that he had tested positive for the HIV virus he knew he would have to tell his mother. He had to have faith that his mother could live with the facts regarding his life choices. Mr. C had not understood how to be more separate and express differences. Mr. C's focus was on his spiritual life. Part of becoming more compassionate was about knowing more about his brothers' and his uncles' and mother's lives. The relationship with his mother had been positive, but distant; the disagreements went underground. Finally, he found the courage to talk about his sexual orientation and his relationship with Mr. G. As he explained his mother said, "I knew about your relationships all along." Her position was that it was his to put on the table and not hers, as it was his "private" life. She was shocked to hear he had the HIV virus, as he looked so healthy. After this talk, Mr. C was relieved and then found it easier than he had feared to talk to his brothers. They were more open and deeply supportive and encouraged him to tell others in the family.

When asked about how Mr. C would explain Mr. G's having serious symptoms while he was currently free from them, he offered the following ideas: both had family and professional loss in the 1980s, around the time they became infected. In 1981, Mr. C had left a high-paying job with the Corps of Engineers to set up a business with a firm in Miami. By 1983 that firm went bankrupt. At the same time, Mr. G invested in a restaurant with a new partner. This partner made Mr. G's life miserable. Under this increasing pressure, Mr. G acted out the tension with sex and drugs. Mr. C. then found a new job in Washington, DC, and moved back in with Mr. G. As the relationship's stress increased, Mr. C became more shut down physically and withdrew from the relationship. There was no way to deal with the way his partner was behaving. The emotional distance and increasing tension almost led to their breakup. But when a friend of theirs died from AIDS in 1984, they became aware that each of them might test positive. They decided to join the SHARE group at Johns Hopkins. This was a volunteer effort to test and track gay males in high-risk groups. One year later in 1985, the program let people know what their test results were. Both tested as HIV positive. Mr. C. was the calmer one and functioned in the role of the caretaker for Mr. G. This had been his role, but now he was conscious of trying not to control Mr. G. Instead he wanted to maintain his curiosity as to how Mr. G would take care of himself. Mr. C tried to not be so sensitive to Mr. G's critical comments and to then automatically withdraw. He tried to stay in conversation about his sensitivity. Most of the time he defined his effort to change himself and stay on the path of spiritual growth. As far as his medical treatment went, he noted that survivors are misfits. The physicians did not know how to explain that as of June 23, 1987, his T-cell count had gone up. T cells were 250 a year ago. Now they were 605. Perhaps this was due to a combination of belief in God and more focus on steadying himself. Mr. C thought that another variable was that there was less turmoil in his extended family than in Mr. G's family.

Preparing for Death

Overall, Mr. C used his spiritual life to deal with the dependency and worry as to the health of others. His spiritual orientation gave him the courage to prepare for his own death. Clearing up relationship blocks was a priority. This effort resulted in a more open relationship with his maternal uncle's son. He also became close with this cousin's daughter. Eventually, she moved to DC just to care for him. Toward the end of his life, Mr. C asked the researcher/coach to give his eulogy at Trinity Church in Washington, DC. The ceremony was a celebration of his life, his many kindnesses to those in the gay community, his church family, and his own family.

Defining a Self and Reconnecting With Family

Initially, people with HIV/AIDS did not know they had a problem in being distant or cut off from family. As individuals in the Whitman Walker support group heard that people's T-cell count went up as they had the courage to define self to others, a few more began contacting family members. People knew from listening to others that they had to be ready to risk being rejected or blamed and not react. Not everyone could do that. The hypothesis was that if one person was willing to reconnect and to be in better contact, while still being self-defined, the reactivity would diminish, and the immune system would improve. If one could relate without feeling sorry for self or others and/or attacking others, then the symptomatic person could increase his life span, when compared to predictions made for average life expectancy by using the T-cell count.

Family members might get symptoms after being told the news of the diagnosis, but this often had a positive effect. By altering the anxious focus from the one diagnosed with HIV/AIDS to others in the family, the anxiety would be absorbed by those better able to recover. The family unit was adapting to increasing anxiety by spreading it out. An emotional shock wave was defined by Murray Bowen, MD, in 1976 as an increase in symptoms among family members in the two years before or after the death of an important person in the family. Often illness and death were not discussed and the anxiety traveled underground. Could talking about illness and death more thoughtfully avoid symptoms? Anxiety might be redirected cognitively rather than acted out. Verbalizing difficult issues is challenging; one needed the courage to talk, be more aware of past emotional upsets, all without blame. It was a risk to say, "I am gay." But it opened the door to talk about practical matters like when, where, and how would one choose to die. Some could talk about wills, a funeral, where to be buried and other personal issues, and could then be more open. People reported a calming effect after being open with family members. This correlated with an increase in survival time. Those who had more open communication relationships improved their health in comparison to those diagnosed with AIDS who had no contact with family members and were isolated. Those who were hostile and/or who had negative relationships often died sooner than predicted. There appeared to be a bell-shaped curve in which at one end families were highly reactive and negative, while at the other end were those willing to be more open and caring. Distance and cutoff are effective strategies in the short term but not in the long term. Emotional cutoff arises from instinctive-like emotions and are often not subject to rationality. Those with less fear could alter relationships. This appeared to influence the immune system.

What allowed individuals to live longer? The researcher/coach consulted with Candace Pert, PhD, who was developing a drug, peptide T, that blocks the virus's ability to enter the T cells. Dr. Pert offered the following explanation: Having the courage to define a self in family relationships could lead to better immune system functioning, as any act of courage could activate more of the naturally occurring vasoactive intestinal peptide (VIP) hormone (found in the gut), thus blocking the T-cell receptors so the HIV virus could not enter. She speculated that those who had open relationships had more "guts" and were producing more VIP hormone (Pert, personal communication). Measuring VIP required a blood test and was too expensive and risky. Nevertheless, pathways for the influence of relationships on immune functioning can be known (Pert, Hill, & Ruff, 1986). Social support systems have been useful in maintaining health, but little research has been done to show how family relationships affected health (Olsen et al., 1991). For example, could an increase in family members with symptoms be an indicator of improving health? Were relationship changes, being more open, the main factor in those individuals who lived longer than average? Were there other differences: in one's diet, belief system, exercise, the intensity of emotionality within the family unit, the support system, job status, and the intensity or relative openness in relationships with family, friends, and even relationships with the medical professionals affecting immune functioning? Did their attitudes or behaviors enhance immune system functioning, or was it just randomness or luck that some individuals were living longer than others?

Findings

To answer this question a survey was developed with the help of Susan Wiegert, PhD, who wrote the computer code and did the statistics on the questionnaires. A computer-scored questionnaire had 353 questions. By 1992, the researcher/coach had seen over 37 individuals; some had died and others dropped out. Only seven individuals who were in the research were still living. Another 19 individuals volunteered to be interviewed for the survey. They were recruited from an AIDS support group in Fredericksburg, Virginia. Statistically, a most unusual finding was that one could predict who was in stage 2 or had AIDS just by the number of symptoms reported in family members. An expected finding was that the relationship system was more supportive of the HIV-infected person after the HIV diagnosis. Lastly, intact families had a greater probability of experiencing an emotional shock wave than a fragmented family (defined as a death in the nuclear family before the individual was 20). Perhaps it is counterintuitive, but those from a more intact family were vulnerable to more symptoms. One possible reason might be that since they had not experienced an early death, they were more vulnerable as they lacked experience. One might think that an intact family would do better than a fragmented family, but if someone lost a parent before they had reached the age of 20, they might be more "prepared" for a loss. Previous experience may be a protective factor. Research suggests that most people return to their happiness level two years after a loss (Bonanno, 2010).

What Have We Learned From the AIDS Crisis?

Without thought, individuals, families, and society react to fears and act in emotional ways. Thinking takes longer than reacting. If we have time, we can sort out the difference between these two states. Fear states, as we saw in the beginning of the AIDS crisis, drive people into polarized states and are difficult to overcome with simple facts. Becoming more differentiated enables people to be more separate from fear and to develop strategies to improve relationships. The emotional programming—to fall back into the automatic behaviors associated with distance, conflict, reciprocity, and projection—can be understood as reactivity. The automatic nature of reactivity leads to fewer choices as the threat of death or death itself can lead to an emotional shock wave throughout the family. Thoughtfulness leads to greater openness and cooperation among family members. Once people see the family as an impersonal unit, with its way of managing anxiety with automatic behaviors, then motivated individuals can alter their health status. Bowen (1978) wrote that it was necessary to first think of the family as a unit and to be reasonably successful at relating to the family unit before it was possible to treat the family as a unit.

Individuals are temporary members. The family emotional unit goes on replicating the sensitivities and often the values of the past. With awareness, individuals can relate thoughtfully to distant and/or disconnected family members. Without knowledge of the emotional guidance system, it is challenging to alter one's habitual ways of responding, especially when under stress. Bowen theory offers a road map to improving relationships, affecting generations to come, by offering innumerable ways to manage self in any emotional system.

REFERENCES

Avert.org. (2017, February 20). *History of HIV and AIDS overview.* Retrieved from www.avert.org/professionals/history-hiv-aids/overview

Benson, H. (1975). Reissue edition (2000, November 7). *The relaxation response.* New York, NY: Harper Torch.

Blank, M., Himelhoch, S., Walkup, J., & Eisenberg, M. (2013, December). Treatment considerations for HIV-infected individuals with severe mental illness. *Current HIV/AIDS Reports, 10*(4), 371–379. doi:10.1007/s11904-013-0179-3. Retrieved from www.ncbi.nlm.nih.gov/pmc/articles/PMC3857330/

Bonanno, G. (2010). *The other side of sadness: What the new science of bereavement tells us about life after loss.* New York, NY: Basic Books.

Bowen, M. (1976). Family reaction to death. In M. Bowen (Ed.), *Family therapy in clinical practice* (pp. 321–335). New York, NY: Jason Aronson.

Bowen, M. (1978). *Family therapy in clinical practice.* New York, NY: Jason Aronson.

Crowe, S. M. (1990, August). Fighting the opportunist infection of AIDS. *Scientific American.*

France, D. (2016). *How to survive a plague: The inside story of how citizens and science tamed AIDS.* New York, NY: Alfred A. Knopf.

Global Health Observatory Data. (2017). Retrieved from www.who.int/gho/hiv/en/

Koolhaas, J. M., de Boer, S. F., Buwalda, B., & van Reenen, K. (2007, September 18). Individual variation in coping with stress: A multidimensional approach of ultimate and proximate mechanisms. *Brain, Behavior and Evolution, 70*(4), 218–226. Epub abstract © 2007 S. Karger AG, Basel. doi:10.1159/000105485

Nickerson, Raymond S. (1998, June). Confirmation bias: A ubiquitous phenomenon in many guises. *Review of General Psychology, 2*(2), 175–220. doi:10.1037/1089–2680.2.2.175

Olsen, R. B., Olsen, J., Gunner-Svensson, F., & Waldstrøm, B. (1991). Social networks and longevity: A 14-year follow-up study among elderly in Denmark. *Social Science & Medicine, 33*(10), 1189–1195. Retrieved from https://doi.org/10.1016/0277-9536(91)90235-5

Pert, C. B., Hill, J. M., & Ruff, M. R. (1986, December). Octapeptides deduced from the neuropeptide receptor-like pattern of antigen T4 in brain potently inhibit human immunodeficiency virus receptor binding and T-cell infectivity. *Proceedings of the National Academy of Science, 83*(23), 9254–9258.

Plous, S. (1993). *The psychology of judgment and decision making.* New York, NY: Alfred A. Knopf.

Seeman, T. (1996). Social ties and health: The benefits of social integration. *Annals of Epidemiology, 6*(5), 442–451. doi:10.1016/S1047–2797(96)00095–6

Stoecklein, V., Osuka, A., & Lederer, J. (2012). Trauma equals danger—damage control by the immune system. *Journal of Leukocyte Biology, 92*(3), 539–551. doi:10.1189/jlb.0212072, PMCID: PMC3427603

Whetten, K., Reif, S., Whetten, R., & Murphy-McMillan, L. (2008). Trauma, mental health, distrust, and stigma among HIV-positive persons: Implications for effective care. *Psychosomatic Medicine, 70*(5), 531–538. doi:10.1097/PSY.0b013e31817749dc

Whitman Walker Health: Our History (2017). Retrieved from www.whitman-]walker.org/our-mission-values/our-history

Woodward, W. (1999, November 8). *Can you explain AIDS and how it affects the immune system? How does HIV become AIDS?* Retrieved from www.scientificamerican.com/article/can-you-explain-aids-and/

18

A RIVER OF SILENCE

A Son Defines Himself in Relation to His Dying Father

Kendall Baker

Introduction by Katharine Gratwick Baker

Kendall was almost 36 years old and single in the summer of 1994, when he learned that his father's advanced prostate cancer was entering its final stage. Kendall was a sculptor with an MFA from Yale who had taken the summer off from teaching to work with a professional builder on an island in Maine, constructing a vacation cabin his father had designed. When he heard that his dad was rapidly going downhill, he got on a plane and flew back to his family home in Washington, DC, where he spent the next two weeks offering gentle massage and relaxation to his father during the dying process. Excerpts from Kendall's journal form the body of this chapter.

The journal is also indirectly an account of the way one family functioned during the death of a significant member. A death is a moment in time, a punctuation point, in the ongoing history of a family, but it has powerful meanings and reverberations.

John Baker graduated from Yale in 1949, received a master's degree in political science from the Institute des Hautes Etudes in Switzerland, and then joined the U.S. Foreign Service in 1951. He had diplomatic assignments to five European and East European countries, as well as Washington, DC, over a 35-year career, and along the way got a PhD in international relations.

John married Sally Bragg in 1955, and they had three sons, Jack, Kendall, and Andrew, in rapid succession in 1957, 1958, and 1959. After the third birth, Sally developed a postpartum psychosis and never fully recovered from it. In September 1962, while they were living in Rome, she took her own life, and John became a single parent, moving back to the United States a year after Sally's death so that his parents could help him raise his three small sons.

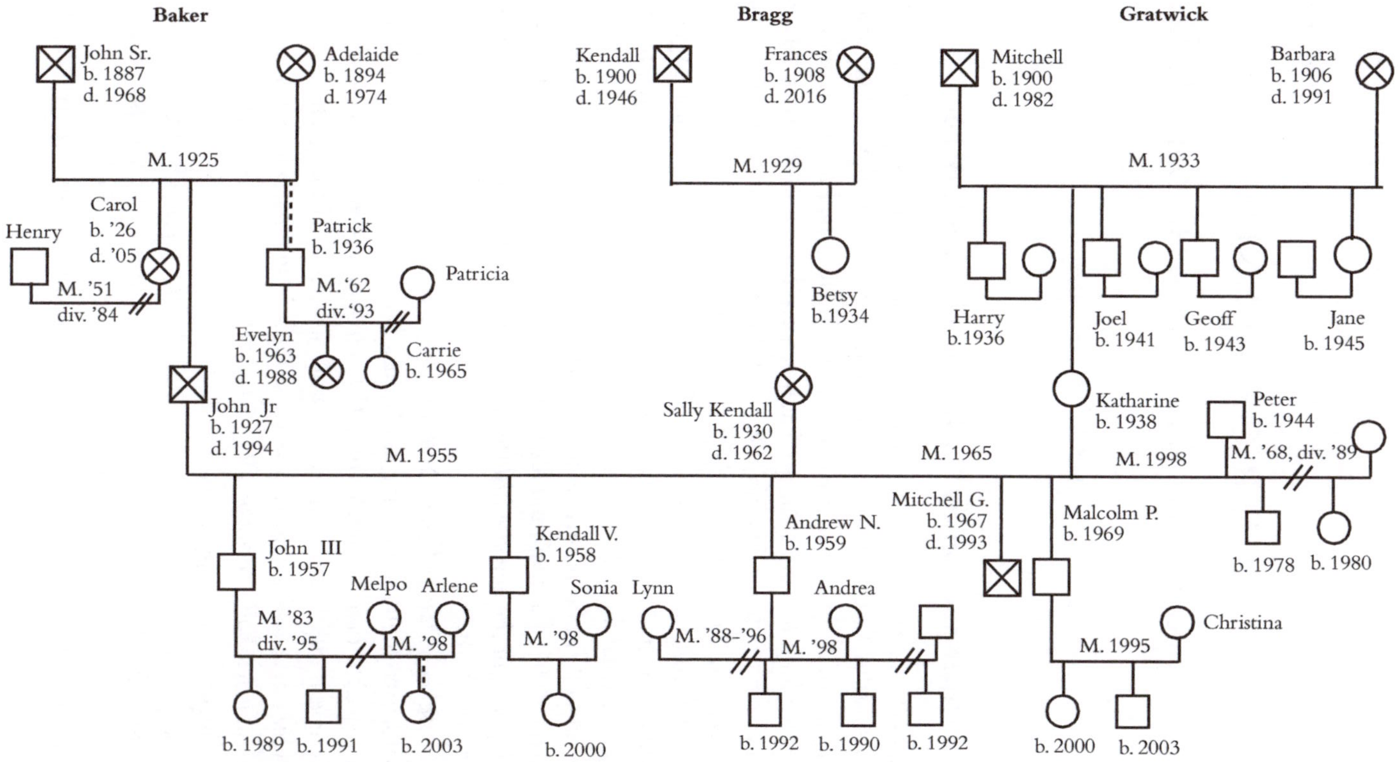

Figure 18.1 The Baker Family

John did not talk much about Sally in the years following her death, and his young sons did not openly ask him questions about her, fearing that he would be upset. This inevitably led to emotional distance between him and them as they grew up. Kendall's relationship with John was further complicated by the fact that he strongly resembled his mother in coloring and facial features, so he was the recipient of considerable anxious projection from his father and grandparents after Sally's death.

In 1965 John married me, and we had two more sons, Mitchell and Malcolm, in 1967 and 1969. We were then a family with five boys, following John's Foreign Service career as we lived sequentially in Washington and two European cities over the next 25 years. He was the primary wage earner and the dominant parent of the boys, teaching them to swim, ice skate, play tennis, ski, climb mountains, and paddle their own canoes. In high school the three older boys tried at various times to talk with their father about Sally's death, but John continued to guard himself from this area of intense vulnerability, became upset, and they backed off.

When John was diagnosed with advanced metastatic prostate cancer in 1987, the idea of his having a life-threatening illness came as a shock to the whole family. By then his older three sons had graduated from college and were self-supporting. The oldest son had married in 1983 and was in medical school. His fourth son was in college, and his youngest son was a senior in high school. Their expectation had been that their father would have many years of healthy productive life ahead of him as they got on with their own independent young adult lives.

John undertook management of his illness as he had undertaken most other challenges in his adult life. He wanted to deal with the anxiety generated by this serious illness by being in charge of it. He explored a wide variety of treatment options, read medical journals sent to him by his physician son, and shared experiences with colleagues and friends who had prostate cancer. He went on a strict macrobiotic diet that he maintained for the seven years of his illness, and he continued to be deeply engaged in his professional life. People closest to him noticed that he began to develop a gentler mellowness in his family relationships that was new for him. He never directly acknowledged that his life was coming to an end, but said he was determined to live it as fully as possible for as long as possible.

Six years before John died, his niece Evelyn committed suicide as the culmination of many years of depression. Five years later, and one year before John died, Mitchell, his fourth son (and my first), a jazz musician, took his own life while staying with the family in Washington and trying to cope with depression. These deaths were devastating for John and for the whole family, and they reawakened memories of Sally's death in 1962. But we tried to handle them differently, talking about them, asking questions, sharing our thinking, and openly expressing our grief.

During John's final dying days, his sons, their partners, wives, and I were together with him in our family home in Washington. He did not want to be in a hospice program, so each family member took on particular individual functions. The oldest son, a physician, had medical responsibility for his care and was the liaison to a visiting nurse. Kendall provided the massage described in his journal. Others prepared food, handled phone calls and visitors, and kept the household going. I worked to sustain a calm nurturing environment for the whole family. We also had functions we took on together: We cooked, ate, sang John's favorite songs, laughed, talked, took dog walks, and reminisced. One son wanted John to participate in planning his funeral, but John refused, pronouncing that "I won't be there, so do whatever you like. Funerals are for the living anyway."

After his death we stepped up: One son wrote John's obituary, others washed his body and prepared him for cremation. Together we planned two memorial services—one in Maine for the family, and one in Washington for a broader circle of friends. And then we went on with the task of grieving together and individually, while rebuilding our lives without the central family member that John had been.

Both overfunctioning and underfunctioning can bind anxiety in families, and when important family members die, the survivors sometimes experience what Bowen called a "shock wave" effect, as symptoms ripple out from the family's disrupted emotional center and down through the generations. The family tries to find new ways to fill in the gaps, both functional and emotional. Although we thought we had prepared ourselves for John's death and continued to talk about it for years afterwards, a "shock wave" effect did happen in our family. And it was intensified because it also followed the shocks generated by Sally's, Evelyn's, and Mitchell's deaths.

We had to learn how to get along without John, as the family had somehow learned to survive without Sally, Evelyn, and Mitchell, and it wasn't a smooth process. After John's death, two of his sons divorced, and three sons later contracted serious illnesses.

Eventually, however, they recovered; John's two divorced sons remarried, I remarried, and by 1998 all four surviving sons (including Kendall) were in solid marriages and serious professional careers. Four more grandchildren were born who wanted to learn about their grandfather. The five older grandchildren who had known him grew up. Two step-grandsons joined the family. And the family went on into its next generations.

Excerpts From a Journal

Late in July I called to say that I was coming home. The Maine vacation cabin I had been building for two summers with my father was nearing completion. I still had the wild hope that he would return to spend the traditional August weeks here, but in my heart I feared it couldn't be.

Packing my things for the trip down to Washington, my thoughts raced over memories of my father's long illness. His demise had seemed imminent for seven years. I had shared his trials, often at some distance, updating the list of hospital phone numbers, watching him rise and fall as he struggled to overcome the disease. I knew implicitly that his strong life-force could not continue to persist against advanced metastatic cancer, yet so far he had miraculously brokered the massive imbalance. A brilliant navigator, he had held his own against the storm for so long, that it was impossible not to join with him in his unyielding vision. He would reach remission.

Going home for a prolonged visit would be different. I didn't know what I would find, but I longed for the closure and release that come with direct experience. I was going there to confirm everything I was afraid of admitting. All summer I'd been anticipating the trip, but didn't want to arrive prematurely and end up hanging around conspicuously, waiting to see if this was the show's final act. Now I was buying my ticket to the mainland. This was it. Within minutes the ferry was churning past a familiar stretch of granite-bound shoreline. The ridge of the new cabin stood quietly obscured behind a cluster of spruce trees, strong and well-built. Leaving the bright island, it seemed impossible to believe that there wouldn't be more time, more summers there with my father.

During that first week at home I began giving him regular massages and found an intimacy in the act that changed everything. The touching of his body completed a long-broken circuit that arched back across years, bridging a distance no broader than the sound of a breath or the thickness of skin.

Without having intended to, I began writing a journal and taking photographs a few days after my arrival in Washington. I let the words come out of a need to see them on the page and to confront my disbelief at the truth of the experience. I wrote while sitting with him, looking across the yard or the living room where I had grown up and seen so many events unfold. Memories of the family and of my own development, past and present, fused with this moment of dying. He slept and woke. A lot was usually going on in spite of what seemed like long intervals of silence. There were trips to the bathroom, drinks to be prepared, and the continual shift from bed to porch and back again—according to the hour and the weather. Each move came with the snarled oxygen line, catheter, nephrostomy tubes, and omnipresent phone cord for maintaining contact with all his projects and programs.

I wrote in the present tense. Sometimes I addressed him directly, writing "You," and sometimes I wrote indirectly about "Dad":

Nothing seems real or true. The breath, the energy, the blue light? Am I full of shit or is this the self-consciousness of documentation? These events that I'm witnessing are in some ways the communion I've always wanted with you. The father–son fantasy trip. Now we touch at this peculiar intersection between life and death.

Three days ago Mom and I spoke frequently about the prospect of getting you up to Maine, to get out of the swelter of DC and into the new cabin. You weren't interested, even though it was a plan that had been in the making all summer and one you both had your hearts set on. But it would mean long hours traveling—car, plane, ferry—and then having only limited medical services available at the little clinic on the island. You will choose. But I was anxious and I tried playing hardball and joked about kidnapping you. You fixed your eye on me sternly and said, "Don't make a mistake, Kendall. Don't make a mistake."

"Do you think I would do anything against your will?" I said stuttering, and then threw out, "You're running the show." As soon as the words left my throat, I knew how bitterly untrue that was. The show was really running you now and you were gearing up for the final battle. I hadn't fathomed the degree of helplessness and loss of control you felt from the aching horizontality of your bed.

Maine and the cabin are forgotten now, along with my notions about what should happen in the coming days. Mom continues to organize piles of "Maine things," just in case the spirit in him shifts. But she knows better than I do not to try and push anything onto him. This is the Marshall Award–winning man after all, who strategizes for the twenty-first century . . .

The bone pain is intense. Dad slept well last night for the first time in a while, but as he's helped up out of his porch chair, his nephrostomy tube is accidentally pulled out. Dad's anger and frustration with this whole situation, his struggle, his continual decline, just explodes. We're a little shaken by the outburst, but it's one of the many risks of home health care. This morning Dad's in the hospital getting the tube replaced.

Coming back from Georgetown Hospital, Mom calls me to help you climb the steps from the car. The tubes are in and urine is moving again. Grasping both my arms, you lift your body and urge your feet forward. We struggle to the railing. "My legs are so heavy," you say. And this is so plain to see. The skin is tight and firm like the skin of a water balloon. Full and stretched taut, it gives the flesh a youthful look.

Dawn, the home health care nurse, comes by to give you shots and change your Groshong dressing. She has this really irritating habit of excluding you from conversation while you're present. Are you somehow "not there" that she can refer to you in the third person? Perhaps these are the side effects of trying to balance compassion and efficiency. "God bless him," she says, while changing the dressing that requires you to sit up and lean forward for 15 minutes. This puts terrific pressure on your swollen belly, making you groan some and wince. We all know you feel far more than you express.

"How does he seem to you?" I ask Dawn later, when we're alone in the kitchen.

"Not good. Very weak, but he's a trooper." She says this so readily. Almost glibly. It stings my ears to hear the truth rattled off this way. I'm rapidly learning how to blind myself to the truth about your condition. How else to face you without feeling the pain of your decline? This reflex is so subtle and automatic. And you have never mentioned death directly. But I think you know . . .

Mom is at work today and I'm alone with you for the day. Being alone with you has never been easy and I'm inwardly anxious. I'm more aware now of how much she's been doing to look after you, helping with your needs, your body, your pain. Everything is a major production. Getting to the bathroom, eating, changing clothes. A few weeks ago the oncologist, Dr. M., had told Mom, "There's nothing we can do for him at the hospital that you can't do better at home." And while this is true, it's a massive amount of work . . .

Going through a massage with you I watch my hands move across your skin, pressing, tracking the arches and crests of your jaw, cheekbones, and sunken eye sockets. This suchness is your body.

I'm the stern-man this time. The battered aluminum canoe lies propped in the gravel run against the back fence. My thoughts drift and I can hear the gnawing groan as icy rocks score into the soft metal. We're reckoning the options ahead of us as we flush downriver, and I feel the nervous vibrations of the hull as you stand, balancing in the stern, correcting, making the call. The scars and creases of that old canoe glint softly beyond the porch trellis, and the gray patina is burnished like the sky, a brilliant overcast, now dropping in over Friendship Heights.

I'm in the stern now, working you through this last stretch. We're falling slowly through the riverbed into an approaching noise, a babbling fullness. Fast, so imperceptibly fast. Temples, jaw, forehead, fleshless neck, all corded sinew hauled out and fastened with double knots at the shoulders. I'm not going to pretend, recalling the vital man you once were. The strength gone, your mind still plunges, pulling with deep strokes, leaning against the sweeping wash. The air, the lungs filling, releasing, becoming again with another round. I'm holding you.

To be grateful and still profoundly saddened by loss. Is this a contradiction? The two can fit easily in the scope of our relationship. By grateful I don't mean relieved by the merciful cessation of your suffering. I'm grateful for the sense of release I will feel from the spell you've woven into my character. I'm thinking of those early trials after losing Sally.[1] You inevitably became superhuman in those months and intervening years when we were alone together against fate. Now I can see how much I long to outgrow my need for you. But will I? You are a giant and still manage to tower over me from your bed.

We made a contract, in those early years, signed with the ink of an unnamable fear. All I had to do was give my will over to you. I thought I could fuse myself into your acts and manners, carving a place for myself from your superhuman flesh. With my child's will to survive, I wanted only for you to endure, and imagine I gave up my independent voice to please you. I was so happy to say your words and align my body with your movements. When our grip on each other is finally loosened, who will I become?

I can't tell you any of this now. This is my story, my stuff, and very likely the coded song of human generations. We can't solve this. I either deal with it or pass it down the line. You have so much else to offer and I'm just learning how to listen . . .

Drugged. You've been sleeping through the morning doped on morphine in order to buy some rest from the waking struggle. Earlier this morning I massaged your head, arms, and shoulders. Maybe this makes it more clear now why I am here at this time. It's the nature of "bridging" life and death that feels etched into my character. This is what gives me a sense of place. I am a bridge. Meeting you so fully at this crossing invokes so many unforgotten hopes. What will be revealed and redeemed in these diminishing days?

It's clear that there isn't much time left. When Mom gets back from work, we'll see about plans for the final family circle. You know that there isn't any more that can be done. I'm sitting here writing all of this down as I watch your hands dancing and bobbing in the air, guiding your spirit through the changes that must now be sifting within you. It helps me to keep from moving away, from removing myself from the present. I keep thinking, "Dad, you're going to be out of my life, you'll be dead in another four or five days."

Perhaps in your universe there is nothing to be said that isn't already apparent. The "corner has been turned," as you feared it would be, and now the time, the hours and days, pass in ways you have never experienced before. There is just time to be. I'm overwhelmed and yet entirely with you too. This is where we find each other.

What brought me here early? I could have gone on with my work in Maine and come down for the final days to say goodbye. But I had little choice in the matter. No, it was something else. To give something back to you? To have reached toward an understanding together through your body? We have met here in the amazingly physical substance of being. Touching, caressing, lifting, smoothing, pressing, guiding your mind into relaxation and deep into the blue lumina of the breath. It was just to be . . .

As much as I want to I still haven't gotten down to the simple act of saying "goodbye," of speaking those words to Dad without expecting him to respond in kind. I don't think his psyche's constitution would allow for that. It's not part of his vocabulary. Still, I think I have to say it tonight. Can I tell him that I will miss him? That he's been such a strong and enriching part of my life? That finding a way to reach each other in this time has been really important for me?

He slips in and out of clarity, and I'm certain that he's not reachable. Then Mom comes out onto the porch and casually asks him what to do with the River Road[2] water bill. He opens his eyes and lays out a solution. He is right there . . .

What was it like when your father died? I was about to ask Mom since you were still asleep. But I think I already know. You told me once about the disappointment you felt at not being able to be with him when he died. You had a job to do. We were all in Prague and it was 1968. Your plate was full. Besides, Grandpa had reached his time, at age 80. Nothing was out of place. There's a pain and a recognition that the cycles of life move on, and you have already anticipated and embraced the changes. On and on . . .

Only Mitchell's death seems to hurt more now. It's the contrast between the way Dad has hurled himself towards life in such a determined way (something on the molecular level) and the way Mitchell hurled himself from the bridge towards death in an equally determined if senseless fashion. Recognizing the weight of either choice, I feel like a witness frozen on the yellow line between lanes of traffic.

During dinner you are so awake and present. We sit under the yellow porch light, talking about a *New Yorker* article on FDR and Eleanor. Mom remembers how you once met Eleanor through a connection with Grandma. Mom prompts you with questions, engaging you. You're with us, but not really part of the conversation. Pain, exhaustion, confusion? You always rise to any occasion, but economy of effort is everything at this point . . .

This morning Mom describes an article in the paper about coup plotters in the ex-Soviet Union who were acquitted. She asks you if you want to read the article. I pull you up in the bed and we locate your glasses. What are you thinking, Mom? He hasn't been able to read in the last couple of days. His eyes roll up and drift into the absent zone of policy negotiations. But I'm impressed. Mom has always tried to encourage optimum functioning. She doesn't take over for him with unsolicited care and preemptive accommodation. There's no giving in . . .

The home will change tonight when the brothers all arrive. Malcolm returns from Boston. Jack, his medical practice covered by a partner, will leave Lansing this afternoon. Lynn[3] calls from Maine to let me know that Andrew is aboard the 11:30 ferry and headed for Portland, reaching here late tonight. I talk with Mom in the kitchen. Traced in her face and particularly her eyes is a nervous welter of confusion; she's clinging to the reassurance of my father's survival while moving towards acceptance of the great changes spelled out by his immediate condition. There's too much to say but most of it is already understood, implicit.

I'm beginning to grasp the signs myself. Somewhere in the distant present my father is dying. The resistance to admitting this is so strong. Half of my divided will wants to categorize the experience in some abstract framework of nature and cycles. The other half wants to strip away the names and identities from all concerned and abandon days, dates, and hours, and engage with the "now." This is the opposite of the abstract and conceptual, but at the same time it can only be shown abstractly, if it can be shown at all. A large family and all the gyrating activity would normally keep me from bringing anything together and would limit the dwellingness here . . .

I think that, like many of us, myself included, you have a predominately mechanistic view of the body: the magnificent and nearly comprehensible machine. It's a deeply embedded paradigm before which modern science and doctors all bow. It's what we think . . .

Light rain this morning moistens the porch tiles. Cool breezes wander through the house. There have been many massages today. A thought comes to me during the massage about how this physical contact has been so entirely different from all other experiences I have ever had with you in my lifetime. This isn't simply a special effort to comfort you in this difficult time. When I find myself standing behind you with your forehead slipping beneath the pressures of my palms, I know that I've crossed a once inviolate distance. This has been a traversing that was previously unimaginable. What a journey.

Did you think your love was going to be entrusted to a phrase or left in some kind of wording to sustain me in the years after your passing? For you it was never an issue. Instead I've been given your body, even in its sadly deteriorated form, to grip and knead with my hands and eyes. What is this? The word love doesn't have any meaning without a context. You've said it from time to time and meant it, implied it, and written it. But from early on I longed for it to be spelled out in direct contact, something that I could be certain of, something palpable that would give the words a value. Now, at this penultimate threshold it isn't you who are reaching out. Instead it's you who are letting me reach you, letting me in. I've been at the door for so long . . .

Your brother Pat calls and I put him through to you. You acknowledge with your voice, measured but weak, that "the time will be coming soon, I'm afraid."

Your nephrostomy tube must be clogged with sediment. Dawn said this would happen and there's apparently not much to be done about it at this point. I look over the thick ocherous fluid and think "clogged." Death is a clogged drain.

Haven't I been saying goodbye to you every time I've seen you over the past seven years? Cancer is a taking away, a diminishing, as it grows and blossoms, exploding endlessly into all our lives. Looking at your chest rising and falling, and hearing the reassuring sound of your breath, I'm already missing you . . .

Last night I went out with my old girlfriend, Marty. We went to her health club to work out and took in a movie: *La Vida Loca.* When I got back, Malcolm and Jack had arrived and you had gone into your own *Vida Loca* of heavy dissociation. Jack gave you some Haldol to calm your raging confusion.

The house is full now and my writing only recaptures recent events. I'm no longer witnessing the moment, keying in the action from long mornings and afternoons alone with you. Family dynamics are taking over, and I can see myself like a ball on a pool table. Whose turn is it?

Talked late last night with the brothers. Jack is nervous and changes the subject quickly. Andrew and I end up in the hot kitchen, clocking into languid discussion at floor level where it's cooler. Malcolm and Jack are slouched into familiar conversations nearby. Malcolm's Olympic-sized body upholsters the couch. Beyond the door in the dark living room, my parents sleep cradled by the spasmodic melody of the oxygen pump. Mom is on a mattress on the floor. Dad is in the hospital bed. We're all here. We've all gathered. There is a mythic sort of comfort—a belonging, however diminished, that comes with this massing of the brothers. Awkward in our uselessness, we're all off-balance, uncorrected, leaning heavily into the hours. Waiting, perhaps, to be told what to do . . .

In the morning you become restless and want to move again, this time to the car. Why? Are you serious? What does serious mean? Do I challenge your will? I can't remember a single irrational decision in a lifetime of acts and choices. I decide it will be better to try and let it pass, and thankfully Mom appears. Mom leans over to hug you, whispering in your ear. You put your arm around her head the way you've been doing to lift your body out of the chair. "What are we doing?" she asks. "Pulling you down to me," and the two of you embrace and kiss. You notice her perfume. "I put it on to attract your attention," she says pouting coyly. "It worked," you say smiling, and your eyes lift with a brightness to meet her gaze. The confusion has evaporated.

The tenderness of your relationship is so moving. Seeing the way you have become a part of one another, sharing and growing, yet distinct; clearly separate in your spheres and movements, and yet twined like bright vines supporting and traveling through the ordeals and adventures. When she's with you I can feel the bond shaped by so much love and communion, and the sacrifices you've made for each other. Mutual respect prevents the crossing of personal boundaries. She would never presume to give you any pills without first identifying them to you and neither will you accept any pills without having a clear sense of what each one is. Lying there with your hand in hers the lacing weaves between you in limpid strands of his trust . . .

Stored-up heat shed by the walls leaves glistening sweat lines on our faces in the night light. Mom, looking at the floor, mentions how much she expects to see Mitchell now that the family is circled. "Mitchell could walk in the door any minute with a sheepish smile on his face and a long, elaborate story for why he's so late." I let her know I've been thinking of him as well. I can't mention the anger that burns with his memory. Fresh as ever. We come and go more easily than we can know . . .

Malcolm, Jack, Christina,[4] and I go down to the park to play tennis. It's good to get out of the house. Exercising reminds me that I'm in fact alive and not dying, even if a big part of my life is passing with this giant. The four of us hang out afterwards, as you sleep off the Haldol. I catch up on bills and writing. Mom and Christina go to the gym. Andrew begins working up a draft for the obituary. The obituary. I'm shocked for a moment before I realize how much there will be to do. This is the kind of planning you'd have taken care of. Did you write Sally's obituary? Most likely. But it didn't contain what we'd lost. I'm glad your obituary is Andrew's job. I'm unable to think methodically enough to summarize a life in a few paragraphs. I guess it's like writing an outline, and someone has to decide what's really important. In my own life's outline your dying and your death will have a large heading. This is important, maybe more so than any other event in my life. This is one for "before and after" shots.

Jack and Malcolm are in the back room grappling with the trust set up to defer taxes. Division of labor is the great payback for the youthful chaos of a large family. Jack reassures all of us with his medical acumen, and together with Malcolm he goes over the paperwork that lives on long after the body is gone. Death is in the other room watching over my father as he "sleeps," gazing at the ceiling and groaning as he builds things with his hands in the air above him, working and making shrewd adjustments. Bone deep . . .

I've lost track of the time. Day? Hour? The family moves in a slow eddying motion through the rooms. We're all in a dreamlike state, sleepwalking. Not wanting to wake up to the clinical truth of death and dying, we continue circulating through the rooms, fusing with the furniture and intervening spaces that curl around us, inventing ourselves perfectly together with each passage. We are the house, and our bodies are growing out of its memory. My body longs to be folded into the walls and darkening windows . . .

Death. The very personalized death, the one that is yours only, Dad, is present with you. Nearby. Close. Your body, weaker now, can't refuse its charms. Neurological functions affecting your swallowing make it harder for you to take fluids. And I'm still not ready. You have such a presence for one who is in a sense already dead. Much of you has left already, and believing in recovery now would be no less than complete fantasy. Still, you manage to fill up the house tonight, weaving in the threads of a Gordian knot that we will be picking at indefinitely.

Before going upstairs for the night I'm drawn back to your bedside. There is a specific weight or gravity of the dying, I think, that slants and curves the space around it. I stand for a moment with my hand on your shoulder. I don't know exactly why I am here. Your eyes are closed though I have a feeling you are aware of me. I think I'm here to hold onto you; to remind myself of what it is that I am losing as I strain against the anticipated fragmentation of your wholeness.

My own eyes soften and weep, tears dropping past the bed frame into the mechanical chassis. Your eyes open and you see me. Worried, unable to prevent the pain in me, I bury your gaze, furrowing my fingertips into your brow and temples because I know. In the heart of your eye I become Sally's life and energy. Matched through genes and history, you and I live out a relationship that has been dying since her death and yet being constantly reborn in our attempts to remember and invent her. Unsure how to acknowledge my role, I'm nervous. I am her, I am me. There is a strength and depth in this anima's presence. Possibly I'm even so accustomed to it that it's only externalized experiences like this that surprise me.

Sally's invisible presence is a big part of me, and along with this man's death will go his living memory of her. The secret and complete knowledge of my mother will be gone and, I think, we'll be burying her with him. We have fragments, extracted in pain from him, and we have the genes that carry on through us. A cellular memory, both more visible and more inscrutable. Dying young she was gone before we knew her. Leaning over his body, working the tired tissue, I'm glad to be bringing her to him; we complete the rippling circles of the loved and the lovers . . .

Jack seems to think that this will be the last night. You're so agitated and restless. Sitting beside you, I feel the spasms and parched utterances that stress your exhausted body. We look at each other in a long gaze. Where do you see from? I don't know my place here in this curious gathering. Jack says that your sight may be gone because you no longer focus anywhere. As true as this may or may not be, I think we see each other well enough. The less we see and speak, the more is understood and communicated.

You're still not ready to go, to step through the doorway. Who would be when filled with such a massive will for life and living? You never believed in any afterlife. "This is it," as Mom said while we were eating something, perhaps breakfast. Malcolm and I pump your heavy, fluid-filled legs, and I massage the bones and deeper tissues while you grimace with the discomfort, irritated by the body's failure. Turning to me, Andrew says, "What about singing?" My first reaction is that the "noise" will disturb him. Waking up a little, I remember what it might mean to him. A break from the pain.

So we go through the old guitar numbers, reminding me of childhood when my eyes were glued to the theatrical expressions of your face as the tragic plots unrolled in "Little Joe the Wrangler," "Streets of Laredo," "The Golden Vanity," and others. Then, in the middle of that restless circle, as we reach the chorus of "The Golden Vanity," your voice joins ours and lifts with the music. Hearing your voice recasts the whole event, braiding strands of nostalgia and grief into a lead rope or a lifeline, stretching forward into time, into the present. You sing only two or three notes, but it is more than enough to be certain that you are there, parched mouth and all, joining the party. We aren't singing for you after that. We are simply joined together again in our routine, doing the typical family stuff, even if it will be the last time . . .

In the living room that morning Jack was reading poems to you from Grandma's poetry book, *To Mark the Time.* Jack was marking this time with you by bridging the generations through verse—finding you, your mother, and perhaps himself in the continuity of her words.

I'm so blessed. There have been many things—multiple dissatisfactions—distorted views of childhood struggles and adult misconceptions—that I imagined were strapped to my shoulders for a longer haul. Here beside you I feel your legacy and so much unexpected resolution filtering through these final hours. In each return to the bed that your body ballasts, I see a keel moving well through the last bends of a tide-bound river.

We circle the bed again singing lullabies. Later the singing gets a little wild and I'm making up absurd verses to "Camptown Races." Harmonizing to "Molly Malone" at anyone's deathbed is a little odd. But none of us has done anything or experienced anything like this before, this dying, and so if no one objects, it seems anything goes. Why not enjoy ourselves? There will be plenty of time for sadness. Lynn has also arrived today and completes the circle. We sing "My life flows on." Jane[5] has also arrived and her voice adds shimmering harmonics.

It's late and time for bed. Mom, who has been sleeping on the floor by your bed, prepares for what might be the last night together with her husband. In looking at her I see her alone for the first time since she appeared in my child's world as the stranger who became my mother. She has no illusions, and the trials of loss, having been reeled in for years, are not going to be a shock. But the anticipation of solitariness drifts like an unwanted recognition in the uncertainty of her gaze.

We say goodnight and hugs go all around. I can hear in Mom's exhausted, yet slightly steeled voice, "Sleep well. See you in the morning," that she senses tomorrow will begin without you. Lying on the bed in Mitchell's room, my face and hands feel impossibly removed from the touch of sheets and pillowcases. I'm not really here—this isn't real. Time freezes and thaws, and I leave the light on. What is this place, this house, this room, this stuff? There's no way to know anything now. This is the edge of the grid. I want to pray and can't. I feel excited, lost, empty . . .

Death, August 16, 1994. The end of the road and the beginning. Mom heard you release your last breath just before first light. Shortly after, she woke Jack who was sleeping in the next room. The knock on the door. It is Jack, waking us to the event. It's over, I say to myself, it's finally over; in my mind the words plummet and rise, unable to settle, leaving me shaken and giddy. I get up and wash. I know it will be a long morning and I want to be clean. There will be a body downstairs. It is like Christmas inverted; something has been taken away and something left behind. Odd. I am stunned and full of curiosity. What is this going to be like? A body that was once a giant in my life. Lifeless. Ended. Dead. Turning the corner from the stairs into the living room I am not surprised to see you lying on the bed. Lynn had suggested moving your bed into the middle of the room the night before so that your "beautiful bride," as you dubbed Mom this past year, could lie beside you on the couch. The head of the bed is elevated and in the dim light of the new day I can see your eyes, cloudy blue, unblinking. I stand gazing at your spirit's house, knowing that you left it only recently. Your spirit must have drawn up and left the body and all your will and energy with it because what is left is so small. The rise and fall of your chest has been the engine of hope and the tirelessly unrealistic determinations to overcome the disease that had found you. It was more than an hour before the projected image of your moving chest burned through. The measure of life-as-will is so clear. In you, in me, in everything.

Mom asked me if I would like to recite the words I had spoken to Dad during our daily massages. Holding his head in my hands and stroking the still-warm skin around the half-opened eyes, I feel the words move with the same rhythm that carried me through all the changes of the past few weeks. It's real now. My own voice and cycles of breath echo back to me off his stillness. I feel the reassurance of images I'm certain had reached and soothed him through his trial. It isn't until later that I weep and feel the wrenching hollowness. But the heaving tension and release from the gut is welcome. The mind is given an opportunity to empty itself into solid feeling. The vast dimensions of death dissolve into the familiar here-and-now. Finally.

Sunlight has risen up above the windowsill and inched across the room. We join hands together and Mom says something about the endurance of the family and of his joy in what the family has been for him. We sit in silence. Andrew sits at his side holding his hand. Jack sits at the head with Mom and me on the couch. Malcolm and Christina sit farther away, and I feel a need to link Malcolm closer to the circle. Maybe the older brothers use up too much psychic space. Maybe our need to hold onto this last blood parent has pushed him into the margins. Mitchell used to be the front man for the second set of brothers, and Malcolm hasn't gotten used to the new arrangement. The family is smaller and maybe there's more room too for us to get bigger. I stare across the room as the light and clouds scatter patterns on the floor. It's clear that time has not stopped and this, for the moment, seems odd.

Gradually, as the day wears on we each begin to move. Jane has made muffins and coffee. Carol[6] and Pat are called to phone-tree all the Baker relatives. Jane goes next door to phone other relatives . . . Jack tries to phone the police, but gets a busy signal for 911. It's a busy day for them too. Jack warns that we may not be able to keep the body for long this morning if the police interfere. This pisses me off. Whose body is it? Death isn't for us to sort out and examine? I put off eating breakfast and make sure there's enough time to prepare and clean the body. Jack makes arrangements with Vince, our MD friend, to come over and officially confirm the death. He also makes a call to Gawlers' Funeral Home.

The foremost thing on my mind is what to do with the body. I want to wash and oil him. I'm surprised by the power of this purpose. I feel inclined to just do it and not ask. Whose decision is it? Part of me thinks it's a job for the "women," as if this is some Greek tragedy. So when Lynn mentions that she would like to wash him too, it becomes completely natural. Andrew then joins us and we collect washcloths and bowls of warm water. Somewhere among the medications, the "Ganges" massage oil is found.

The body has cooled substantially in the last couple of hours and rigor mortis has set in, making it hard to remove his shirt. Each shift and adjustment of the body logs an understanding of death, of being and nonbeing, into my consciousness. Touching the body. The need to handle, to feel the weight, evaluate the material, literally the "remains." Among many mammals death is accompanied by nuzzling, guarding, touching, and smelling the body. The subtle and yet massive shift from animation to stasis requires an investigation. What happened? Dwelling with the body, drawn into its space and time, takes you out of your world and reveals the first few stairs of a longer flight into the other. The first step is stillness. Stasis, Jack informs us, is the medical term for the change that takes place in the blood shortly after death. Lynn asks if the body will bleed when we pull the tubes out. Jack explains, while he's removing the Foley catheter from the body, how the blood coagulates and turns into a kind of jelly. Using a syringe he deflates the bulb of the bladder, releasing the rubber tube that has been in place for so long. His pubic area is nude from the side effects of fluamide. His penis, shrunken from what was once an impressive organ, appears whole again without the snaking tube that was forever getting snagged on furniture and doorknobs.

The Groshong port is next. Removing the shirt we pull one arm at a time through the sleeves. The stiffened joints make this routine operation strangely comical. You're not "helping." I get the strangest sensation from pushing your body around, rolling and twisting it about on the mattress. It's just a body, I keep telling myself. The owner is out of town. Finally the shirt is off and the body lies there so impressively motionless. I can't get over this.

Below the skin on your upper chest a tiny hose snakes upward toward your neck where it disappears into the artery. Jack tugs hard on the hose until I point out the tracing of a patch that seems to fasten it to the collarbone. The body is no different than a thawed chicken, inert, senseless. Why are we so careful? Are we afraid he'll wake up? The dead body is like a child's. There is a wholeness to it that's to be respected. Then I think what I would do if I were alone.

Looking down at your body, so little has changed. The arms and hands and fingers are the same now, only still, free from effort. How many times did you raise yourself up in bed, hanging from my neck with all your waning strength?

We place bowls of water and washcloths beside you on the sheets. Spilling isn't a problem now. The dripping and splashing sounds of the water rinsed into the bowls makes it all real and immediate. Turning you to the side to wash your back, we discover the cruelly macerated skin that has broken down from the long confinement. It's hard to believe you endured this with such fortitude. I don't think you ever complained. After cleaning and working the fine oil into the cooling skin, we dress your body. A three piece suit? A bathrobe? We decide on your well-worn running outfit and it takes all three of us to get your limbs through the sleeves and legs. I imagine you watching all this, laughing. We lace up your sneakers good and tight and then add a hat. The hat looks completely goofy. We try others and eventually decide that you'll go bareheaded on your last run. Looking at you, I think we're all somewhat stunned by our encounter with the dead body. Our laughter only thinly disguises the wash of fear and wonder condensed in this physical contact with the lifeless material that was once a man—once my father.

Cleaning the house. Removing all the medicines, syringes, tape, oxygen tanks, tubes, hoses, special supplements, and fluid bottles from the fridge. Jack decides he wants to taste the canned liquid food supplement. Malcolm and Christina go around with a trash bag and fill it up with the endless medical paraphernalia that has accumulated everywhere. Home health care requires a vast amount of equipment. There are boxes of syringes, dressings, and bottles. Vince the MD, a policewoman, and a young detective arrive and Jack meets with them. The policewoman's radio squawks with a worldly harshness, ripping through the care-layered atmosphere. Mom asks her to turn off her radio or go outside. The volume is lowered very marginally. The law doesn't respect the event within these walls. To them it's another duty call and they don't make allowances. You're not supposed to die at home and it makes trouble for them. Who knows, maybe we did him in. The phone rings as soon as it's on the hook. Condolences are made. It begins to rain.

The vacuum left by your departure is heard in the voices and shuffling feet as we move in circles around the house, no longer clocked by the rhythms of struggle and of dying. We are all alive and yet we've touched the other world and move suspended and timeless; we're free of your pain just as you are . . .

The estate lawyer arrives, and we find ourselves sitting around the dining room table going over the will procedures and examining the trusts and other things that we don't understand. Clear explanations help me comprehend the details of the complex methods devised to escape probate taxes through trust loopholes.

Jack, Andrew, and I go to Gawlers' Funeral Home to arrange the cremation contract. There's a Fragonard reproduction on the upholstered wall. It's the woman on a swing with a boy looking up her skirts. Life goes on. When the papers are all signed we take the elevator upstairs to see the body. It's just a thing now and cold from the cooler. They've fixed your body up, jaw closed, lips look wrong. Maybe the wire holding the jaws together is too tight. The shroud is made of a paper towel–like material, ripped open neatly to reveal the head. The coffin is made of hardboard with a plywood plinth. Pulling up the shade of the nearest window, the light plays on those sunken cheeks and it's easier to see how small the body is. I have this urge to do something more with your body. Be with it; feel the awkward weight of carrying it down the towpath to the river. Maybe go canoeing and dig a hole for your diminished self up in the red clay banks above the falls.

I feel ripped off and displaced by the carefully sanitized legalities and the overly plush interior of this phony death house. None of this is about death. It's all so nauseatingly homogenized and disrespectfully unoriginal. It's such a scam. There must be some other way. I want to slap somebody. I distract myself taking photos and ribbing the unctuous funeral director about the overdone funeral accessories conveniently on display in the room. Andrew says, "You could go over Niagara Falls in one of these." The metal and wood craftsmanship on the Diplomat coffin is impressive. But you wouldn't have gone for it. You'd have used some of the old carpeting and ceiling tile stored in the garage. Anger and irritation goad me and I take a lot of photos. No reason to hold back . . .

The next morning Jack and Lynn leave, but I'm not ready to go back to my life in NYC. I can't even remember my phone number there. We're planning a family service in Maine. A second service will follow in Washington in mid-September after vacationing friends and associates return . . .

Malcolm leaves the following morning for Boston. Andrew and I remain. Andrew sorts through the wall-to-wall maze of documents spilling out of boxes in Dad's study. I think he's trying to find continuity in sorting, labeling, filing the parquet pattern of mixed papers that cover a lifetime of endeavors. It's his way of dealing with the man's complex and elaborate understandings, fleshed out in bulging files of papers, photos, old letters, and endless cancer cures and protocols.

In the late afternoon I meet Marty to go kayaking on the Potomac above Great Falls. The river is dangerously high and full. Sitting above the rapids after working the eddies and leaning to maneuver, I can see, in the water's unrippled rushing surface, something of you, Dad. Marty asks me what you were like when you and I went canoeing in the early years. I recall that, when spilling into the frigid water, my thoughts wild and shocked, your voice was always calm and measured, if only somewhat more urgent, as we flushed through channels and standing waves behind the boat. The day usually ended with dry clothes and stew cooked on the fire, but rarely any easy chitchat.

You weren't one to retell and relive the exciting moments, working over the events in hindsight. Somehow you were always moving into the future. This was confusing, and it took me some time as a boy and young adult to reconcile this with my own needs. Needs that now don't seem so different from yours. Looking at the broad sweep of the passing water, its surface agitated only by blossoming patterns served up from the river bottom, I can imagine the enthusiasm and delight you took in our trips together. You couldn't be other than you were, in spite of my longings. You were yourself: full, potent, coursing with confluent purposes, designs, and curiosities. An unhesitatingly creative spirit that, in the later years, revealed itself to a wider circle through love, that flowed through eye and hand, to all those whose lives blended with your expanding current.

NOTES

1 Sally was my biological mother.
2 A rental property owned and managed by my father.
3 Andrew's wife.
4 Malcolm's fiancée.
5 Mom's younger sister, a professional singer.
6 My father's older sister.

Appendix I

Males are drawn as squares, females as circles:

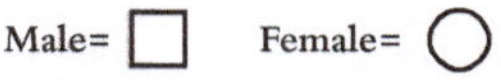

Date of birth and death are written next to the person's symbol. Age may be shown within the square or circle. Death is indicated by an X through the symbol.

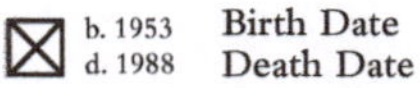

Couples are shown by a line connecting their symbols as follows, with the relevant dates written on the line:

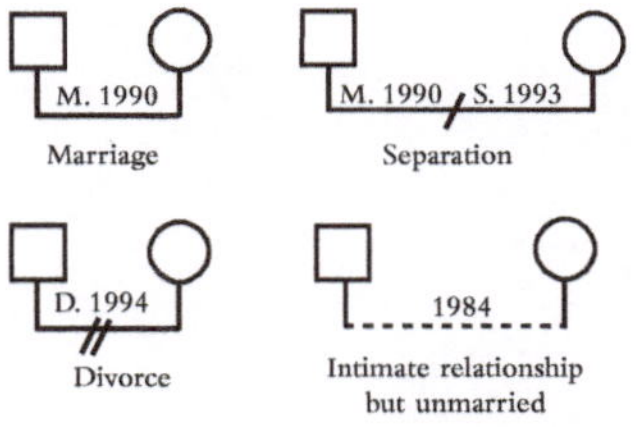

Children are shown left to right, oldest to youngest

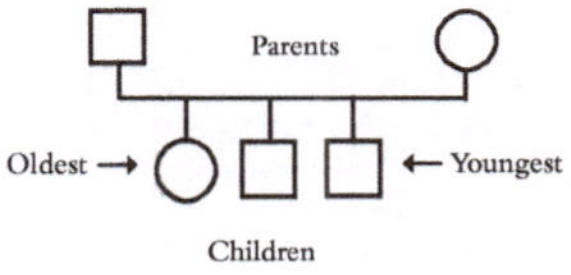

Here is an example of some of the family characteristics you can show:

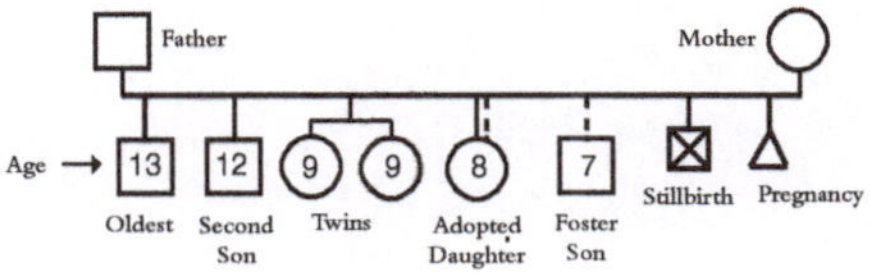

Emotional relationships between people can be indicated by a second set of lines:

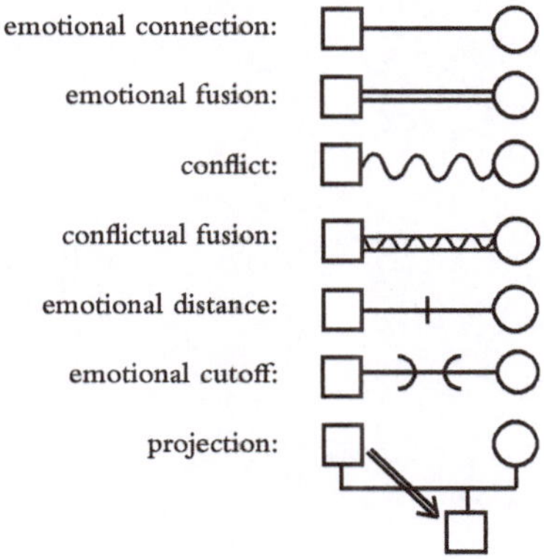

Appendix II

EDUCATIONAL AND TRAINING PROGRAMS IN BOWEN FAMILY SYSTEMS THEORY AND THERAPY

Bowen Center for the Study of the Family

Anne S. McKnight, Director
4400 MacArthur Blvd NW Suite 103
Washington, DC 20007–2521
Phone: 800–432–6882 or 202–965–4400
E-mail: info@thebowencenter.org
www.thebowencenter.org

Bowen Theory Academy

Michael E. Kerr, President
1523 Pripet Woods Lane
Islesboro, ME 04848
Phone: 207–542–6082
www.bowentheoryacademy.org

Center for Family Consultation

Sydney Reed, Director of Training
820 Davis Street Suite 504
Evanston, IL 60201
Phone: 224–567–2888
E-mail: info@centerforfamilyconsultation.net
www.centerforfamilyconsultation.net

Center for Family, Organizational, and Natural Systems Education

Charles M. White, Founder & Principal Associate
Phone: 908–451–5818
E-mail: charlesmwhite@verizon.net
Ellen Rogan, Principal Associate
Phone: 201–218–9812
E-mail: ellenrogandnp@gmail.com
Rutgers University School of Social Work—Office of Continuing Education Clinical Programs in Bowen Family Systems Theory https://socialwork.rutgers.edu/academics/continuing-education/certificate-programs/bowen-family-systems-theory-clinical-certificate

The Center for Family Process

Myrna Carpenter, Partner and Faculty
Mickie M. Crimone, Partner and Faculty
10601 Willowbrook Drive
Potomac, MD 20854
Phone: 410–799–7774 or 301–299–7475
E-mail: contactus@centerforfamilyprocess.com
www.centerforfamilyprocess.com

Center For The Study of Human Systems

Roberta Gilbert, Director
Phone: 703–850–475
E-mail: rgilbert09@gmail.com
www.hsystems.org

Center for the Study of Natural Systems and the Family

Victoria Harrison, Director
724 Rutland
Houston, TX 77007

Phone: 713–790–0226
E-mail: vaharrison@sbcglobal.net
www.csnsf.org

Center for the Study of Natural Systems and the Family Programs at the Border
(El Paso, TX and Ciudad Juárez, Mexico)

Louise Rauseo, Director
10450 Lottsford, Apt, 312
Bowie, Md. 20721–3303
Phone: 443–623–4021
E-mail: louise@rauseos.net
www.csnsf.org/borderprograms

The Family Systems Institute

Jenny Brown, Executive Director
Director, The Family Systems Practice
30 Grosvenor St Neutral Bay 2089
Phone: 02 9904 5600 Fax: 9904 5611
E-mail: jbrown@thesfi.com.au
www.thefsi.com.au
www.thefsp.com.au

The Florida Family Research Network, Inc. / Bowen Theory Postgraduate Training Program of South Florida

Eileen Gottlieb, Education Director
232 SW 28th Avenue
Delray Beach, FL 33445
Phone: 561–279–0861
E-mail: ebgfamilycenter@comcast.net
www.ffrnbowentheory.org

ISS Wofoo Family Institute

International Social Service Hong Kong Branch
Peggy Chan
Yaumatei, Kowloon, Hong Kong
www.isshk.org

Kansas City Center for Family and Organizational Systems

Margaret Otto, Director
3100 NE 83 Street, Suite 2350
Kansas City, MO 64119
Phone: 816–436–1721
E-mail: motto@kcfamilysystems.com
www.kcfamilysystems.com

Leadership Coaching, Inc.

John Engels, President
63 Klink Road
Rochester, NY 14625
Phone: 585–381–9040
E-mail: heidi@leadershipcoaching.com
www.leadershipcoachinginc.com

Leadership in Ministry

Robert Dibble, Coordinator
www.leadershipinministry.org

Navigating Systems

Priscilla J. Friesen, Founder
4545 42nd St NW #201
Washington DC 20016
Phone: 202–262–2478

E-mail: pjfries9249@gmail.com
Phone: 202–966–1145

Living Systems

Randall Frost, Director of Training and Research
Lois Walker, Faculty
209–1500 Marine Drive
North Vancouver, BC V7P1T7
Phone: 604–926–5496
E-mail: info@livingsystems.ca
www.livingsystems.ca

New England Seminar on Bowen Theory

Ann V. Nicholson, Chair
25 Medway Street
Dorchester, MA 02124
Phone: 617–312–8694
E-mail: annvnicholson@gmail.com
www.bowentheoryne.com

Northampton Seminar on the Therapist's Own Family and Clinical Cases

Peter Titelman, Faculty
53 Center Street
Northampton, MA 01060
Phone: 413–584–7733
www.familysystemstherapynorthampton.com

Princeton Family Center for Education, Inc.

Lee S. Gardner, Director
PO Box 331
Pennington, NJ 08534

Phone: 609–203–0162
E-mail: leegardner@verizon.net
www.princetonfamilycenter.org

Programs in Bowen Theory

Laura Havstad, Executive Director
120 Pleasant Hill Avenue N #370
Sebastopol, CA 95472
Phone: 707–823–1848
E-mail: info@programsinbowentheory.org
www.programsinbowentheory.org

Southern California Education & Training in Bowen Family Systems Theory

Carolyn Jacobs, Director
625 Third Ave.
San Diego, CA. 91910
Phone: 619–525–7747
E-mail: info@socalbowentheory.com
www.socalbowentheory.com

Vermont Center for Family Studies

Erik Thompson, Executive Director
65 Leeway Circle
St George, VT 05495
Phone: 802–658–4800
E-mail: info@vermontcenterforfamilystudies.org
www.vermontcenterforfamilystudies.org

Western Pennsylvania Family Center

James B. Smith, Director
733 North Highland Avenue
Pittsburgh, PA 15206
Phone: 412–362–2295
E-mail: info@wpfc.net
www.wpfc.net

INDEX

Page numbers in *italics* indicate figures and in **bold** indicate tables on the corresponding pages.